D1608259

Shoulder Arthroscopy

Springer
New York
Berlin
Heidelberg
Hong Kong
London
Milan
Paris
Tokyo

James E. Tibone, MD
Department of Orthopaedics, University of Southern California,
Los Angeles, California

Felix H. Savoie III, MD
Mississippi Sports Medicine, Jackson, Mississippi

Benjamin S. Shaffer, MD
DC SportsMedicine Institute, Washington, DC; Associate
Professor, Georgetown University Medical Center,
Washington, DC

Shoulder Arthroscopy

With 257 Illustrations in 357 Parts, 306 in Full Color

DVD
INCLUDED

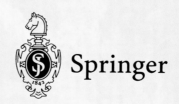

Springer

James E. Tibone, MD
Department of Orthopaedics
University of Southern California
Los Angeles, CA 90033
USA
tibone@usc.edu

Felix H. Savoie III, MD
Mississippi Sports Medicine
Jackson, MS 39202
USA
busavoie@aol.com

Benjamin S. Shaffer, MD
DC SportsMedicine Institute
Washington, DC 20016
and
Associate Professor
Georgetown University Medical Center
Washington, DC, 20007, USA
shaffer@dcsportsmedicine.com

Illustrator: Janice Schwegler, MS, Long Beach, CA, USA

No author has received any benefit for personal or professional use from a commercial enterprise related to the subject of any chapter.

Library of Congress Cataloging-in-Publication Data
Shoulder arthroscopy / editors, James E. Tibone, Felix H. Savoie, Benjamin S. Shaffer.
    p. ; cm.
    Includes bibliographical references and index.
    ISBN 0-387-95363-9 (h/c : alk. paper)
    I. Shoulder joint—Endoscopic surgery.   2. Shoulder joint—Abnormalities—Diagnosis.
    3. Arthroscopy.   I. Tibone, James E.   II. Savoie Felix H.   III. Shaffer, Benjamin.
    [DNLM: 1. Shoulder—surgery.   2. Arthroscopy—methods.   3. Shoulder Joint—surgery.
    WE 8190 S5435 2003]
    RD557.5 S5435 2003
    617.5'72059—dc21   2002030553

ISBN 0-387-95363-9   Printed on acid-free paper.

Printed in Singapore.

9 8 7 6 5 4 3 2 1   SPIN 10852695

www.springer-ny.com

Springer-Verlag New York Berlin Heidelberg
A member of BertelsmannSpringer Science+Business Media GmbH

Foreword

Neither shoulder anatomy nor its potential disorders have changed over the past 2000 years, but the methods of diagnosing and treating shoulder injury most certainly have. Since its clinical introduction in the 1970s, shoulder arthroscopy has continued to expand how we look at, and treat, shoulder dysfunction.

This book and its accompanying DVD provides an invaluable resource for orthopaedic residents, fellows, and surgeons, by describing and illustrating the current state of arthroscopic surgery for the shoulder. The 25 chapters are written by specialists who in many instances have been responsible for the procedures' development. The text and DVD detail nuances of the sometimes technically demanding procedures that are critical for surgical success. Beautiful four-color illustrations complement the text and serve to illuminate the specific techniques in even greater detail.

Asked to write the foreword to what I believe will become the standard in the field is an honor. I have had the privilege of working with these fine editors personally and professionally, and this comprehensive body of work reflects their creativity and perseverance. This book represents an important contribution to our literature because it serves to provide a well-crafted approach to arthroscopic shoulder surgery in 2003. I am confident that this book will assist readers in synthesizing their thoughts and mastering the many challenging and rewarding techniques in operative shoulder arthroscopy.

Frank Jobe, MD

Preface

Few areas in orthopaedics have witnessed the type of exponential growth that has characterized the current field of arthroscopic shoulder surgery. Certainly a debt of gratitude is owed the early pioneers (both open and arthroscopic), whose passion and skill fostered today's phenomenon. Rapid advances in imaging, electronic communication, instrumentation, and implant technology, have "suddenly" permitted arthroscopic access to problems once exclusively the province of the open surgeon. Pioneering work by Lanny Johnson, Dick Caspari, Harv Ellman (and others) further facilitated the application of these emerging technologies into a practical and useful new skill set. Today, with few exceptions, most shoulders requiring surgical intervention can be thoroughly assessed, and in many cases, definitively treated arthroscopically.

Yet, and perhaps a consequence of the rather rapid evolution of these techniques, few single-source references are available for either the "would be" shoulder arthroscopist or the experienced clinician looking to hone his/her arthroscopic skills about the shoulder. The purpose of this text is to address this deficiency and provide the orthopaedic and arthroscopic community with a single definitive "how to" technical reference on operative shoulder arthroscopy. In keeping with this initiative, our goal was to assemble a group of authors who themselves were responsible for developing the techniques described, learning firsthand how "they do it." We are indebted to these contributors for their time and effort, and believe they have provided a wealth of valuable information that will enhance our technical understanding.

The text has been divided into nine major sections, beginning with a section on Anatomy and Technique. Introductory chapters are intended to provide the reader with a basic overview of the two "competing" standards for shoulder arthroscopy (lateral decubitus and "beach-chair" position) and a foundation for normal, variational, and pathologic arthroscopic shoulder anatomy. Subsequent sections are divided into Glenohumeral Pathology, SLAP and Biceps Lesions, Instability, Stiffness, Subacromial Pathology and Rotator Cuff Tears, the AC Joint, Rehabilitation, and Complications. Each chapter addresses management of a specific shoulder problem. Some sections will include more than one method by which the problem can be addressed, in deference to the practical reality that there is "more than one way to skin a cat." Final sections on Rehabilitation and Complications complete the text.

All motor skills (of which arthroscopy is certainly an example) improve with practice, and mastering the techniques described in this book requires more than just reading and/or watching the accompanying video demonstrations. Fortunately, practice opportunities abound, including regional and national courses and workshops, lab at the Orthopaedic Learning Center (Rosement, IL), shoulder models, and in a limited but probably increasingly available capacity, "virtual" computerized shoulder models.

Finally, technological capability and surgical aptitude, by themselves, do not necessarily lead to good patient care, which instead depends upon good judgment and experience.

ACKNOWLEDGMENTS

We are especially appreciative to our contributors, who are true educators. Despite busy clinical practices, competing professional, and compelling personal responsibilities, they labored to provide us with invaluable educational information based on their own hard work and experience, for which we are truly indebted. Jan Schwegler, our medical illustrator, has provided beautiful renderings that clearly illustrate our contributors' intent. Thanks to Rob Albano and his editorial staff at Springer-Verlag, who helped shepherd this book from concept to creation. And finally, thank you to all of our families for your support in bringing this to fruition.

James E. Tibone, MD
Felix H. "Buddy" Savoie III, MD
Benjamin S. Shaffer, MD

Contents

Section One   Anatomy/Technique

Section Two   Glenohumeral Pathology

Section Three   SLAP and Biceps Lesions

Section Four   Instability

Section Eight   Rehabilitation

Section Nine   Complications

Contributors

Jeffrey S. Abrams
Princeton Orthopaedic and Rehabilitation Associates, Princeton, NJ 08540, USA. rxbonz@aol.com

David W. Altchek
Department of Orthopaedic Surgery, Hospital for Special Surgery, New York, NY 10021, USA. altchekd@hss.edu

Robert A. Arciero
Department of Orthopaedic Surgery, University of Connecticut Health Center, Farmington, CT 06034, USA. arciero@nso.uchc.edu

Gregory S. Bauer
Goldsboro Orthopaedic Associates, Goldsboro, NC 27534, USA. gandh98@yahoo.com

Louis U. Bigliani
Department of Orthopaedic Surgery, Columbia Presbyterian/NY Presbyterian Medical Center, New York, NY 10032, USA. lubl@columbia.edu

Theodore A. Blaine
Department of Orthopaedic Surgery, Columbia Presbyterian/NY Presbyterian Medical Center, New York, NY 10032, USA. tb211@columbia.edu

Pascal Boileau
Hôpital de L'Archet, Nice, France 06202. boileau.p@chu-nice.fr

James P. Bradley
Department of Orthopaedic Surgery, UPMC Medical Center, University of Pittsburgh, Pittsburgh, PA 15215, USA. bradleyjp@msx.upmc.com

Stephen S. Burkhart
540 Madison Oak Drive, San Antonio, TX 78258, USA. ssburkhart@msn.com

Scott P. Fischer
280 South Main Street, Orange, CA 92868, USA. spfischer@scottfischermd.com

Evan L. Flatow
Department of Orthopaedic Surgery, Mount Sinai School of Medicine, New York, NY 10029, USA. eflatow@aol.com

Leesa M. Galatz
Department of Orthopaedic Surgery, Washington University School of Medicine, St. Louis, MO 63110, USA. galatzl@msnotes.wustl.edu

Mehrdad Ganjianpour
Tower Orthopaedic and Sports Medicine, Los Angeles, CA 90048, USA. drganj@yahoo.com

Jeffrey T. Gittins
OrthoNeuro, 1313 Olentangy River Road, Columbus, OH 43212, USA.
jtgittins@yahoo.com

Sandra J. Iannotti
North Shore Orthopaedic Surgery, Smithtown, NY 11787, USA.
s_iannotti@hotmail.com

Christopher K. Jones
Southern Center for Orthopaedic and Sports Medicine, LaGrange, GA 30240,
USA. ckj113@yahoo.com

W. Ben Kibler
Lexington Clinic, Lexington, KY 40504, USA. wkibler@aol.com

John J. Klimkiewicz
Department of Orthopaedics, Georgetown University Hospital, Washington,
DC 20007, USA. kajklim@pol.net

Sumant G. Krishnan
Shoulder and Elbow Service, W.B. Carrell Memorial Clinic, Dallas, TX 75204,
USA. sgkrish@attglobal.net

Cyrus J. Lashgari
The Orthopaedic and Sports Medicine Center, Annapolis, MD 21401, USA.
lashgaricl@msn.com

Richard G. Levine
Department of Orthopaedics, Union Memorial Hospital, Baltimore, MD 21218,
USA. lync@helix.org

Mark I. Loebenberg
Department of Orthopaedics, NYU School of Medicine, New York, NY 10003,
USA. loebem01@popmail.med.nyu.edu

Leslie S. Matthews
Department of Orthopaedics, Union Memorial Hospital, Baltimore, MD 21218,
USA. lync@helix.org

Augustus D. Mazzacca
Department of Orthopaedics Surgery, University of Connecticut, Farmington,
CT 06034, USA. mazzocca@uchc.edu

Suzanne L. Miller
UPMC Center for Sports Medicine, University of Pittsburgh, Pittsburgh, PA
15203, USA. slm_10128@yahoo.com

Carl W. Nissen
Department of Orthopaedic Surgery, University of Connecticut Health Center,
Farmington, CT 06034, USA. cnissen@nso.uchc.edu

Wesley M. Nottage
Sports Clinic Orthopaedic Medical Associates, Laguna Hills, CA 92653, USA.
tscwmn@aol.com

Bernard C. Ong
Center for Sports Medicine, UPMC Center for Sports Medicine, University of Pittsburgh, Pittsburgh, PA 15203, USA. ongmd@hotmail.com

Peter M. Parten
Summitt Orthopedics, 1600 St. Johns Boulevard, Maplewood, MN 55109, USA. parten@worldnet.alt.net

Andrew S. Rokito
305 Second Avenue, New York, NY 10003, USA. arokito@aol.com

Anthony A. Romeo
1725 West Harrison Street, Chicago, IL 60612, USA. aromeo@rush.edu

Charles J. Ruotolo
Department of Orthopaedics, Nassau University Medical Center, East Meadow, NY 11554, USA. cruotolo@hotmail.com

Felix H. Savoie III
Mississippi Sports Medicine, Jackson, MS 39202, USA. busavoie@aol.com

Jon K. Sekiya
Center for Sports Medicine, UPMC Center for Sports Medicine, University of Pittsburgh, Pittsburgh, PA 15203, USA. jsekiya@hotmail.com

Robert Sellards
Department of Orthopaedics, Louisiana State University, New Orleans, LA 70112, USA. rsella@lsuhsc.edu

Benjamin S. Shaffer
DC SportsMedicine Institute, Washington, DC 20016; Associate Professor, Georgetown University Medical Center, Washington, DC 20007, USA. shaffer@dcsportsmedicine.com

Ken Shubin Stein
185 West End Avenue, New York, NY 10023, USA. kshubinstein@yahoo.com

Kevin L. Smith
Department of Orthopaedics, University of Washington, Seattle, WA 98195, USA. drsmith@u.washington.edu

Stephen J. Snyder
Southern California Orthopaedics Institute, Van Nuys, CA 91405, USA. snyder@scoi.com

James P. Tasto
6719 Alvarado Road, San Diego, CA 92120, USA. doctas007@aol.com

Armin M. Tehrany
11 Ralph Place, Staten Island, NY 10304, USA. armin@tehrany

Michael A. Terry
Department of Orthopaedic Surgery, Hospital for Special Surgery, New York, NY 10021, USA. terrym@hss.edu

Raymond Thal
Town Center Orthopaedic Associates, Reston, VA 20190, USA.
raythal@aol.com

Kenneth R. Thompson
UPMC, Shadyside Hospital, Pittsburgh, PA 15232, USA.
thompsonkr@msx.upmc.edu

James E. Tibone
Department of Orthopaedics, University of Southern California, Los Angeles,
CA 90033, USA. tibone@usc.edu

Stefan J. Tolan
Oakwood Orthopaedics, Greenville, SC 29605, USA. tolan@charter.net

Gilles Walch
Department of Orthopaedic Surgery, Clinique St. Anne Lumière,
Lyon, France 69008. walch.gilles@wanado.fr

Ken Yamaguchi
Department of Orthopaedic Surgery, Washington University School of
Medicine, St Louis, MO 63110, USA. yamaguchik@msnotes.wustl.edu

SECTION ONE

Anatomy/ Technique

Diagnostic Shoulder Arthroscopy in the Lateral Decubitus Position

James E. Tibone

Arthroscopy of the shoulder has become increasingly popular as a standard diagnostic and therapeutic surgical technique among orthopedic surgeons worldwide. Evolving technology has furthered our understanding of the shoulder and its associated pathology; as a result, progressive advances and improvements in both surgical equipment and technique continue to be realized. Current arthroscopic treatment of common shoulder problems such as instability and rotator cuff tears has led to outcomes that are comparable to those achieved with standard open procedures, yet with less morbidity. Arthroscopy also allows visualization and treatment of certain intra-articular pathology (e.g., SLAP lesions) that are not easily accessible by open means. The single limitation associated with arthroscopic shoulder surgery is the learning curve. Some procedures are technically demanding and may prove challenging to anyone without considerable experience. This chapter presents a basic overview of our simple and reproducible surgical technique for diagnostic shoulder arthroscopy. We outline the operating room setup and patient positioning for arthroscopy in the lateral decubitus position, and also describe the conventional portals utilized in routine diagnostic shoulder arthroscopy.

PATIENT SETUP AND POSITIONING

Arthroscopy of the shoulder in the lateral decubitus position may be performed on a standard operating room table. Many authors believe that the lateral decubitus position offers advantages over the beach chair position in visualization and maneuverability owing to glenohumeral distraction via an adjustable shoulder traction device. A beanbag with an overlying draw sheet should be prepositioned on the operating room table prior to patient positioning, and kidney rests should be readily available.

When the patient has been transferred to the operating room table, an anesthetic is administered. At our institution, we prefer the use of a general anesthetic, although a regional anesthetic such as interscalene block may be utilized as well. After induction of anesthesia, the shoulder should always be examined to document passive range of motion and to determine the extent of glenohumeral translation and laxity. Comparison to the contralateral shoulder should be performed, since laxity in the shoulder is highly variable.

The patient is next placed into the lateral decubitus position. The preplaced beanbag is used to support the patient in position. We do not routinely use a padded axillary roll under the thorax, but instead take measures to ensure that there is no pressure on the contents of the axilla. The patient's torso is rolled or tilted back approximately 20 to 30°, and the patient is also placed into slight reverse Trendelenburg position to place the glenoid roughly parallel to the floor. This creates a standard reference for glenohumeral joint orientation and also allows easier intra-articular manipulation by making the anterior aspect of the shoulder joint more accessible for the arthroscope and instrumentation.

Kidney rests are placed on either side of the beanbag to secure it in place. The posterior kidney rest—where the surgeon will be standing for most of the surgical procedure—should be placed at the tip of the scapula to ensure that it is completely out of the surgeon's way. The contralateral downside arm should be forward flexed approximately 60 to 80° away from the torso and placed on an arm board, with all bony prominences well padded. Care should also be taken to ensure that the peroneal nerve of the downside leg is not subjected to any undue pressure. This can be accomplished by placing a pillow under the slightly flexed contralateral hip and knee, making sure that the fibular head and peroneal nerve are thus well protected.

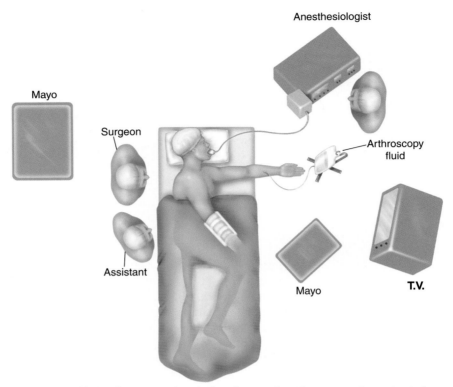

FIGURE 1.1. In this aerial view, the table has been rotated such that the anesthesiologist is at the patient's front, permitting the surgeon complete access to the anterior and posterior shoulder.

Next, two pillows are placed between the legs, and the ipsilateral hip and knee are also slightly flexed. A Velcro or buckled strap may be used around the patient's pelvis to secure both the patient and the bean-bag construct to the operating room table. The operating room table should also be turned to allow the surgeon adequate room to work around the shoulder. The surgeon should have unimpeded 180° access, to be able to walk around the head of the table and to the front of the shoulder. This is extremely important when anterior shoulder pathology (e.g., Bankart lesion, anterior capsular redundancy) needs to be addressed, and to permit diagnostic arthroscopy from the anterior portal (Figure 1.1).

With respect to traction, we prefer an apparatus utilizing an extremity sleeve coupled with a shoulder suspension pulley system, allowing traction in two different directions (Figure 1.2). We use the shoulder traction and rotation (STAR) sleeve system (Arthrex, Naples, FL), which has distinct advantages over a single overhead pulley in that it allows for selective traction in separate planes, facilitating longitudinal traction and glenohumeral distraction. In addition, this system allows intraoperative changes in shoulder positioning to be made easily if necessary (Figure 1.3).

We routinely place the traction tower at the lower end of the table on the same side as the operating surgeon. This allows for greater forward flexion of the involved extremity, which is important in providing visualization of the glenohumeral joint.

The traction tower should then be adjusted to the appropriate height and forward angulation to maintain the arm in the abducted and forward flexed position. Although the least amount of strain on the brachial plexus is present with the arm adducted at the side, some degree of abduction is necessary to allow arthroscopic visualization of the glenohumeral joint. We currently recommend abduction of approximately 45° coupled with forward flexion of 30°. We have found this position to allow easy global access to any pathology within the glenohumeral joint; intraoperative adjustments to forward flexion can be performed to improve visualization. The arm can also be brought into less abduction to relax anterior structures when, for example, one is addressing anterior labral pathology. We do not recommend abduction beyond 60°. We have not found that increasing abduction beyond 45° aids in visualization; in fact, it is our experience that increasing forward flexion is more beneficial. If greater abduction is deemed necessary, forward flexion and

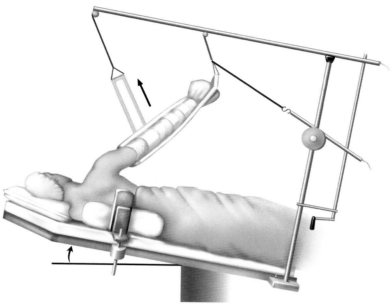

FIGURE 1.2. The STAR distraction system permits arm suspension and glenohumeral distraction for optimal exposure in the lateral position. The table has been placed in a slight reverse Trendelenburg position to orient the glenoid parallel to the floor.

internal rotation of the glenohumeral joint should be performed concomitantly, to decrease brachial plexus tension.

The entire shoulder–upper extremity is prepped first, and the arm is then positioned and secured in the traction apparatus. The foam extremity traction sleeve can be placed on the patient's forearm in a sterile fashion. Care should be taken to ensure that the sleeve is of the appropriate length by cutting off any excess so that the sleeve is just long enough to extend above the elbow.

After the patient has been draped, ensuring adequate exposure to the anterior and posterior aspect of the shoulder, the traction sleeve is secured into position in the overhead pulley system. For diagnostic arthroscopy of the glenohumeral joint, we generally employ 10 lb of traction on the lateral component of the traction apparatus and 5 lb on the longitudinal component. When arthroscopy of the subacromial space is performed, we merely switch the weights on the pulleys so that more traction is placed in the longitudinal direction to distract the humeral head from the

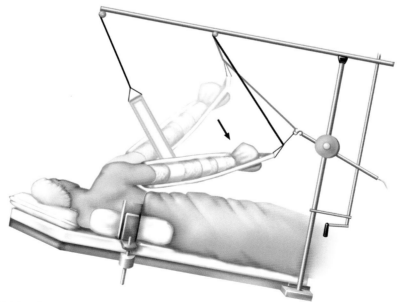

FIGURE 1.3. The STAR traction setup permits easy intraoperative adjustment of arm position.

undersurface of the acromion (Figure 1.3). We do not employ traction beyond 15 lb, since any increased weight places additional strain on the brachial plexus and increases the potential for neurological injury.

SURGICAL PERSONNEL AND INSTRUMENTATION SETUP

The surgeon and the operating room personnel should position themselves around the operating room table in a fashion that allows free access to the joint. The surgeon stands directly posterior to the shoulder, with the operating room personnel and back table positioned at the foot of the table on the same side as the surgeon. Additional assistants may stand on either side of the primary surgeon (Figure 1.1).

Surgical instrumentation and equipment need to be properly set up and arranged on the operating room table. The arthroscopy cart, containing the video monitor, a camera and video control box with an appropriate light source, and a mechanical shaver power source, is routinely set up directly opposite the surgeon at the level of the torso on the other side of the patient. This positioning provides for excellent visualization of the monitor and allows the various cables and tubing to be arranged in an orderly fashion so as not to interfere with the surgical procedure.

A Mayo stand should contain the basic and most frequently used instrumentation—the arthroscope and a shaver with various blades. A second Mayo stand may be placed behind the surgeon to hold other instruments that need to be at the surgeon's disposal: 11-blade scalpel, spinal needles, blunt trocars and sleeves for the arthroscope, switching sticks, and various cannulas. The back table is positioned within easy reach of the operating room personnel at the foot of the table and should hold the other instruments needed for arthroscopy.

A continuous gravity inflow of 0.9% normal saline or Ringer's lactate solution from elevated 3 L bags is utilized throughout the procedure. One ml of epinephrine (1:1000) is mixed in the first three bags. Inflow should be set up opposite the surgeon, and accessible to nursing.

PORTAL PLACEMENT

The posterior portal is established first. This portal is placed approximately 2 cm inferior and 1 cm medial to the posterolateral corner of the acromion (Figure 1.4). The spine of the scapula can usually be felt even in heavyset individuals, and this can be followed to the posterolateral corner of the acromion. Joint dis-

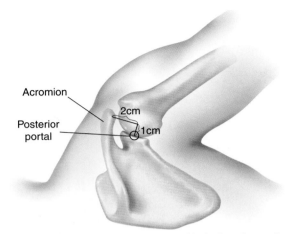

FIGURE 1.4. The posterior portal is established in the "soft spot," approximately 2 cm distal and 1 cm medial to the posterolateral acromion.

tension before arthroscope insertion is unnecessary. After the skin incision has been made, the arthroscope sheath with blunt trocar is inserted through the deltoid and infraspinatus muscle to the posterior capsule. With a blunt-tipped obturator, a step-off can be felt between the posterior glenoid rim and the humeral head. If a step-off is not felt, the position of the portal may be too low or too medial and should be repositioned. Arm rotation facilitates confirmation of the glenohumeral joint, palpating through the blunt obturator. Upon confirmation of appropriate position, gentle, manual, longitudinal traction is applied, and the trocar is directed toward the coracoid process. With gentle pressure, the capsule is penetrated and the joint entered.

Once inside the glenohumeral joint, inflow tubing and suction are connected to the dual-inflow arthroscope sheath. Arthroscopy is initiated with identification of the biceps insertion on the superior labrum, which serves as a landmark for orientation. We proceed with arthroscopic inspection systematically, beginning with the biceps tendon. The rotator cuff is then examined out to its humeral head insertion. The articular cartilage of the humeral head and glenoid are visualized. After sweeping down into the axillary pouch and examining the posterior labrum, we reposition the scope at the biceps for anterior examination. The labrum is examined superiorly, anteriorly, inferiorly, and finally posteriorly. Anteriorly, the superior tendon border of the subscapularis can easily be visualized, as well as the glenohumeral ligaments (superior, middle, and inferior glenohumeral ligaments). There are many anatomical variants in the anterior superior labrum, as well as different configurations of the middle glenohumeral ligament. These must be appreciated to avoid confusing a normal anatomic variant with a pathological lesion (see chapter 3).

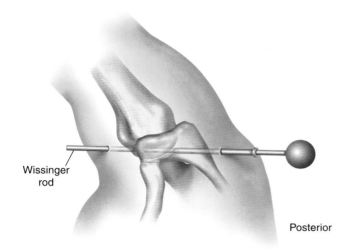

FIGURE 1.5. Anterior arthroscope portal is established by use of a Wissinger rod, passed bluntly, anteriorly, through the rotator interval. The tip must be directed lateral to the coracoid process.

The anterior portal is then established; both inside-out and outside-in techniques can be used to establish the anterior portal. The inside-out technique is usually performed with a Wissinger rod. The arthroscope is pushed anteriorly just above the superior border of the subscapularis tendon in the rotator interval. A Wissinger rod is then inserted through the arthroscopy sheath and pushed through the capsule anteriorly until it tents the skin just superior and lateral to the coracoid process (Figure 1.5). A stab incision is made in the skin, and the Wissinger rod is pushed through, followed by the arthroscope sheath. A metal or plastic cannula is then mated onto the protruding arthroscopic sheath tip and retrograde delivered back into the glenohumeral joint, thereby establishing the anterior portal (Figure 1.6).

Alternatively, an outside-in technique may be used to establish an anterior portal. While the surgeon is viewing from the posterior portal, finger palpation anteriorly will show the area where a portal will be established in the rotator interval. If a line were drawn from the tip of the coracoid to the anterolateral corner of the acromion, an 18-gauge spinal needle inserted from the middle of this line in a posterior and slightly inferior direction into the glenohumeral joint would approximate this portal (Figure 1.7). The spinal needle usually enters the joint inferior to the biceps in the center of the rotator interval. After confirmation of proper needle placement, a skin incision is made, and a metal or plastic cannula inserted parallel to the spinal needle. The anterior portal is first used for probing and palpating the labrum and other structures. When completed, scope portals are exchanged by means of switching sticks, permitting the scope to be placed anteriorly and the working (probe) portal posteriorly.

A complete diagnostic arthroscopy should include visualizing the glenohumeral joint and its structures from the anterior portal as well as the posterior portal. From the anterior portal, the arthroscope can be placed in the subscapularis bursa, a common location for occult loose bodies. The glenohumeral ligaments can easily be seen from this portal, as well as the rotator cuff, the posterior labrum and glenohumeral ligament.

Before the arthroscope is placed in the subacromial space, the arm abduction angle is usually lowered. This allows distraction of the arm more inferiorly, which facilitates visualization of the subacromial space. Upon completion of the diagnostic glenohumeral arthroscopy, the arthroscope is reintroduced through the same posterior portal into the subacromial space. The arthroscope sheath with obturator is angled superiorly toward the anterolateral corner of

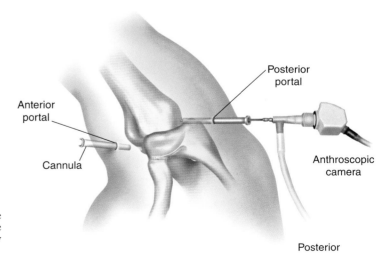

FIGURE 1.6. Posterior and anterior portals after use of the Wissenger rod (or "outside-in" technique): the arthroscope is posterior and the anterior disposable cannula permits easy instrumentation.

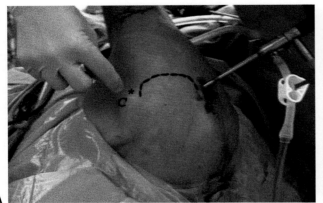
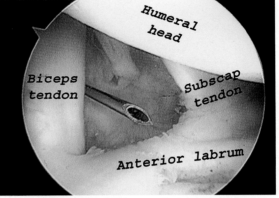

FIGURE 1.7. (A) An anterior portal is established through an "outside in" percutaneous approach. A spinal needle (*) is introduced midway between the coracoid (C) and the anterolateral acromion. (Right shoulder, lateral decubitus position.) (B) Arthroscopic view demonstrating the entrance of the needle in rotator interval when placed using an "outside in" percutaneous technique. (Right shoulder, lateral decubitus position.)

the acromion. The arthroscope should pierce the posterior "veil" of the subacromial bursa, which extends posteriorly parallel to the posterior aspect of the acromioclavicular joint. The coracoacromial ligament and the bursal side of the rotator cuff can be easily seen. Additional anterior or lateral portals can be used for probing or removing the bursa to aid visualization.

Upon completion of the diagnostic arthroscopy, portals are closed with simple nylon sutures and Tegaderm, or a simple absorbent dressing is applied. The arm is placed in a sling.

Recommended Reading

Caspari RB. Instrumentation and operating room organization for arthroscopy of the shoulder. In: McGinty JB, ed. *Arthroscopic Surgery Update: Techniques in Orthopaedics.* Rockville, MD: Aspen Systems Corp; 1985:15–24, 155–160.

Matthews LS, Zarins B, Michael RH, et al. Anterior portal selection for shoulder arthroscopy. *Arthroscopy* 1985;1: 33–39.

Stanish WD, Peterson DC. Shoulder arthroscopy and nerve injury: pitfalls and prevention. *Arthroscopy* 1995;11:458–466.

2

Diagnostic Shoulder Arthroscopy Technique: Beach Chair Position

Michael A. Terry and David W. Altchek

Beach chair positioning for shoulder arthroscopy was introduced in 1986 as an alternative to the lateral and modified lateral positions for shoulder arthroscopy.[1] Most shoulder arthroscopic procedures are possible with either the lateral or the beach chair position.

The beach chair position offers several distinct advantages. First, the patient is positioned anatomically. This more "anatomic" positioning permits better orientation and understanding of shoulder anatomy. Examination under anesthesia is facilitated in this position by the greater ease of stabilizing the scapula.

Second, traction is rarely necessary during beach chair positioning. Disadvantages of traction include the somewhat cumbersome setup and the potential for transient or permanent nerve damage.[2,3] Skin and soft tissue damage at the site of traction application have also been reported, including skin slough. Instead, simple inferior distraction in the plane of the scapula facilitates visualization and access to the subacromial space when necessary. Humeral rotational control, not easily attained in the lateral position, is easily accomplished for procedures such as arthroscopic rotator cuff repair, either manually or with an "arm holder." Gentle lateral humeral translations with the arm adducted provide easy access to the axillary region of the glenohumeral joint, which can be useful during arthroscopic stabilizations and release procedures.

Third, conversion to an open surgical procedure from the beach chair position is seamless, avoiding the need to either reposition or redrape the patient. The ease of such a conversion can, at times, influence surgical decision making.

Finally, the beach chair position complements either general or regional anesthesia. In contrast, regional anesthesia can be uncomfortable and is not well tolerated by the patient in the lateral decubitus position. Two common and extensive arthroscopic procedures, arthroscopic anterior stabilization and arthro-

scopic rotator cuff repair, deserve special mention regarding the use of the beach chair position. Successful arthroscopic anterior stabilization requires that two criteria be met. First, the anterior portal must allow insertion of anchors on the glenoid neck inferior to the 4 o'clock position (the inferior quarter of the glenoid). Second, the surgeon must be able to distract the humerus laterally to allow sutures to be placed in the anterior inferior capsule. The beach chair position facilitates achieving these two objectives. At the completion of the diagnostic arthroscopy, the arm is adducted and internally rotated. This "releases" the superior tendon of the subscapularis, allowing the surgeon to effectively place the anterior working portal more inferiorly, fulfilling the first criterion. Second, this position removes tension from the anterior capsule. The assistant can then laterally distract the humerus, fulfilling the second criterion, and allowing the surgeon access to the anteroinferior pouch.

Visualization of the rotator cuff is imperative for arthroscopic rotator cuff repair. The mobility of the upper extremity during arthroscopy in the beach chair position allows visualization of the posterior rotator cuff structures with internal rotation and visualization of the anterior rotator cuff structures with external rotation of the humerus. This mobility also facilitates the operative procedure itself. The structures visualized with the above-described maneuvers are also more easily accessed via the same motions. Inferior humeral distraction in the scapular plane also makes rotator cuff repair easier by increasing the volume of the subacromial space.

INDICATIONS/CONTRAINDICATIONS

The beach chair position can be used whenever diagnostic or operative arthroscopy of the shoulder is indicated. These indications include treatment of labral injuries with or without instability, rotator cuff disease with or without subacromial impingement, adhesive capsulitis, glenohumeral arthritis, biceps tendon lesions, and infection. The beach chair position may be preferred when one is concerned about traction or when conversion to an open procedure is likely. In our institution, beach chair is the preferred position for all arthroscopic procedures of the shoulder.

PREOPERATIVE PLANNING

Preoperative planning for diagnostic shoulder arthroscopy is similar to that for any operative procedure and includes creation of an operative plan after a careful history and physical exam, and interpretation of appropriate radiographs and imaging studies. The operative plan for a diagnostic shoulder arthroscopy in the beach chair position includes anesthesia and analgesia, patient positioning, creation of appropriate portals, the diagnostic arthroscopy and other indicated procedures, wound closure, and postoperative care.

SURGICAL TECHNIQUE

Positioning and Setup

Planning for shoulder arthroscopy in the beach chair position differs from planning for the lateral position with respect to positioning equipment. Equipment that should be available for positioning and securing the patient includes a full-length moldable beanbag with suction activation, appropriate patient padding, a standard operating room table with an attachable footplate, and, in our institution, an arm-positioning device clamped to the operating table. Standard arthroscopic equipment includes an arthroscopic camera sheath with inflow cannula attachment, an arthroscopic pump, and a video camera with image capture capability. Probes and instruments for establishing secondary portals must also be available.

Before anesthesia is administered, the patient is placed supine on the operating room table with a full-length, suction fitted, moldable beanbag in place. Regional anesthesia or general anesthesia may be utilized with this technique, but at our institution the overwhelming majority of shoulder arthroscopies are performed under interscalene block regional anesthesia (with 1.5% mepivacaine). Before the patient is positioned, a footboard is placed perpendicular to the leg portion of the operating room table (Figure 2.1). The table is then manipulated into the beach chair position, with the patient carefully supported. The table is flexed at the hip region and knee region. The torso is angled approximately 70 to 80° to the floor. The thighs should be approximately perpendicular to the torso, and the knees are positioned at an angle of approximately 70° of flexion (Figure 2.2). All bony prominences should be well padded. A foam head support is used for all shoulder arthroscopy. The inferior corner on the operative side of the foam head support is routinely torn away prior to positioning to allow increased exposure of the shoulder and neck (Figure 2.3).

The beanbag is then molded to the patient and held in place during inflation. Molding the beanbag around the hips, head, and neck of the patient is important (Figure 2.2). The entire scapula on the operative side should be visible and free of obstructions, permitting complete access to the entire shoulder (Figure 2.4). If necessary, after the beanbag is firm and has been appropriately molded, the patient may be moved laterally with the beanbag so that the scapula is exposed off the lateral edge of the table (Figure 2.5). The table may be slightly tilted (airplaned) away from the operative side to position the patient's center of gravity more securely over the table. Generally, the head is

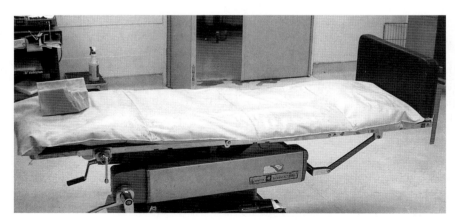

FIGURE 2.1. A footboard is secured perpendicular to the operating room table.

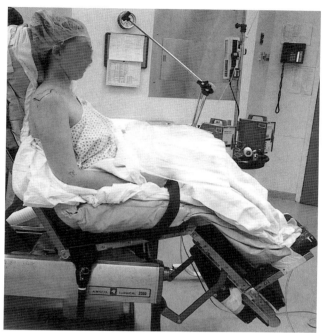

FIGURE 2.2. The operating room table is positioned such that the torso is approximately 70 to 80° from horizontal. The hips and knees should be flexed as shown, and the patient should be secured to the table and well padded.

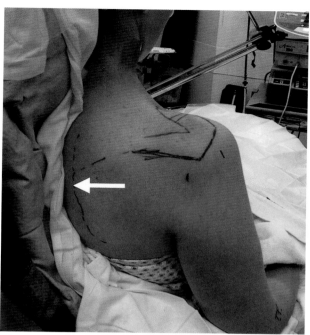

FIGURE 2.4. The medial border (arrow) of the scapula should be freely accessible after the beanbag has been evacuated.

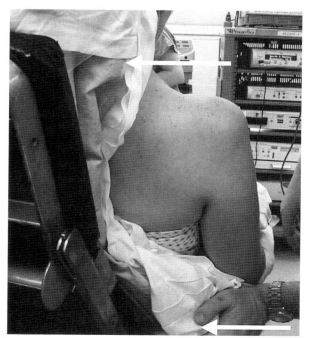

FIGURE 2.3. It is imperative to mold the beanbag around the hips, cervical spine, and head of the patient (arrows) prior to final positioning.

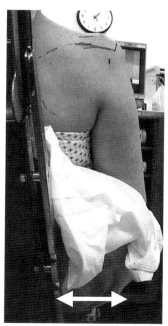

FIGURE 2.5. After the beanbag has been evacuated, the patient and supporting beanbag are moved laterally, toward the operative side, leaving approximately 8 in. of the patient off the table (arrow).

secured with tape to the foam pillow and the bean-bag, taking care to avoid direct shear on the skin of the forehead or pressure on the eyes.

An alternative to the use of a beanbag for the beach chair position is use of the "OR Direct" or similar positioning table. This device can be placed on the operating room table and padded prior to the patient arrival. After anesthesia has been obtained, the positioning table is brought to the upright position. Care is again taken to ensure proper padding of the lower extremities, head, and neck. Removing the shoulder support from the operative shoulder allows adequate shoulder exposure.

With the patient secured to the table and anesthesia obtained, but before the patient has been draped, a thorough examination is performed. Evaluation of passive range of motion is usually easily accomplished and documented. The exam continues with an evaluation of glenohumeral stability in both the anterior and posterior directions, using a modified Hawkins load-shift maneuver. We use the grading system of 1 to 3 plus translation as described elsewhere[4] to rate glenohumeral instability. Inferior stability of the shoulder is evaluated by using the sulcus sign test. During the examination under anesthesia it is essential to stabilize the scapula. In the beach chair position, the molded beanbag provides excellent scapular stability, facilitating an accurate examination.

The patient's shoulder girdle is then prepared free. Half-sheet drapes are put in place, followed by U-drapes superiorly and inferiorly. Care is taken during the draping process to avoid limiting the operative field. The appropriate borders for draping are the neck medially and 3 to 4 cm distal to the axilla inferiorly. This ensures that the coracoid and lateral two-thirds of the scapula are in the operative field. An ether screen is generally placed from the contralateral side of the patient to prevent the drapes from lying directly on him or her and to permit patients who are awake to watch the procedure on an arthroscopic monitor.

An articulated forearm-positioning device (McConnell Universal Positioner, Greenville, TX) may be utilized with the beach chair position, and the base should be attached before the patient is prepared and draped. The arm is positioned in the arm holder after the patient has been draped (Figure 2.6).

Instrumentation

Standard arthroscopic instrumentation is used. A camera sheath with an inflow portal is used. A standard 4.5 mm diameter, 30° lens is used with an arthroscopic camera. Probes, disposable cannulas, and other operative tools are similar to those used for knee arthroscopy. A pump with centralized pressure control is also utilized.

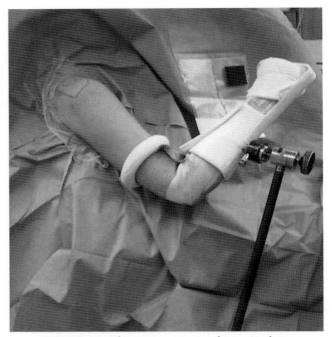

FIGURE 2.6. The arm-positioning device in place.

Surgical Technique

After the patient has been prepared and draped, anatomical landmarks are defined and carefully marked, including the scapular spine, acromion, acromioclavicular joint, clavicle, and coracoid. The posterior portal popularized by Andrews and coworkers[5] is utilized for the camera and inflow for most of the visualization of the glenohumeral joint during diagnostic arthroscopy. The posterior portal is generally located approximately 2 cm inferior to the acromion and approximately 1 to 2 cm medial to the lateral corner of the acromion (Figure 2.7). The exact position will vary and can be determined by palpating the posterior glenohumeral joint line. Placement can also be facilitated by grasping the proximal humerus and translating the humeral head anteriorly and posteriorly, indicating the exact site of the joint line.

The glenohumeral joint is first distended with 20 to 30 mL of a 1:300,000 epinephrine–saline solution prior to capsule penetration with the trocar. The posterior portal sites are infiltrated with 0.25% bupivacaine prior to skin incision. Because the posterior portal sites occasionally are incompletely anesthetized by the regional block, we routinely infiltrate these sites prior to skin incision. After incising the skin, the surgeon creates the posterior portal, using a blunt trocar to penetrate the capsule, aiming anteriorly toward the coracoid process. Entry into the joint can be facilitated with the adduction distraction maneuver[6] or with gentle lateralization of the humeral head. The camera is

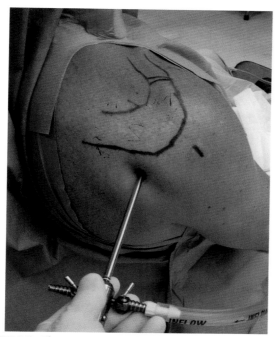

FIGURE 2.7. The posterior portal with inflow and camera sheath.

inserted into the camera sheath, and the arthroscopic fluid under pump control is connected to the capula-side port (Figure 2.7). Inflow is allowed just long enough to confirm intra-articular placement, after which free flow is permitted.

The anterior portal is then created. This portal should enter the glenohumeral joint just inferior to the long head of the biceps tendon through the rotator interval. Exact portal placement will vary depending on the procedure. For most diagnostic arthroscopies, this portal is established in the center of the interval. A spinal needle helps in "outside-in" portal localization (Figure 2.8). A scalpel is used to incise skin prior to creation of the portal with a standard arthroscopic canula. A probe is then utilized through the cannula during the diagnostic arthroscopy.

Diagnostic arthroscopy proceeds systematically. The synovium is visualized primarily. The superior labral anchor of the biceps tendon is inspected and probed. The anterior labrum is examined carefully, beginning superiorly and continuing inferiorly. The rotator interval, a common site for synovitis and loose bodies, is carefully visualized. The size of the rotator interval is noted, although it is difficult to objectively assess, particularly in patients with chronic instability. The superior tendon of the subscapularis should be easily visualized and can be followed laterally to its insertion on the lesser tuberosity.

As the arthroscope is moved inferiorly, the anterior labrum is visualized in its entirety. At the level

of the glenoid equator, the arthroscope is then advanced anterior to the labrum and into the anterior capsular pouch. Ability to easily advance the scope past head and labrum anteriorly is known as the "drive-through" sign, which is often present in anterior and multidirectional instability patterns. The middle and inferior glenohumeral ligaments (GHLs) are visualized, including the anterior band of the inferior GHL. The arthroscope is directed inferiorly into the anterior inferior pouch, and its size is noted. The humerus is then gradually externally rotated from its neutral position, and the responses of the anterior band of the inferior glenohumeral ligament and the axillary pouch are observed. Both should tighten up with external rotation, often forcing the scope out of its viewing position.

Prior to evaluation of the rotator cuff and the lateral biceps tendon, the humerus is placed in 45° of external rotation, and inferior traction is applied in the plane of the scapula via the arm-positioning device or by a surgical assistant. The lateral aspect of the biceps tendon is then inspected as it disappears from the glenohumeral joint. The rotator cuff is inspected from anterior to posterior. To facilitate cuff visualization, the humerus can be internally and externally rotated as needed in the arm-positioning device. Moving the probe superior to the biceps tendon facilitates probing and inspection of the rotator cuff. The probe is used to lift the cuff away from the humeral head and inspect the insertional anatomy. The articular surfaces

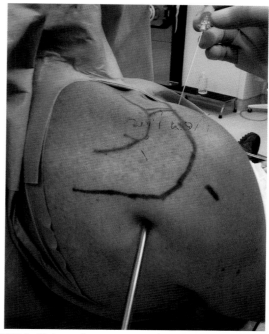

FIGURE 2.8. Using arthroscopic visualization via the posterior portal to localize the anterior portal with a spinal needle.

of the humeral head and glenoid are evaluated carefully.

Although seen from the posterior portal, the posterior glenohumeral structures are better visualized from an anterior perspective. We therefore place the camera through the anterior portal for evaluation of the posterior structures.

Diagnostic arthroscopy is incomplete without a subacromial exam. Evaluation of the subacromial space utilizes the same skin incision used for the posterior shoulder portal. The arthroscopic sheath and obturator are redirected anteriorly into the subacromial space while gentle inferior traction is maintained. Upon penetration of the space, the trocar should move freely in the horizontal plane. The trocar is then exchanged for the arthroscopic camera. A lateral subacromial portal is next established. This portal is made approximately 1 cm posterior to the anterior acromial border and 2 cm inferior to the lateral aspect of the acromial border (Figure 2.9). The skin is divided with a scalpel, and a disposable cannula is inserted.

Structures identified arthroscopically in the subacromial space include the bursa, the bursal side of the rotator cuff, and the fat and synovium underlying the acromioclavicular joint. The condition of the bursa is noted, and a bursectomy is occasionally necessary for accurate evaluation. Rotator cuff inspection

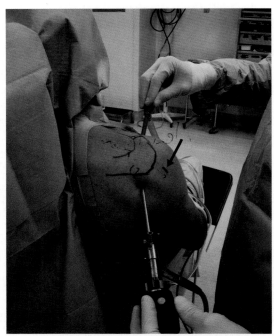

FIGURE 2.9. Posterior view during diagnostic arthroscopy of the right shoulder using the beach chair position. Note use of probe through anterior (arrow) portal and skin marking over intended lateral subacromial working portal.

is facilitated by internal and external rotation. This completes the diagnostic shoulder arthroscopy.

POSTOPERATIVE MANAGEMENT

The portal sites are closed and a dressing is applied. Postoperative analgesia and or anti-inflammatory medication may be injected into the glenohumeral joint and/or the subacromial space as needed. The patient is carefully repositioned onto a flat operating room table. When the patient is in a stable position, the beanbag may be decompressed and the operating room table adjusted to a flat position to facilitate transfer of the patient from the operating room.

Postoperative physical therapy regimen and any splinting and immobilization are individually tailored.

RESULTS/OUTCOME

The beach chair position offers numerous advantages and is the preferred technique for all our patients. These advantages include more natural anatomical orientation, improved manipulation of the arm intraoperatively, good visualization and access, and ease of conversion to an open procedure when necessary. Complications and difficulties associated with traction are avoided.

COMPLICATIONS

Complications of shoulder arthroscopy are reported elsewhere (see Chapter 25). Complications more specific to the beach chair position include nerve injury, pressure problems, possible cardiac problems, and intolerance to positioning under a regional anesthetic.

Complications related to positioning are avoided only with meticulous positioning and padding of all patients, and frequent reevaluation of that positioning during the procedure.[7] Transient or permanent nerve injuries have been described in postoperative patients secondary to lack of attention to positioning and padding. Prolonged regional anesthesia may increase the incidence of injuries of these types in patients whose peripheral nerves remain compressed during sugery.

One complication that has been reported to be specific to the beach chair position is a transient hypotension and bradycardia seen when the patient is positioned upright after interscalene block anesthesia. This is thought to occur secondary to the Bezold–Jarisch[8] reflex and has been reported in greater than

20% of patients who undergo shoulder arthroscopy in a sitting position under interscalene block anesthesia. Onset of symptoms has been generally reported to occur between 30 and 100 min after regional blockade. Symptomatic treatment of this problem is generally all that is required, and the phenomenon is usually transient. Prophylactic use of metoprolol immediately after the block is obtained has also been shown to be effective in preventing this phenomenon.[9]

References

1. Skyhar MJ, Altchek DW, Warren RF, et al. Shoulder arthroscopy with the patient in the beach-chair position. *Arthroscopy* 1988;4(4):256–259.
2. Klein AH, France JC, Mutschler TA, Fu FH. Measurement of brachial plexus strain in arthroscopy of the shoulder. *Arthroscopy* 1987;3:45–52.
3. Pitman MI. Arthroscopic research. In: *Abstracts on Sports Injuries and Rehabilitation, 19–21 November 1987, Roosevelt Hotel, New York.*
4. Altchek DW, Skyhar MJ, Warren RF. Shoulder arthroscopy for shoulder instability. *Instr. Course Lect* 1989; 38:187–198.
5. Andrews JR, Carson WG, Ortega K. Arthroscopy of the shoulder: technique and normal anatomy. *Am J Sports Med* 1984;12:1–7.
6. O'Brien SJ, Gonzalez DM, Wright JM, et al. The adduction distraction maneuver. *Arthroscopy* 1997;13(4): 530–532.
7. Stanish WD, Peterson DC. Shoulder arthroscopy and nerve injury: pitfalls and prevention. *Arthroscopy* 1995;11(4):458–466.
8. D'Alessio JG, Weller RS, Rosenblum M. Activation of the Bezold–Jarisch reflex in the sitting position for shoulder arthroscopy using interscalene block. *Anesth Analg* 1995;80:1158–1162.
9. Liguori GA, Kahn RL, Gordon J, et al. The use of metoprolol and glycopyrrolate to prevent hypotensive/bradycardic events during shoulder arthroscopy in the sitting position under interscalene block. *Anesth Analg* 1998; 87:1320–1325.

Recommended Reading

Andrews JR Carson WG. Arthroscopic surgery of the shoulder. In: Parisien JS, ed. *Arthroscopic Surgery.* New York: McGraw-Hill; 1988:231–241.

Altchek DW. Arthroscopic shoulder stabilization using a bioabsorbable fixation device. *Sport Med Arthrosc Rev* 1993;1(4):266–271.

Matthews LS, Fadale PD. Technique and instrumentation for shoulder arthroscopy. *Instr Course Lect* 1989;38:177–185.

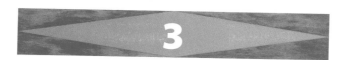

Arthroscopic Shoulder Anatomy

Cyrus J. Lashgari, Leesa M. Galatz,
and Ken Yamaguchi

A firm grasp of shoulder anatomy is requisite to ensure the best possible outcome and to avoid complications of arthroscopic shoulder surgery. Enthusiasm for minimally invasive shoulder surgery has fostered many studies on arthroscopic shoulder anatomy. This chapter focuses on the arthroscopic rather than open anatomy of the shoulder. An emphasis is placed on appreciating normal anatomy and its variants as distinguished from true pathology of the shoulder. The chapter is organized into the following sections: superficial anatomy, the long head of the biceps tendon, the rotator interval, the glenoid labrum, the glenohumeral ligaments, the rotator cuff, bony anatomy, neurovascular structures, and the subacromial space.

SUPERFICIAL ANATOMY AND PORTAL PLACEMENT

The palpable bony landmarks are important in creating safe, accurate, and reproducible portals. These landmarks are outlined before the procedure begins. The acromion is outlined in its entirety with focus on three important points: the posterolateral corner, the anterolateral corner, and the confluence of the distal clavicle and scapular spine. The posterolateral corner of the acromion is often the easiest landmark to feel, because the overlying posterior deltoid is thin. The anterolateral is more difficult to palpate secondary to the thickness of the overlying deltoid in this area. The anterolateral corner is in line with the distal clavicle anteriorly. Awareness of this relationship is helpful in avoiding confusion with the greater tuberosity of the humeral head. The third landmark is the supraclavicular fossa at the confluence of the distal clavicle and scapular spine. This point marks the posterior aspect of the acromioclavicular (AC) joint and is just lateral to the "Neviaser" supraclavicular portal.[1] When appropriately marked, these three points should approximate an equilateral triangle (Figure 3.1). The distal clavicle, AC joint, coracoid tip, and lateral acromial border are outlined to complete the orientation.

The posterior portal for initial arthroscopic viewing is located in the "soft spot," approximately 2 cm medial and 2 cm below the posterolateral corner of the acromion. This portal is considerably superior to the axillary nerve, whose anterior branch courses with the posterior humeral circumflex through the quadrangular space (bordered by the teres minor superiorly, the teres major inferiorly, the long head of the triceps medially, and the surgical neck of the humerus laterally) and passes anteriorly along the deltoid's undersurface. The nerve is found an average of 5.5 cm distal to the lateral edge of the acromion, but it can be as close as 3.1 cm.[2]

The anterior portal is usually made after initial arthroscope placement. Whether established "inside out" with a Wissenger rod, or "outside in" with a spinal needle, the portal is located within the rotator interval. Arthroscopically this triangle is bordered by the glenoid, the biceps long head, and the subscapularis tendon's upper border[3] (Figure 3.2). Externally, the portal is usually 1 to 2 cm inferomedial to the anterolateral acromion. One must be lateral to the coracoid tip, a critical landmark in safely establishing this portal. The brachial plexus and axillary vessels lie medial and inferior to the coracoid. When introduced lateral to the coracoid tip, a spinal needle is directed inferiorly and medially to enter the joint. Once needle position has been deemed satisfactory, an incision is made and the anterior cannula placed parallel to the needle.

Additional portals during shoulder arthroscopy depend upon the pathology encountered. The anterolateral portal is used for procedures in the subacromial space. This portal is located approximately 1 cm posterior to the anterolateral acromion and 2 to 3 cm distal to its lateral edge. As with the anterior portal, an 18-gauge spinal needle can help localize the ideal position during viewing in the subacromial space. This portal is relatively safe because the anterior branch of

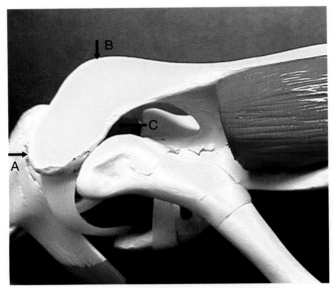

FIGURE 3.1. Aerial view demonstrating the superficial anatomy of the shoulder. Points A and B represent the anterolateral and posterolateral borders of the acromion, respectively. Point C represents the supraclavicular fossa and marks the posterior extent of the acromioclavicular joint. These three points approximate an equilateral triangle.

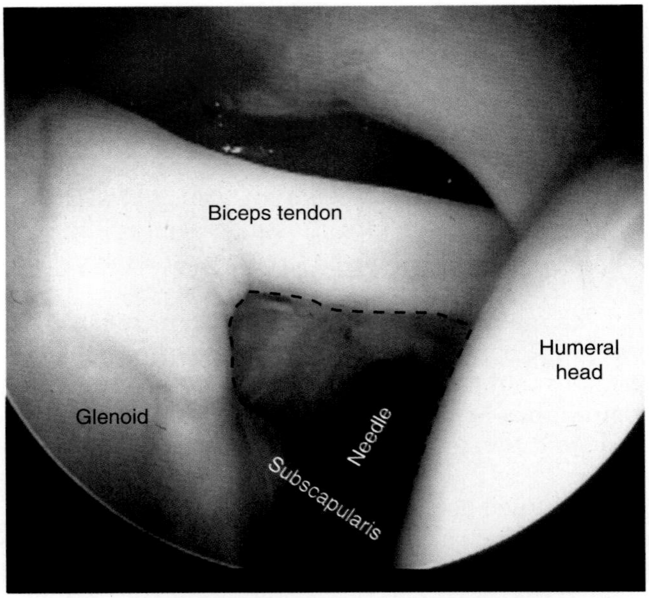

FIGURE 3.2. Intraoperative photograph of the rotator interval in a right shoulder in the beach chair position, as viewed from the posterior portal. The glenoid is located to the left and the humeral head is to the right. The needle is in the arthroscopic triangle formed by the biceps tendon superiorly, the subscapularis inferiorly, and the glenoid.

the axillary nerve is found an average of 5 cm distal to the anterolateral corner.

The anterior inferior portal, used during anterior arthroscopic stabilization procedures, was described by Davidson and Tibone[4] and provides direct access to the anterior inferior glenoid rim (the location of capsulolabral detachment in patients with anterior instability). This portal is created under direct visualization from "inside out" by passing a blunt-tipped Wissinger rod through the anterior capsule and soft tissue until it tents the skin. The rod is directed to the leading edge of the anterior band of the inferior glenohumeral ligament. With the arm adducted, the rod is directed as laterally as possible. This portal passes lateral to the conjoint tendon and through the lower third of the subscapularis muscle. The minimum safe distance between this portal and the axillary nerve has been shown to be 14 mm. The minimum safe distance from the musculocutaneous nerve was 12 mm. Abduction of the shoulder decreases both these distances.

THE LONG HEAD OF THE BICEPS TENDON

In initial viewing from the posterior arthroscopic portal, the long head of the biceps tendon is usually the first recognizable structure seen. Nowhere in the shoulder is there more normal variability than at the biceps origin and the anterior superior labrum. The long head originates from the posterosuperior labrum and the supraglenoid tubercle. The tendon is widest at its origin and progressively narrows as it approaches its muscle belly. The origin of the long head is variable. Habermeyer et al. described the long head origin as completely labral in 50% of specimens, with only 20% arising solely from the supraglenoid tubercle. The remaining 30% of specimens had a dual origin from the two structures.[5] The tendon had a mean length of 9.2 cm and was 8.5 mm by 2.8 mm wide at its origin. Vangsness et al.[6] showed that 40 to 60% of the specimens arose from both the labrum and supraglenoid tubercle, with the remainder originating from the labrum alone. They classified the labral attachment into four types: type I, the labral attachment is entirely posterior (22%); type II, the majority is from the posterior labrum with some fibers originating anteriorly (33%); type III, equal posterior and anterior contributions (37%); and type IV, most of the origin is from the anterior labrum (8%) (Figure 3.3). Regardless of exact labral origins, when the articular cartilage of the superior glenoid rim is extended, it always blends superiorly with the biceps tendon origin.

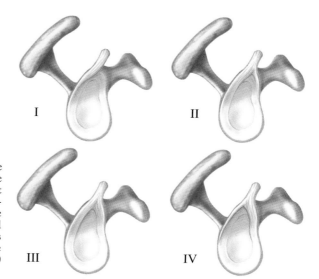

FIGURE 3.3. Schematic drawings of the variations in the biceps origin. Type I: the labral attachment is almost entirely posterior; this is seen 22% of the time. Type II: most of the labral contribution is posterior with a small amount of anterior contribution; this is seen 33% of the time. Type III: equal contributions from both the anterior and posterior labra; this is seen 37% of the time. Type IV: most of the labral contribution is anterior, with only a small posterior contribution; this is seen 8% of the time. (Reprinted from Vangsness CT, Jorgenson SS, Watson T, Johnson DL. The origin of the long head of the biceps from the scapula and glenoid labrum. An anatomical study of 100 shoulders. *J Bone Joint Surg Br* 1994;76:951–954.)

From its origin, the long head of the biceps arches anteriorly over the humeral head to exit the joint encased in a synovial sheath beneath the transverse humeral ligament. The synovial sheath ends as a blind pouch at the end of the intertubercular sulcus (also referred to as the bicipital groove). Therefore, the long head of the biceps is intra-articular but extrasynovial. Pathological changes are commonly found along the portion of the biceps tendon that lies within the bicipital groove. This part of the tendon can be examined by placing traction on the intra-articular portion in an inferior direction with a probe through the anterior portal, pulling a few centimeters of tendon into the joint (Figure 3.4). Alternatively, an Allis clamp may be inserted through the anterior portal and clasped around the tendon. Spinning the clamp in either direction pulls the extra-articular tendon into the joint.

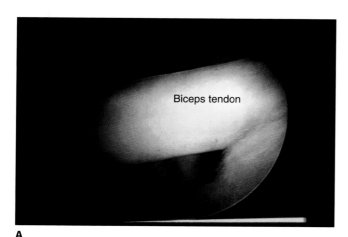

A

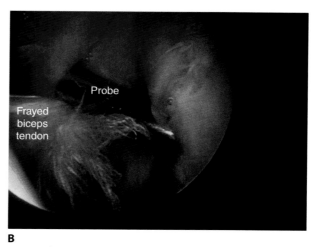

B

FIGURE 3.4. Intraoperative photos of the long head of the biceps tendon viewed from the posterior portal (left shoulder, beach chair perspective). (A) Normal appearing intra-articular biceps tendon. (B) Extensive degenerative fraying of the same tendon when the portion in the bicipital groove is pulled into the joint.

THE ROTATOR INTERVAL

The rotator interval, an area of intense interest and current investigation, lies between the anterior border of the supraspinatus and superior edge of the subscapularis muscle. It extends medially to the coracoid and laterally to the bicipital groove. The superior glenohumeral ligament (SGHL), the coracohumeral ligament (CHL), the joint capsule, the biceps tendon, and the superior aspect of the middle glenohumeral ligament all lie within the interval (Figure 3.5).

A recent study by Jost et al. describes the anatomy in detail.[7] The interval is divided into a medial portion composed of two layers, and a more lateral portion composed of four layers. The medial portion consists of the more superficial CHL, the deeper SGHL, and the joint capsule. Laterally, the first, most superficial layer consists of the superficial fibers of the CHL that extend lateral to the insertions of the subscapu-

laris and supraspinatus. Layer 2 consists of tendon fibers of the subscapularis and supraspinatus that cross each other at the insertion point and blend with the CHL. Layer 3 consists of the deep fibers of the CHL that insert into the greater tuberosity and to a lesser extent the lesser tuberosity. The deepest layer consists of the SGHL and capsule. Externally, the CHL can be seen to originate as a band 1 to 2 cm wide from the proximal third of the dorsolateral aspect of the coracoid process, which travels anterior and superficial to the biceps tendon to insert into the tuberosities (Figure 3.6). Jost described the CHL to be a well-developed ligament, not just a reinforcement of the joint capsule. Other studies, however, have described the coracohumeral ligament as a capsular reflection, not a true ligament.[8]

Tetro et al. studied the anatomy of the rotator interval from an arthroscopic perspective to guide surgeons when performing an arthroscopic release for ad-

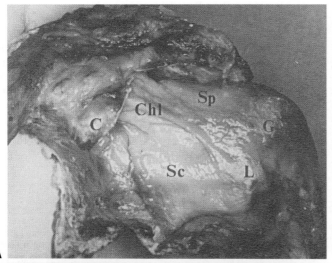

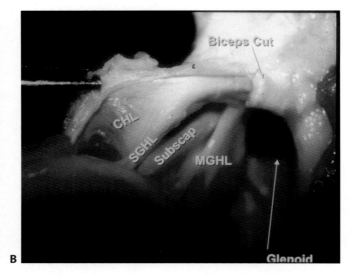

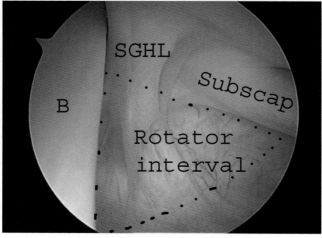

FIGURE 3.5. (A) Cadaveric dissection demonstrating external anatomical features of the rotator interval (left shoulder, viewed from anterior): C, coracoid; Chl, coracohumeral ligament; G, greater tuberosity; L, lesser tuberosity; Sc, subscapularis tendon; Sp, supraspinatus. (B) Cadaveric dissection of the deep surface structures of the rotator interval (left shoulder, viewed from posterior). The biceps tendon has been cut to reveal the relationships of the subscapularis tendon, the middle glenohumeral ligament (MGHL), the superior glenohumeral ligament (SGHL), and the coracohumeral ligament (CHL). Notice how the SGHL and CHL form a sling for the biceps as it exits the glenohumeral joint: B, biceps. (C) Intraoperative photograph of arthroscopic equivalent of deep surface of rotator interval: right shoulder, lateral decubitus orientation. Note biceps (B) tendon on the left and subscapularis tendon on the right. Spanning the interval and forming the inferior border of the bicipital sheath at its exit is the superior glenohumeral ligament (SGHL).

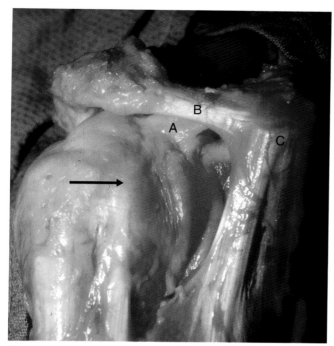

A

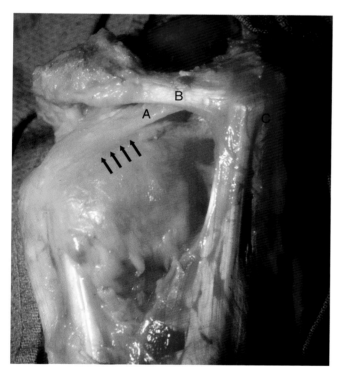

B

FIGURE 3.6. (A) Cadaveric specimen revealing external surface of rotator interval structures and the relationship between the coracohumeral and coracoacromial ligaments (right shoulder, anterior view). Note the CHL A arising from the coracoid C and passing deep and inferior to the CA ligament B. In neutral and internal rotation, the CH ligament (arrow) is barely discernible (B). In external rotation, the CH ligament A becomes prominent and stands out in relief as a distinct structure contributing to the interval (arrows).

hesive capsulitis.[9] The depth of release, however, had not been previously described. Tetro observed that the fibers of the CHL are extra-articular medially but laterally become interlaced and indistinguishable from those of the capsule and SGHL. He noted that to completely release the interval, the fibers of the coracoacromial ligament must be visualized at the completion of the release. The measured distance from the rotator interval to the coracoacromial ligament averaged 3.5 mm in this cadaveric study. In patients with adhesive capsulitis, the capsule has thickened and hypertrophied and internal tissue is even more prominent, markedly increasing the depth of tissue requiring release.

The lateral extent of the rotator interval is critical in providing stabilization of the biceps tendon at its exit into the intertubercular groove. The superior glenohumeral ligament, the medial head of the coracohumeral ligament, and the insertion of the subscapularis tendon become confluent and support the biceps tendon as the medial sheath at the proximal aspect of the intertubercular groove (Figure 3.7). The subscapularis tendon inserts onto the lesser tuberosity just inferior to the articular cartilage and medial to the SGHL/CHL complex. The fibers of the subscapularis and the SGHL/CHL complex interdigitate in this area. The lateral head of the CHL crosses the bicipital groove to insert with the fibers of the supraspinatus onto the greater tuberosity. Shoulder elevation and internal rotation allow visualization of these supporting structures.

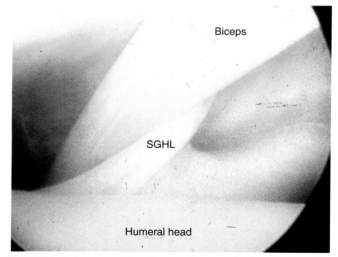

FIGURE 3.7. Intraoperative close-up photograph of a right shoulder, beach chair perspective, showing the biceps tendon as it exits the glenohumeral joint. Together, the coracohumeral and superior glenohumeral ligaments form a medial buttress preventing biceps tendon subluxation. This ligament complex is the most important stabilizer of the biceps tendon: SGHL, superior glenohumeral ligament.

THE GLENOID LABRUM

The labrum is an ovoid rim of fibrocartilage tissue attached to the margin of the glenoid fossa, which both deepens the fossa and serves as an attachment site for the glenohumeral capsule–ligament complex. Evaluation of this structure is complicated by the number of normal variants that have been described. Knowledge of normal variability is crucial in assessing and treating pathological lesions.

Although somewhat variable, the labrum is peripherally continuous with the joint capsule and the periosteum of the scapular neck. Centrally, the labrum is in continuity with the hyaline cartilage on the surface of the glenoid fossa (Figure 3.8). Most of the labrum is attached both centrally and peripherally, but there is considerable variation in its size, morphology, and mobility. Variations are best described regionally based on location: superior, anterior, inferior, and posterior.

The superior labrum is a unique and important structure because of its close association with the biceps tendon and its involvement in superior labral anterior–posterior (SLAP) lesions. This area also demonstrates the greatest degree of variability in normal anatomy. The superior labrum is contiguous with the insertion of the biceps tendon long head at the supraglenoid tubercle. Usually triangular, similar to the knee's meniscus, the labrum has been classified into two types by Detrisic and Johnson.[10] The most common type is the "central detachment" type, seen in 60% of specimens. In this variant, the labrum is secured peripherally, but centrally at its free margin, a probe can be insinuated between its edge and the superior glenoid rim (Figure 3.9). The key to distin-

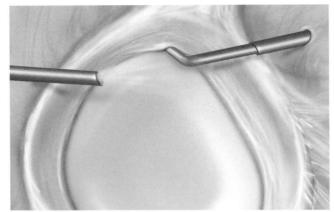

FIGURE 3.9. The more common variant of the superior labrum, in which there is some mobility of the labrum's free edge, which permits insinuation of a probe between it and the superior glenoid rim.

guishing this normal variant from a true "SLAP" lesion is to recognize the presence of normal hyaline articular cartilage extending over the glenoid's superior rim and smooth transition to the labral undersurface. The labrum may appear to be "loose" and in fact is often quite mobile, but this is entirely normal and should not be confused with a SLAP lesion.[11] In the remaining 40%, the labrum is "centrally attached," with seamless continuity from the superior glenoid rim to the labrum (Figure 3.10).

True labral pathology superiorly is recognized by fraying, tearing, displacement, or instability of the superior labrum/biceps tendon complex (Figure 3.11). Distinguishing pathological findings from normal variants is aided by clear tissue damage, loss of normal articular transitional continuity, abnormal mobility, or the presence of dynamic instability of the

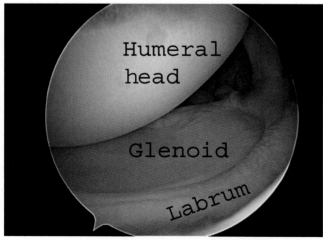

FIGURE 3.8. Arthroscopic view of labrum, left shoulder, lateral decubitus position, viewing from posterior scope portal. The labrum is circumferentially secured at articular margin interface.

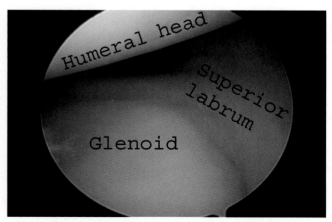

FIGURE 3.10. In this arthroscopic photograph of a left shoulder (lateral decubitus perspective, looking from posterior portal), there is no "seam" between the superior glenoid and the articular surface and one can see the normal transition between these two structures.

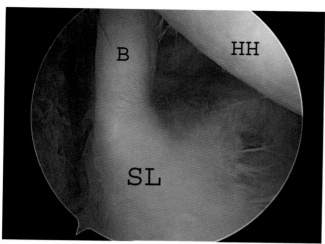

FIGURE 3.11. Arthroscopic photograph of right shoulder, lateral decubitus perspective, shows degenerative fraying of free edge of superior labrum: HH, humeral head; B, biceps; SL, superior labrum.

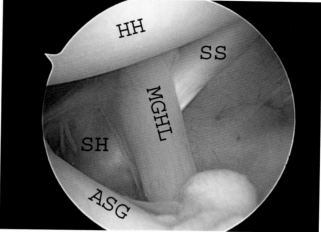

FIGURE 3.12. In this close-up arthroscopic view of a left shoulder (lateral decubitus perspective) note the "sublabral hole" formed by the cordlike middle glenohumeral ligament (MGHL) attached to the superior glenoid: HH, humeral head; MGHL, middle glenohumeral ligament; SH, sublabral hole; ASG, anterior superior glenoid.

complex. For a thorough review of superior labral pathology, the reader is referred to Chapter 7 on SLAP tears.

Although not considered a true "SLAP" tear, a "peel-back" injury has been recently described by Burkhart, in which the biceps–superior labrum complex "peels back" medially along the glenoid when the arm is placed in the throwing position (abduction/external rotation). Only through dynamic assessment can this pathological variant be recognized, and this phenomenon may well account for cases of suspected subtle instability, in which no other dramatic arthroscopic findings are visually evident.

The anterosuperior labrum is a difficult area to evaluate because it also has a significant amount of normal variability. Like the superior labrum, the anterosuperior labrum demonstrates a meniscal pattern. There can be a firm attachment directly to the glenoid, although studies have shown this to be the exception rather than the rule. In a relatively common variant, present in an estimated 12% of shoulders, the labrum above the midglenoid notch is absent. This so-called sublabral hole, formed by the absence of labrum between the anterior superior glenoid and the overlying middle glenohumeral ligament (MGHL), is a normal variant, not indicative of pathology (Figure 3.12). In a unique subset of patients with a cordlike glenohumeral ligament, the MGHL arises directly from the superior labrum, and there is no anterior–superior labral tissue present between the attachment and the midglenoid notch. Reported as occurring in 1.5% (3/200) of shoulders, this "Buford complex" represents a normal variant (Figure 3.13) that should not be confused with a traumatic detachment of the labrum.[12]

If the Buford complex is mistakenly reattached to the neck of the glenoid, as illustrated in our case example, severe painful restriction of rotation and elevation may result. In general, "labral deficiency" "north" of the glenoid notch rarely reflects true pathology. The typical Bankart lesion seen in patients with anterior instability is found "south" of the notch.

The anterior and inferior labra are more consistent in appearance and relationship with surrounding structures. The labrum in these areas is typically attached both centrally and peripherally (Figure 3.8), and appears as a thickened band of capsule, rounded, in contrast to the triangular meniscal morphology of the

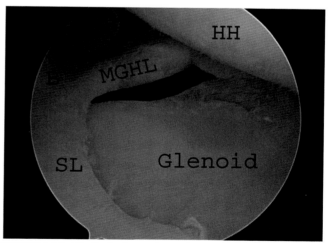

FIGURE 3.13. The Buford complex in fact represents a normal variant, here seen as a consequence of a cordlike MGHL meeting the biceps at the superior corner of the glenoid, with no intervening labrum along the glenoid rim: B, biceps; HH, humeral head; SL, superior labrum; MGHL, middle glenohumeral ligament. (View from right shoulder, lateral decubitus perspective.)

superior glenoid. The anterior band of the inferior glenohumeral ligament is intimately attached to both the glenoid and the labrum at the 4 o'clock position (Figure 3.14). Fraying or detachment in this area is considered to be pathological.

The posterior labrum has not been the subject of extensive anatomical dissection and evaluation. There is a gradual transition back to a more loosely attached labrum from the 6 o'clock to the 12 o'clock position (Figure 3.15). In one study there was a sublabral hole at the 8 o'clock position in 4 of 11 specimens.[13] The significance of this variation is unknown, and further studies are needed to clarify its significance. The mobile labrum is anchored to the glenoid at the 10 o'clock position. Separation of the labrum from the articular margin probably has the same significance posteriorly as it does anteriorly (Figure 3.16).

The capsular attachment to the labrum has also demonstrated variability. The most significant variation is the relationship of the inferior glenohumeral ligament (IGHL) attachment to the labrum. In a study of 52 fetal and embryonic shoulders, 77% were found to attach directly to the capsule, and 23% attached medially to the scapular neck with a freestanding labrum, creating an anterior pouch.[14] This observation is important in demonstrating that not all inferior glenohumeral ligaments arise from the labrum directly, and some may normally arise from more medially along the neck itself (Figure 3.17).

The most common pathology findings include degenerative fraying and tissue attrition. Other findings include flap tears (Figure 3.18), bucket handle tears,

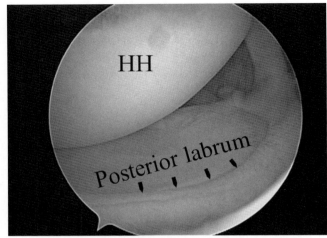

FIGURE 3.15. The posterior inferior labrum is normally a slightly prominent structure, seamlessly connected both centrally and peripherally to its adjacent articular margin (left shoulder, lateral decubitus perspective, scope posteriorly): HH, humeral head.

SLAP lesions, internal impingement, and labral detachments. The most common labral detachment of course is the Bankart lesion, in which the labrum and/or inferior glenohumeral ligament has been avulsed from the anterior–inferior glenoid rim (typically from 3 to 6 o'clock in a right shoulder) (Figure 3.19). In an ALPSA (anterior ligamentous periosteal sleeve avulsion) lesion, the IGHL–labrum complex has been avulsed and has healed in a displaced position medially along the anterior inferior glenoid neck (Figure 3.20).[15]

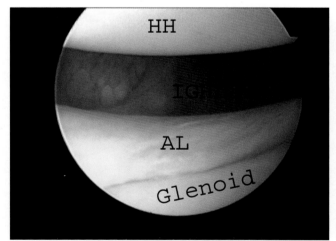

FIGURE 3.14. This close-up arthroscopic view of the anterior inferior labrum demonstrates the normal appearance of insertion of the inferior glenohumeral ligament (IGHL), whose leading band is seen to attach directly to the anterior labrum at about the equator of the glenoid: HH, humeral head; IGHL, inferior glenohumeral ligament; AL, anterior labrum. (Vew from right shoulder, lateral decubitus perspective.)

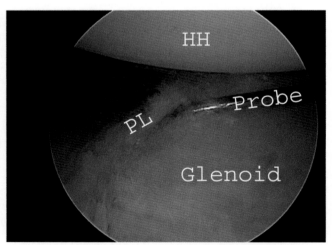

FIGURE 3.16. Probe from anterior portal (viewing from posterior portal, left shoulder, lateral decubitus position) shows easy insinuation in Bankart equivalent in this patient with a posterior labral (PL) detachment and recurrent posterior shoulder instability symptoms: HH, humeral head; PL, posterior labrum.

encompass™

HOME HEALTH & HOSPICE

P: 817.737.4300   F: 817.737.4305

FORT WORTH

www.ehhi.com

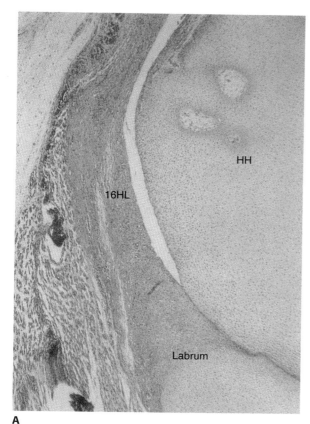

A

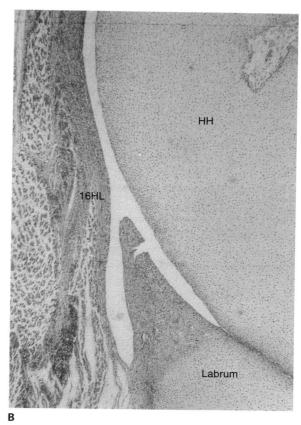

B

FIGURE 3.17. Cutaway embryo sections demonstrating the variability in normal anterior capsular attachments. (A) The presumed normal attachment, in which the inferior glenohumeral ligament (IGHL) is in continuity with the labrum: HH, humeral head. (B) An alternative variant of normal, in which the labrum is a distinct structure, separate from the IGHL, which attaches medial to the labrum along the glenoid rim. (From Ref. 14.)

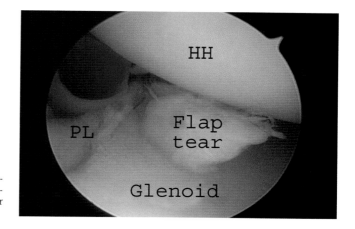

FIGURE 3.18. Viewing from anterior portal (right shoulder, lateral decubitus perspective), a large flap tear of the posterior labrum is insinuated between the humeral head (HH) and the glenoid: PL, posterior labrum.

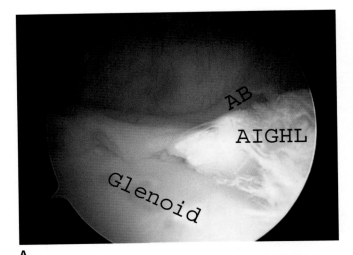

A

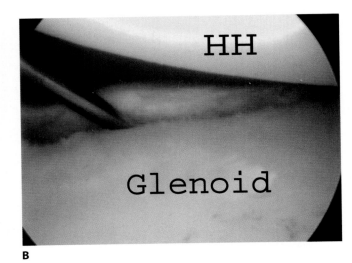

B

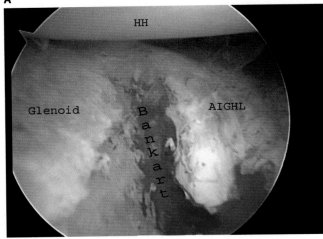

C

FIGURE 3.19. (A) Bankart lesion seen with fraying at site of torn anterior inferior glenohumeral ligament (AIGHL) along anterior–inferior glenoid rim (view from posterior portal, right shoulder, lateral decubitus perspective). (B) A probe from the anterior superior portal palpates the interface between the labrum and the glenoid rim. (C) The Bankart lesion is seen more clearly as the scope has been positioned in the anterosuperior portal of a left shoulder (lateral decubitus perspective). The hemorrhage, which occurred during labral mobilization and glenoid debridement, marks the lesion interface: HH, humeral head; AB, anterior band.

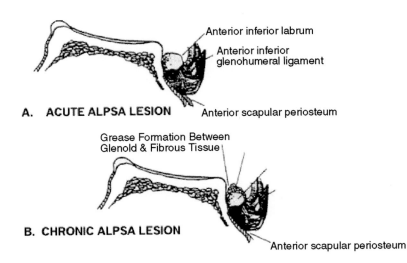

FIGURE 3.20. The ALPSA lesion shown schematically in acute (A) and chronic (B) forms represents an avulsion of the labrum as a periosteal sleeve anteriorly and must be considered in the absence of an obvious Bankart lesion in the patient with instability. [Reproduced with permission from Neviaser, TJ. The anterior labroligamentous periosteal sleeve avulsion lesion: a cause of anterior instability of the shoulder. *Arthroscopy.* 1993;9(1):17–21.]

THE GLENOHUMERAL LIGAMENTS

The superior, middle, and inferior glenohumeral ligaments play a critical role in glenohumeral stability. When viewed externally, the glenohumeral capsule is featureless. But when its internal surface is examined, the deep capsule has discrete thickenings, the glenohumeral ligaments, which are defined by their humeral insertions as superior, middle or inferior, and have been shown through selective cutting studies to provide specific functional contributions to glenohumeral stability. Like the labrum, these ligaments demonstrate significant normal variations that must be recognized if appropriate treatment strategies are to be formed (Figure 3.21).

The superior glenohumeral ligament (SGHL) arises near the supraglenoid tubercle and inserts just superiorly to the lesser tuberosity, crossing the capsular portion of the rotator interval (Figure 3.5C). It is the primary restraint to inferior translation in the adducted shoulder. In addition to providing some stability to the arm in the adducted position, it also resists posterior and inferior humeral head displacement. The smallest of the glenohumeral ligaments, it is quite consistent, present in 97% of specimens examined by DePalma. It is often obscured behind the biceps tendon, and may be buried within the synovium and not discretely recognizable.

Variations in the SGHL have to do with its origin. It has been described as originating from the superior glenoid tubercle, anterior to the long head of the biceps tendon origin. It has also been described as arising solely from the glenoid labrum at approximately the 1 o'clock position of a right glenoid, possibly sharing a common origin with the middle glenohumeral ligament. It inserts on the lesser tuberosity in close association with the coracohumeral ligament, forming an anterior band around the biceps tendon. This is the main restraint to medial biceps subluxation. The superior glenohumeral ligament is almost always present (94–100%) but varies in thickness. The SGHL is usually found superior to the long head of the biceps but may be obscured by the biceps as it courses laterally. The SGHL can be difficult to identify if it is thin and rudimentary. It is best visualized with the arm in adduction and external rotation (Figure 3.22).

The middle glenohumeral ligament (MGHL) arises from the glenoid labrum immediately below the origin of the SGHL or from the adjacent glenoid neck and inserts just medial to the lesser tuberosity, crossing over and occasionally blending into the subscapularis tendon. It is an important restraint to anterior translation in the the midrange of shoulder function, especially if the inferior glenohumeral ligament has been damaged. It is not seen as consistently

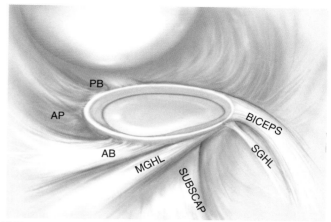

FIGURE 3.21. Cutaway illustration (viewed from anteriorly, right shoulder, lateral decubitus perspective) demonstrates the glenohumeral ligaments. The superior (SGHL) lies under cover of the biceps tendon and is the most commonly present. The middle (MGHL) crosses the subscapularis at an oblique angle and is easily identified interoperatively based on this relationship. The inferior (IGHL) complex consists of the anterior (AB) and posterior (PB) bands and intervening axillary pouch (AP).

as the SGHL, though it is significantly larger and more variable in size. It also has the greatest number of normal variants among the three ligaments. The ligament is present 85% of the time, averaging 3.6 mm in diameter and 18 mm in length.[16] However, it can be a thin wisp of tissue or as thick as the biceps tendon. Arthroscopically, the middle glenohumeral ligament consistently crosses deep to the subscapularis at an oblique angle and is best seen in its midportion, where it obliquely crosses the rolled upper tendon edge of the subscapularis at approximately 60° (Figure 3.23). In approximately 9% of the population, the MGHL is "cordlike" and may contribute to the misperception that the labrum is deficient[12] (Figure 3.13).

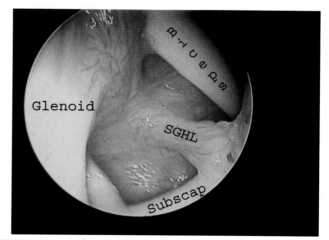

FIGURE 3.22. The superior glenohumeral ligament (SGHL), which is best observed with the arm in adduction and internal rotation, is shown running parallel to and under cover of the biceps tendon. (View from posterior portal, right shoulder, beach chair position.)

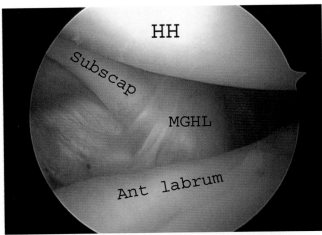

FIGURE 3.23. The middle glenohumeral ligament (MGHL) runs obliquely across the subscapularis tendon and has the most variability of the glenohumeral ligaments. Here the ligament appears as a sheet of tissue. (View from posterior, right shoulder, lateral decubitus): HH, humeral head.

The inferior glenohumeral ligament (IGHL) is a complex consisting of an anterior band, a posterior band, and intervening axillary pouch (Figure 3.24). It originates from the glenoid, the labrum, or the neck of the glenoid just adjacent to the labrum.[17] The anterior band originates between the 2 and 4 o'clock positions, while the posterior band originates between the 7 and 9 o'clock positions. As a complex, the inferior glenohumeral ligament originates between the 3 and 8 o'clock positions in over 90% of shoulders. A distinct ligament is found in 72%, a thickening of capsule in 21%, and no ligament or thickening in 7%. The ligament inserts in one of two configurations onto the anatomical neck of the humerus either as a collar just inferior to the articular margin or as a "V" with the axillary pouch inserting distal to the articular cartilage. The presence of the ligament is best demonstrated arthroscopically with the arm in an abducted position. The posterior band becomes prominent with internal rotation and the anterior band becomes prominent with external rotation. The inferior glenohumeral ligament complex is the main static contributor to glenohumeral stability with the arm in the adducted position.

The Bankart lesion, which is the most common manifestation of anterior instability, can involve the glenohumeral ligaments themselves and/or the labrum, along the anterior inferior glenoid rim. Uncommonly, instability can be due to avulsion of the IGHL from the lateral insertion along the tuberosity. This finding has been coined the "HAGL" lesion, standing for humeral avulsion of glenohumeral ligament, and has been described as occurring in up to 9.3% of arthroscopically examined shoulders.[18] This lesion is best seen either from an anterior portal or with use of a 70° scope from the traditional posterior portal. Remember it when an unstable shoulder has an unexpectedly normal-looking anterior inferior glenoid rim–labrum interface.

Finally, as an observation, there really is no single "normal" pattern of development or insertion of the glenohumeral ligaments. Recognize then that there are variations in the individual size, shape, and insertion of each ligament, as well as collective differences in their pattern. The ligaments have been evaluated and classified with respect to their general appearance.

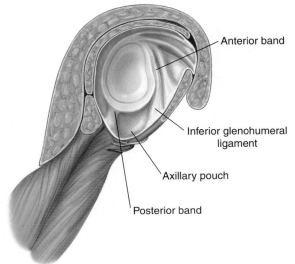

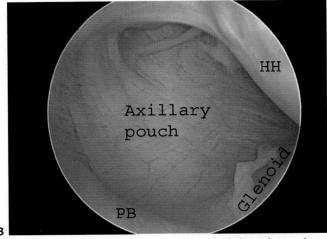

FIGURE 3.24. (A) Cutaway view of the inferior glenohumeral ligament complex, composed of anterior and posterior bands, and intervening axillary pouch. (B) Note the arthroscopic appearance of the axillary pouch and the posterior band of the inferior glenohumeral ligament (scope in posterior portal, lateral decubitus perspective, left shoulder): PB, posterior band; HH, humeral head.

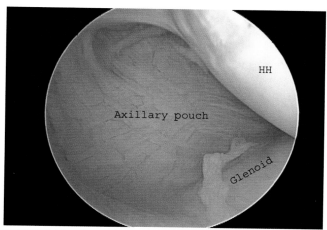

FIGURE 3.25. This arthroscopic view (scope posterior, left shoulder, lateral decubitus perspective) demonstrating the capacious axillary pouch found in patients with generalized laxity and those with multidirectional instablity: HH, humeral head.

In the "classic" pattern, seen in 66% of shoulders, each ligament (SGHL, MGHL, and IGHL) is distinct, with recesses or synovial reflections between them. Seven percent of shoulders demonstrate a pattern of "confluence" in which the MGHL and IGHL are confluent as one ligament without an intervening recess. Eight percent have no discernible ligaments, and when viewed externally, the anterior capsule appears as a confluent sheet without reflections or recesses. Patients with multidirectional instability often have no specific pathological finding but are noted to have a positive "drive through" sign and to demonstrate a capacious axillary recess (Figure 3.25).

THE ROTATOR CUFF

The rotator cuff is formed by four distinct muscles that coalesce to form a "cuff" that inserts on the proximal humerus. The subscapularis forms the anterior cuff. The posterior cuff is composed of the supraspinatus, the infraspinatus, and the teres minor. These three tendons insert together as a continuous sleeve along the greater tuberosity. The posterior rotator cuff insertion extends medially from the articular margin to the lateral extent of the greater tuberosity. Because each cuff tendon is approximately 2 cm in width, estimating the extent of involvement of each tendon in full-thickness cuff tears is fairly straightforward. More challenging is the accurate assessment of the extent of partial-thickness cuff tears.

The subscapularis is a multipennate muscle arising from the subscapularis fossa. It is separated from the other muscles of the rotator cuff by the coracoid process. The superior two-thirds of the muscle inserts as a tendon onto the lesser tuberosity, and the inferior third has a direct muscular attachment along the surgical neck. The distal 1.5 cm of the subscapularis is tendinous. The most superior tendon fibers interdigitate at their insertion with the supraspinatus as these muscles send fibers to both the lesser and greater tuberosities.[11] From an arthroscopic perspective, the superior tendinous edge of the subscapularis is visible, forming the inferior border of both the rotator interval and the arthroscopic triangle (Figure 3.23). The subscapularis bursa is a structure separating the glenoid from the subscapularis tendon and lined with synovial membrane. It is best seen from an anterior arthroscopic vantage and can be the site of loose bodies.

The supraspinatus originates from the supraspinatus fossa and passes through the supraspinatus outlet to insert on the superior facet of the greater tuberosity. It consists of a large anterior fusiform muscle belly and a smaller unipennate posterior belly. The anterior muscle has a thicker tendon (3.1 vs 2.5 mm) and contributes the majority of the contractile force.[19] This part of the tendon, therefore, may be the most important during rotator cuff repair.

The anterior tendon fibers blend with the subscapularis to insert onto the lesser tuberosity. These fibers envelop the biceps tendon at the entrance to the bicipital groove, forming a fibrocartilaginous lining. A tendon slip from the supraspinatus forms the roof of the sheath. The floor is formed by tendon fibers passing from the subscapularis to the supraspinatus tendon. The posterior tendon fibers of the supraspinatus merge with the tendon of the infraspinatus approximately 15 mm from their insertion; these two tendons are arthroscopically indistinguishable at the junction.

The infraspinatus is a bipennate muscle that arises from the infraspinatus fossa. It is separated into superior and inferior portions by a raphe. Distally, its tendon becomes confluent with both the tendons of the supraspinatus and teres minor to form a common insertion on the greater tuberosity.

The teres minor is a fusiform muscle that originates from the inferolateral border of the scapula and inserts onto the greater tuberosity. Like the subscapularis, its tendinous insertion is supplemented by a direct muscular attachment onto the surgical neck.

Proximal to the terminal rotator cuff insertion is a thickened, capsular structure known as the rotator cable. It extends from the biceps anteriorly to the inferior border of the infraspinatus posteriorly and runs perpendicular to the rotator cuff tendons. This cable defines the rotator crescent, which spans the insertions of both the supraspinatus and infraspinatus (Figure 3.26). In a study by Burkhart et al. the size of the crescent averaged 41mm in its anteroposterior di-

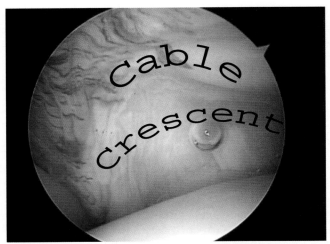

FIGURE 3.26. Undersurface of the rotator cuff demonstrates the "cable" of the cuff, with its intervening "crescent" between cable and tuberosity attachment site. The synovial vasculature of the undersurface of the rotator cuff stops at the rotator cable

mension and 14 mm in its mediolateral dimension, while the cable itself was 12 mm by 4.7 mm thick.[20] The cable is formed by the deep extension of the coracohumeral ligament. The synovial vasculature of the undersurface of the rotator cuff stops at the rotator cable (Figure 3.26). The thinner rotator crescent appears avascular. The relationship of a rotator cuff tear to these anatomical landmarks may influence clinical symptoms and repair strategies.

Partial-thickness tears are sometimes difficult to assess in terms of depth (Figure 3.27). The amount of partial-thickness tearing of the tendon can be deter-

mined by estimating the distance of the residual cuff insertions to the articular margin. For example, if the rotator cuff insertion is seen to be 5 mm lateral to the articular surface, then because the rotator cuff footprint averages 1 cm, approximately 50% of the tendon's thickness has been torn.

GLENOHUMERAL SKELETAL ANATOMY

The glenohumeral articulation is congruent with the radii of curvature of the glenoid and humeral head, deviating less than 1%.[21] Articular cartilage thickness varies on the two surfaces, with the glenoid cartilage thickest at the periphery and the humeral head slightly thicker centrally.

The articular surface of the glenoid has a relatively thin layer of cartilage in the center. This thin area should not be mistaken for early osteoarthritis or chondromalacia (Figure 3.28). Further inspection of the glenoid along the anterior edge reveals a normal indentation. Found just superior to the glenoid's midpoint, this indentation marks the point of fusion between the two ossific nuclei of the glenoid and gives the glenoid its "inverted comma" shape seen on gross inspection[22] (Figure 3.29). The glenoid is superiorly tilted 10 to 15° relative to the medial border of the scapula and is retroverted an average of 4°. The supraglenoid and infraglenoid tubercles, located at the superior and inferior poles of the glenoid, are the origins for the long head of the biceps and triceps, respectively.

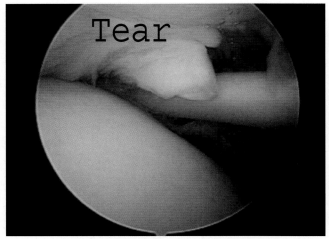

FIGURE 3.27. Arthroscopic view (scope posteriorly, left shoulder, beach chair perspective) shows undersurface cuff fiber failure in vicinity of anterior supraspinatus, immediately posterior to biceps tendon long head.

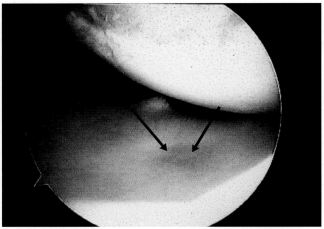

FIGURE 3.28. Arthroscopic photograph (scope posterior, right shoulder, lateral decubitus perspective) showing the normal area of relative chondral thinning (arrows) in mid to inferior third glenoid.

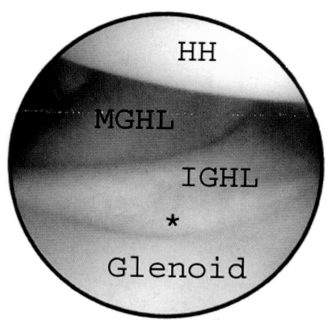

FIGURE 3.29. Arthroscopic photograph (scope posterior, right shoulder, lateral decubitus perspective) of inverted anterior notch at glenoid rim denoted by asterisk (*): HH, humeral head; MGHL, middle glenohumeral ligament; IGHL, inferior glenohumeral ligament.

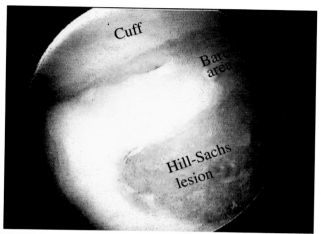

FIGURE 3.31. Scope photograph of large Hill–Sachs lesion in which the chondral surface has been damaged from repeated anterior instability episodes. Note that there is a small area of normal intervening cartilage between the Hill–Sachs lesion and the normal bare area.

The humeral head articular surface is ovoid. The humeral head should appear smooth without evidence of chondromalacia except for the posterior lateral aspect of the head, which is normally devoid of cartilage and has been termed the "bare area." The bare area can appear quite irregular on inspection, but it has a smooth transition with the articular cartilage surface (Figure 3.30). This area should not be confused

with a Hill–Sachs lesion, which is also found posteriorly but more medially than the "bare area" (Figure 3.31).

THE NERVOUS ANATOMY

The nerves at risk during shoulder arthroscopy include the axillary, the suprascapular, and the musculocutaneous. The axillary nerve is a terminal branch of the posterior cord of the brachial plexus. It arises posterior to the coracoid process and travels along the subscapularis passing inferior to it, 3 to 5 mm medial to the musculotendinous junction.[23] The axillary nerve is then in intimate contact with the inferior shoulder capsule.

Uno et al. studied the anatomy of the nerve from an intra-articular perspective.[24] In 12 cadavers, the nerve was held to the capsule by loose areolar tissue between the 5 and 7 o'clock positions. The nerve was in close proximity to the anteroinferior glenoid with the shoulder in a neutral position, with internal rotation, and with extension. The nerve displaced anteriorly with external rotation, and laterally with abduction or perpendicular traction.

Anterior to the long head of the triceps, the nerve branches into anterior and posterior branches. The posterior branch divides into the superior lateral brachial cutaneous (SLBC) nerve and the nerve to the teres minor. Although the anterior branch, which provides muscular innervation to the lateral and anterior deltoid, is of primary concern during open or miniopen procedures around the shoulder, the posterior branch is more at risk during complete arthroscopic

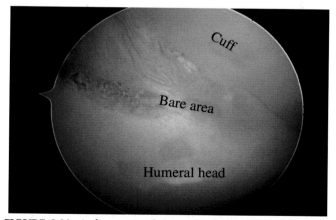

FIGURE 3.30. Arthroscopic photograph of normal "bare area" in which there is distinct area just distal to cuff insertion fibers where articular cartilage is absent.

procedures. The posterior branch lies more medial and superficial than the anterior branch of the axillary nerve. Procedures such as thermal capsulorrhaphy or suture capsular imbrication in particular can cause injury to the posterior branch. Deficits caused by an injury to this branch include lack of sensation in the lateral deltoid as well as a functional deficit to the teres minor.

After branching, the nerve to the teres minor courses medially along the posterior aspect of the inferior glenoid rim for a distance of 18 mm before entering the muscle at its inferior border. The SLBC courses inferiorly deep to the posterior deltoid. It becomes superficial by passing around the medial border of the muscle to provide cutaneous sensory innervation, 8.7 cm inferior to the posterolateral corner of the acromion.

The anterior branch of the axillary nerve passes with the posterior humeral circumflex artery through the quadrangular space. This space is formed by the teres minor superiorly, the teres major inferiorly, the long head of the triceps medially, and the surgical neck of the humerus laterally. The nerve then passes anteriorly on the undersurface of the deltoid. The nerve is found on average 5.5 cm distal to the posterolateral corner of the acromion, but it can be as close as 3.1 cm.[2] The nerve is found an average of 5 cm distal to the anterolateral corner. A cadaveric study found that 20% of the specimens had an axillary nerve closer then 5 cm from the acromion at some point in its course. This distance was narrowed by almost 30% in an abducted position.[2]

The suprascapular nerve arises from the upper trunk of the brachia plexus. The nerve passes below the transverse scapular ligament to innervate the supraspinatus. The nerve is 3 cm from the supraglenoid tubercle as it passes below this ligament. It then passes inferiorly and laterally around the spine of the scapula to innervate the infraspinatus. The nerve lies 1.8 cm from the posterior glenoid rim at this point.[25]

The musculocutaneous nerve is a terminal branch of the lateral cord. It courses obliquely to enter the coracobrachialis muscle an average of 5.6 cm from the tip of the coracoid. The nerve may have more than one branch with the smaller branches entering the muscle an average of 3.1 cm from the tip.[26]

THE SUBACROMIAL SPACE

The subacromial space is a potential space lined by the subacromial bursa. This bursa is found under the anterior half of the acromion. The bursa extends anteriorly and laterally to form the subdeltoid bursa and

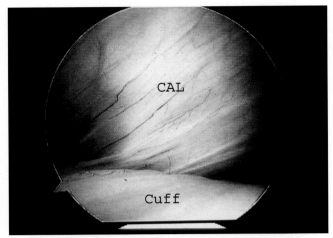

FIGURE 3.32. Arthroscopic view of the subacromial space demonstrating normal anatomy, with the coracoacromial ligament (CAL) covered by a layer of synovium and the bursal side of the cuff inferiorly (scope in posterior portal, right shoulder, beach chair perspective).

extends medially to the acromioclavicular joint. The acromion, the bursal side of the rotator cuff, and the coracoacromial (CA) ligament are visualized within the subacromial space (Figure 3.32).

Acromial morphology has been classified into three types: type I, a flat acromion; type II, a curved acromion; and type III, a hooked acromion.[27] Subacromial spurs are usually found anterolaterally at the site of the insertion of the coracoacromial ligament. Preoperative radiographs help identify the presence and degree of spurring.

The anatomy of the coracoacromial ligament, like the acromion, has been the subject of multiple anatomical studies.[28–30] The ligament arises from the lateral aspect of the coracoid and courses lateral and superior to the anterior edge of the acromion. The insertion extends to the lateral acromion for a distance of 2 cm from the anterolateral corner. Holt and Allibone have described the ligament as quadrangular (48%), Y-shaped (42%), or consisting of one broad band (8%).[28] One specimen in their study had three bands of the ligament, with the third band arising from the inferomedial aspect of the coracoid. In a subsequent study by others, this third band was described as occurring in 14.5% of 124 cadavers.[29] The band was found posteromedial, and the authors suggested that incomplete release of this band could cause failure of the subacromial decompression. The CA ligament is readily detached anteriorly from the acromion without disturbing the fibers of the anterior deltoid. The CA ligament attachment along the lateral acromion, however, is adherent to the deltoid fascia starting at the junction between the anterior and middle deltoid.[30] Care must be taken when releasing the ligament in this area to prevent detachment of the deltoid.

SUMMARY

Understanding the arthroscopic anatomy of the glenohumeral joint and subacromial space is critical in performing effective and safe surgery. Familiarity with normal anatomy will provide the foundation for the study and treatment of pathological conditions of the shoulder. Emphasis should be placed on differentiating the many normal variations from true pathological lesions.

References

1. Neviaser TJ. Arthroscopy of the shoulder. *Orthop Clin N Am* 1987;18:361–372.
2. Burkhead W, Scheinberg R, Box G. Surgical anatomy of the axillary nerve. *J Shoulder Elbow Surg* 1992;1:31–36.
3. Matthews L, Zarins B, Michael R, Helfet D. Anterior portal selection for shoulder arthroscopy. *Arthroscopy* 1985;1:33–39.
4. Davidson PA, Tibone JE. Anterior–inferior (5 o'clock) portal for shoulder arthroscopy. *Arthroscopy* 1995;11:519–525.
5. Habermeyer P, Kaiser E, Knappe M, Kreusser T, Wiedemann E. Functional anatomy and biomechanics of the long biceps tendon [in German]. *Unfallchirurgie* 1987;90:319–329.
6. Vangsness CT Jr, Jorgenson SS, Watson T, Johnson DL. The origin of the long head of the biceps from the scapula and glenoid labrum. An anatomical study of 100 shoulders. *J Bone Joint Surg Br* 1994;76:951–954.
7. Jost B, Koch P, Gerber C. Anatomy and functional apsects of the rotator interval. *J Shoulder Elbow Surg* 2000;9:336–341.
8. Cooper DE, O'Brien SJ, Arnoczky SP, Warren RF. The structure and function of the coracohumeral ligament: an anatomic and microscopic study. *J Shoulder Elbow Surg* 1993;2:70–77.
9. Tetro A, Bauer G, Hollstien S, Yamaguchi K. Arthroscopic release of the rotator interval and coracohumeral ligament: an anatomic study in cadavers. *Arthroscopy* 2002;18:145–150.
10. Detrisac, D.A.; Johnson, L.L. *Arthroscopic Shoulder Anatomy: Pathological and Surgical Implications.* Thorofare, NJ: Slack; 1986:74.
11. Snyder SJ, Karzel RP, Del Pizzo W, Ferkel RD, Friedman MJ. SLAP lesions of the shoulder. *Arthroscopy* 1990;6:274–279.
12. Williams MM, Snyder SJ, Buford D Jr. The Buford complex—the "cord-like" middle glenohumeral ligament and absent anterosuperior labrum complex: a normal anatomic capsulolabral variant *Arthroscopy* 1994;10:241–247.
13. Cooper DE, Arnoczky SP, O'Brien SJ, Warren RF, DiCarlo E, Allen AA. Anatomy, histology, and vascularity of the glenoid labrum. An anatomical study. *J Bone Joint Surg Br* 1992;74:46–52.
14. Uhthoff HK, Piscopo M. Anterior capsular redundancy of the shoulder: congenital or traumatic? *J Bone Joint Surg Br* 1985;67:363.
15. Neviaser TJ. The anterior labroligamentous periosteal sleeve avulsion lesion: a cause of anterior instability of the shoulder. *Arthroscopy* 1993;9(1):17–21.
16. Steinbeck J, Liljenqvist U, Jerosch J. The anatomy of the glenohumeral ligamentous complex and its contribution to anterior shoulder stability. *J Shoulder Elbow Surg* 1998;7:122–126.
17. O'Brien SJ, Neves MC, Arnoczky SP, et al. The anatomy and histology of the inferior glenohumeral ligament complex of the shoulder. *Am J Sports Med* 1990;18:449–456.
18. Wolf EM, Cheng JC, Dickson K. Humeral avulsion of glenohumeral ligaments as a cause of anterior shoulder instability. *Arthroscopy* 1995;11(5):600–607.
19. Roh M, Wang V, April E, Pollock R, Bigliani L, Flatow E. Anterior and posterior musculotendinous anatomy of the supraspinatous. *J Shoulder Elbow Surg* 2000;9:436–440.
20. Burkhart S, Esch J, Jolson R. The rotator crescent and rotator cable: an anatomic description of the shoulder's "suspension bridge." *Arthroscopy* 1993;9:611–616.
21. Oslowsky LJ, Flatow EL, Bigliani LU, Mow VC. Articular geometry of the glenohumeral joint. *Clin Orthop* 1992;285:181–190.
22. Snyder S. *Shoulder Arthroscopy.* New York: McGraw-Hill; 1994.
23. Loomer R, Graham B. Anatomy of the axillary nerve and its relation to inferior capsular shift. *Clin Orthop* 1989:100–105.
24. Uno A, Bain GI, Hehta JA. Arthroscopic relationship of the axillary nerve to the shoulder joint capsule: an anatomic study. *J Shoulder Elbow Surg* 1999;8:226–230.
25. Bigliani LU, Dalsey RM, McCann PD, April EW. An anatomical study of the suprascapular nerve. *J Arthrosc Relat Surg* 1990;6:301–305.
26. Flatow EL, Bigliani LU, April EW. An anatomic study of the musculocutaneous nerve and its relationship to the coracoid. *Clin Orthop* 1989;244:166–171.
27. Bigliani LU, Morrison D, April EW. The morphology of the acromion and its relationship to rotator cuff tears. *Orthop Trans* 1986;1:228.
28. Holt E, Allibone R. Anatomic variants of the coracoacromial ligament. *J Shoulder Elbow Surg* 1995;4:370–375.
29. Pieper H, Radas C, Krahl H, Blank M. Anatomic variation of the coracromial ligament: a macroscopic and microscopic cadaveric study. *J Shoulder Elbow Surg* 1997;6:291–295.
30. Edelson J, Luchs J. Aspects of coracoacromial ligament anatomy of interest to the arthroscopic surgeon. *Arthroscopy* 1995;11:715–719.

Recommended Reading

Arnoczky S, Soslowsky L. Anatomy of the shoulder: form reflecting function. In: McGinty J, Caspari R, Jackson R, Peohling G, eds. *Operative Arthroscopy.* Philadelphia: Lippincott-Raven; 1996:603–624.

Bennett W. Visualization of the anatomy of the rotator interval and bicipital sheath. *Arthroscopy* 2001;17:107–111.

Robertson D, Yan J, Bigliani L, Flatow E, Yamaguchi K. Three-dimensional analysis of the proximal part of the humerus: relevance to arthroplasty. *J Bone Joint Surg Am* 2000;82:1594–1602.

Warner JJP, Deng X-H, Warren RF, Torzilli PA. Static capsuloligamentous restraints to superior–inferior translation of the glenohumeral joint. *Am J Sports Med* 1992;20: 675–685.

4

Arthroscopic Knot Tying in Shoulder Repair Surgery

Scott P. Fischer

Recent reports have demonstrated that arthroscopic repairs of Bankart lesions can have success rates equivalent to open repairs for recurrent anterior instability of the shoulder.[1,2] Similarly, arthroscopic rotator cuff repair techniques have resulted in high degrees of patient satisfaction and clinical success.[3,4] Increasing interest in these and other shoulder repair techniques has led to an emphasis on the importance of adequate arthroscopic knot-tying technique. This chapter presents the basic information and skills necessary to tie arthroscopic knots in a simple, reliable, and reproducible manner.

TERMINOLOGY

An understanding of knot-tying vocabulary is necessary to ensure accurate communication. The following terms are used in this chapter.

Alternating posts The process of alternating the function of "post suture strand" from one suture strand to the other as successive loops of the knot are tied. This results in the interlocking of the two suture strands as the knot is tied, affording greater resistance to knot slippage.

Lockable sliding knot A sliding knot that can be deformed and locked in place by pulling back on the wrapping strand after the knot has been fully seated at the repair site. (Deforming the knot in this fashion produces increased internal friction within the knot and increased resistance to slippage.)

Locking half-hitch A half-hitch loop that is tied after a sliding knot to lock it in place and prevent it from loosening.

Non-sliding knot A knot that is tied or constructed inside the joint by pushing or pulling half-hitch loops down to the soft tissue repair site. The suture does not slide through the tissue as the knot is tightened.

Overhand half-hitch loop A half-hitch loop tied by wrapping the wrapping strand over, around, and then under the post strand.

Past pointing The action of tightening a knot by pushing the tip of the knot pusher past or beyond the knot being tied. This results in the two suture strands being oriented 180° away from each other at the knot, which allows the surgeon to apply maximum tension to both suture limbs simultaneously.

Post suture strand The suture strand that is held straight and under tension while another suture strand is wrapped around it to construct a knot.

Pulling knots When a knot pusher is used to pull a half-hitch loop down to the repair site, the device is placed onto the wrapping strand and then advanced down to the repair site, pulling the loop down the post strand behind it.

Pushing knots When a knot pusher is used to push a half-hitch loop or a sliding knot down to the repair site, the device is placed onto the post suture strand; then the knot or loop is pushed down the post in front of the knot pusher.

Repair site suture loop The loop of suture passing through the tissue at the repair site which, when tightened, will pull the tissue margins together.

Reversed half-hitches The process of tying successive half-hitch loops in opposite directions (i.e., an overhand loop followed by an underhand loop).

Sliding knot A knot that is tied around the post strand, outside the joint, and then pushed down into position within the joint. The suture slides through the tissue as the knot is tightened.

Underhand half-hitch loop A half-hitch loop tied by wrapping the wrapping strand underneath, around, and then over the post strand.

Wrapping suture strand The suture strand that is wrapped around the post to construct a knot.

FACILITATING KNOT TYING

The following are offered as aids in improving facility in knot tying.

Patient Positioning

During arthroscopic shoulder repairs, it is helpful to visualize the joint and place instruments from either the anterior or posterior aspect of the shoulder as needed. Rotating the operating room table 90 to 180° away from the anesthesiologist allows easy anterior, superior, and posterior access to the shoulder and facilitates the repair process.

Visualization and Hemostasis

The need for clear visualization during arthroscopic shoulder procedures is obvious. The combination of low-pressure joint distension with a fluid pump, hypotensive anesthesia (when medically safe), and the judicious use of electrothermal hemostasis provides an optimal environment for the successful completion of these procedures.

Accessory Portals

It is easier for the surgeon to manipulate soft tissue, pass sutures, and tie knots when there is direct access to the repair site. Working through arthroscopic portals distant from the repair site can be challenging, especially when one is using straight instruments around a curved surface within a tight joint. To facilitate suturing and knot tying, and to minimize the risk of iatrogenic articular injury, the use of accessory portals is recommended.

Cannula Selection

When sutures are passed and tied without the use of a cannula, soft tissue may become incarcerated between suture limbs within the knot. When this occurs, the tissue entrapped may be damaged, and final knot tightening is jeopardized. The use of clear plastic cannulas is preferred for suture handling during arthroscopic knot tying. Clear cannulas do not obstruct the surgeon's field of view. In addition, a plastic cannula, with its softer edge, is less likely than a metal cannula to abrade and weaken sutures. Cannulas that screw in through the soft tissue, or have a lip at the tip, seem to be less likely to slip out of position while passing instruments for suturing and knot tying.

Suture Considerations

A variety of suture materials are available for arthroscopic repair surgery. Acceptable results have been obtained with both monofilament and braided suture, as well as with permanent and absorbable suture material. Initially, monofilament suture was preferred because it could be easily delivered directly through soft tissue by using hollow-needle suture passers. Subsequent development of new suture-passing techniques has facilitated the passage of braided suture through soft tissue. Although monofilament and braided suture materials have very different handling characteristics, satisfactory arthroscopic knots can be tied with either. Monofilament materials slide readily through soft tissue and can be passed directly through most suture-passing devices without the use of intermediary shuttle devices. The stiffness of these sutures, however, can make the process of tying tight knots somewhat more challenging. It is easier to tie compact, tight knots in braided suture because it is more pliable than monofilament material. Some studies have also suggested that braided suture is less likely to slip with cyclic loading.[5] However, braided suture material may not slide through tissue as easily as monofilament suture and if abrasion or snagging occurs during instrumentation, the suture may be weakened significantly and rupture.

SELECTING THE PROPER SUTURE TO BE THE POST STRAND

In a soft tissue repair, it is always easier to pull the most mobile tissue *to* the least mobile tissue. In general, the post suture should be the suture strand that exits from the more mobile structure. Then, when the post suture is tightened for knot tying, the tension applied to this suture strand will pull the repair together.

When there is little or no tension in the soft tissue at the repair site, the post suture should be selected to ensure that the location selected for final knot placement is the one that will be best tolerated within the joint. (For a labral repair, e.g., the post suture would be the suture strand emerging through the capsulolabral tissue, to ensure that final placement of the knot is off the joint surface and behind the labrum.)

SUTURE HANDLING

When suture strands become twisted around each other at the repair site, the coiled sutures will be interposed between the tissue surfaces, interfering with complete contact between healing surfaces. If the sutures become twisted around each other during knot tying, there may be interference with suture sliding that can impair final knot tightening. For these reasons, it is important to unwind any tangled sutures prior to knot tying. To identify any suture entanglement, always slide a knot pusher down the post suture prior to passing any suture loops.

Excessive handling of a suture strand with suture passers and retrievers can damage and weaken the suture material. To avoid potential suture rupture during knot tying, such handling should be minimized.

When multiple pairs of untied sutures are simultaneously present within a repair site, it becomes difficult to sort out which suture strands should be paired for knot tying. Multiple suture strands in the same field of view may also obscure the surgeon's visualization. To avoid these problems, it is preferable to place only one suture in the repair at a time, tie it, and then place another. If circumstances require the placement of several sutures at the same time, it is advisable to identify suture pairs by using different color sutures. To further isolate the strands used for the various knots, each pair may be withdrawn from a different portal.

KNOT-TYING CONCEPTS

In both open and arthroscopic surgery, sutures tied with knots are the means most commonly used to secure a repair. The pattern in which the two suture strands are wrapped and interlocked around each other characterizes the type of knot tied. All knots rely upon friction between the two suture strands within the knot to prevent suture slippage. Knots with greater degrees of complexity generally have increased resistance to slippage.[5,6] Arthroscopic knots are grouped into one of three categories: sliding knots, lockable sliding knots, and nonsliding knots.

Sliding Knots

Prior to using a sliding knot in a repair, it is necessary to make sure that the suture slides freely through the cannula, soft tissue, and suture anchor (if one is used). If the suture will not slide freely, a nonsliding knot should be used for the repair.

Sliding knots are constructed outside the joint by wrapping the "wrapping strand" around the "post strand." Once the knot has been tied, the surgeon pulls back on the post strand and pushes the knot down the cannula to the repair site with a knot pusher. The knot is securely seated at the repair site after the soft tissue defect has been closed and all excess slack has been removed from the "repair site loop." When a sliding knot is advanced down to the repair site, the post strand lengthens, and the end of the wrapping strand exiting from the cannula becomes shorter (as a result of the suture sliding). If both suture strands are equal in length before the knot is tied, then as the knot is advanced into the joint, the wrapping strand may disappear within the cannula. To prevent this frustrating problem, the surgeon must adjust the lengths of the suture strands before tying a sliding knot. The wrapping strand should be as long as possible, while leaving the post suture long enough to permit comfortable handling during knot tying.

Standard sliding knots, by themselves, can slip backward when the repair is placed under a load. If this occurs, the repair may gap open and fail to heal adequately. To prevent this complication, sliding knots must be locked in place with additional "locking half-hitches." When there is soft tissue tension at the repair site, a sliding knot may slip backward before these locking half-hitches can be placed. To avoid this occurrence, the surgeon can adjust the patient's arm position to reduce the tension at the repair site (i.e., increase abduction when one is tying knots for a rotator cuff repair). Using a grasping forceps or a traction suture to pull the soft tissue into a "reduced" position will further decrease soft tissue tension. Alternatively, loss of knot tension can be avoided while the knot is tied by advancing a half-hitch up to the knot, then advancing the knot pusher past the half-hitch and knot to retension the sliding knot and lock the half-hitch with "past pointing" (see Terminology section, earlier) while pulling back on the locking half-hitch. A Surgeon's Sixth Finger knot pusher (Arthrex Corp., Naples, FL) may also be used to hold the initial knot secure while locking half-hitches are being placed.

Lockable Sliding Knots

The use of lockable sliding knots can reduce the risk of backward slippage associated with regular sliding knots. Once lockable knots are seated at the repair site, they are secured in place by pulling backward on the wrapping strand to deform a portion of the knot. This increases the mechanical "interlocking" of the two suture strands and improves the knot's resistance to slippage. In tying one of these knots, the surgeon must be careful not to tension the wrapping strand while the knot is being slid down the cannula. Such premature tensioning can cause the knot to become locked where it is, preventing further sliding down to the repair site. Some surgeons report adequate knot security without tying additional locking half-hitches after these knots. When tensioned over time, however, such knots can slip backward. To ensure adequate repair security, it is wise to finish all knots with three reversing half-hitches, using alternating posts as suggested by Chan et al.[7]

Any standard sliding knot can be transformed into a lockable sliding knot by tying a simple half-hitch loop onto the end of the knot. This half-hitch loop is left slightly loose as it and the sliding knot are pushed down to the repair site together. When the knot is fully seated, past pointing is used to tension the half-hitch with slightly more tension on the wrapping strand than on the post strand. With practice, this maneuver will cause the half-hitch to deform the post and lock the sliding knot in place. (Caution is essential when one is tensioning the wrapping strand, to avoid pulling the sliding knot backward and loosening the repair.) Correctly performing this maneuver will "alternate the post" from one suture strand to the other between the body of the sliding knot and the subsequent half-hitch loop. Two additional locking reversed half-hitches with alternating posts are applied to finish securing the knot.

Nonsliding Knots

During some arthroscopic repairs, the suture may not slide through the soft tissue with sufficient freedom to allow the use of a sliding knot. When this occurs, using a nonsliding knot becomes necessary. This type of knot is constructed within the joint at the repair site, one half-hitch loop at a time. Because there is little holding strength present with only one half-hitch loop in place, special measures must be used to prevent loosening of the repair while the subsequent half-hitches are being tied. Most often, maintaining tension on the post ensures resistance to slippage while additional half-hitches are tied. A "Surgeons Sixth Finger" knot pusher (Arthrex Corporation) may also be used to secure the first loop of the knot in its place while subsequent half-hitches are tied. Each successive half-hitch must be fully tensioned as it is tied, to construct a tight and secure knot that will not loosen over time. Avoid tying all the half-hitches around the same post suture, for such a knot may loosen over time. In tying nonsliding knots, it is important to alternate the post between the final three half-hitches to provide secure knot-holding strength.[7]

KNOT-TYING TECHNIQUES

There are many serviceable knots available for use in arthroscopic suture repairs. It is not within the scope of this chapter to provide a comprehensive review of all the knots currently being used in arthroscopic shoulder repair surgery. Rather, we present a representative selection of the arthroscopic knots that are commonly used and have been found to be reliable and reproducible. Knots that are not presented here should not be viewed as less secure or less satisfactory than those that are cited.

Duncan Loop: A Sliding Knot (Figure 4.1A)

1. Thread the knot pusher onto the post strand (held in the left hand: Figure 4.1B) and place a clamp on the post. Pass the knot pusher into the joint to ensure that there are no twists in the sutures, nor any obstructing soft tissue between the tip of the cannula and the repair site. Slide the suture so that the post limb is quite "short" and the wrapping strand is "long."
2. Holding both sutures between the thumb and long finger, wrap the long suture over your thumb (creating a loop), and continue by wrapping it over and around both the post and the wrapping strand sutures four times (Figure 4.1C–E). Pass the free end of the wrapping suture through the loop made by your thumb (Figure 4.1F).
3. Remove the excess slack from the loops within the knot by first tensioning the free end of the wrapping suture; then tension the end of this same suture as it passes from the knot toward the joint (Figure 4.1G).
4. Next, pull back on the post suture (Figure 4.1H), and use the knot pusher to push the Duncan loop down toward the repair site until the tissue to be repaired and the suture loop are tight.
5. Maintain tension on the post while tying a half-hitch loop around it with the wrapping strand. Then push this loop down and tighten it to lock the knot in place.
6. Place two or three additional reversing half-hitches on alternating posts to secure the knot.

Tautline Hitch: A Sliding Knot (Figure 4.2)

1. Thread the knot pusher onto the post strand (held in the left hand) and place a clamp on the post. Pass the knot pusher into the joint to ensure that there are no twists in the sutures, nor any obstructing soft tissue between the tip of the cannula and the repair site. Slide the suture so that the post limb is quite "short" and the wrapping strand is "long."
2. Pass the wrapping suture over the post (this creates a loop) and wrap it around the post suture twice, passing the suture through the inside of the loop both times.
3. After the second wrap around the post, bring the wrapping suture up and out of the loop. Wrap the suture over and around the post a third time, but

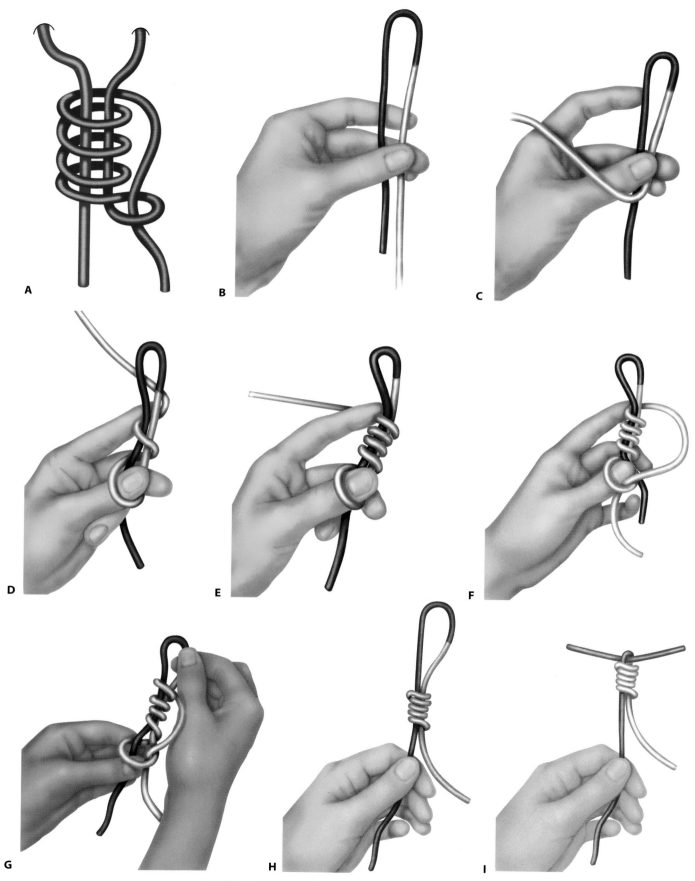

FIGURE 4.1. Duncan loop: (A) the knot; (B)–(I) the steps.

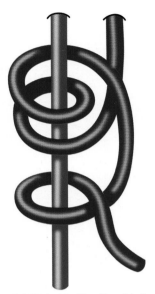

FIGURE 4.2. Tautline hitch.

pass it outside of and proximal to the previous "loop" ("proximal" being closer to you, not closer to the patient). As you make this third wrap, pass the free end of the wrapping suture up through the "new loop" created as the suture was wrapped over the post outside the original loop, as shown in Figure 4.2.

4. Take the excess slack out of the knot by first tensioning the free end of the wrapping suture (taking care not to overtension it and "lock" the knot); then tension the end of this same suture as it passes from the knot toward the joint.

5. Using the knot pusher, push the tautline hitch down the post suture into the joint while pulling back on the end of the post. Slide the knot down to the repair until the tissue and the loop are tight.

6. Place three additional reversing half-hitches on alternating posts to secure the knot.

Tennessee Slider/Buntline Hitch: A Lockable Sliding Knot (Figure 4.3)

1. Thread the knot pusher onto the post strand (held in the left hand) and place a clamp on the post. Pass the knot pusher into the joint to ensure that there are no twists in the sutures, nor any obstructing soft tissue between the tip of the cannula and the repair site. Slide the suture so that the post limb is quite "short" and the wrapping strand is "long."

2. Pass the wrapping suture over, around, and then under the post suture. Bring the end of the wrapping suture outside and over the loop created by the wrapping suture as it passed over the post suture ("outside the loop" being closer to you, not closer to the patient).

3. Wrap the suture over and around the post a second time, but pass it inside the first loop. As you make this second wrap, bring the free end of the wrapping suture up between the post and the wrapping suture as shown in Figure 4.3.

4. Take the excess slack out of the knot by first tensioning the free end of the wrapping suture (taking care not to overtension it and "lock" the knot); then tension the end of this same suture as it passes from the knot toward the joint.

5. Pull back on the end of the post suture strand while using the knot pusher to push the Tennessee slider down to the repair until the tissue and the loop are tight.

6. If locking is desired, maintain tension on the post while slightly overtensioning the wrapping strand to deform the post and lock the knot in place.

7. Place three additional reversing half-hitches on alternating posts to secure the knot.

SMC Knot: A Lockable Sliding Knot (Figure 4.4)

1. Thread the knot pusher onto the post strand (held in the left hand) and place a clamp on the post. Pass the knot pusher into the joint to ensure that there are no twists in the sutures, nor any obstructing soft tissue between the tip of the cannula and the repair site. Slide the suture so that the post limb is quite "short" and the wrapping strand is "long."

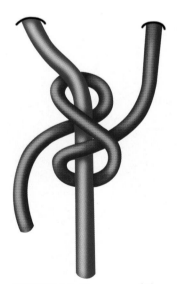

FIGURE 4.3. Tennessee slider.

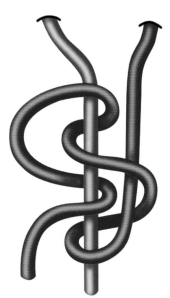

FIGURE 4.4. SMC knot.

2. Hold both sutures between the thumb and long finger. Wrap the long suture over the post and around both suture strands.
3. Wrap the wrapping strand around the post again, but this time bring it up between the post and wrapping strands.
4. Continue by passing the end of the wrapping strand under the post strand a third time and bring it up between the post and the wrapping strand in the interval between the "over" and "under" portions of the first loop of the knot as shown in Figure 4.4.
5. As the suture is pulled through, a loop is created. Place your left index finger into this loop. Remove the slack or looseness from the suture loops in the knot while keeping the index finger in place to avoid tightening this "locking loop" prematurely. Pull on the post strand and use the knot pusher to slide the knot down to the tissue. (Do not pull on the loop strand until the knot is fully seated or the knot will prematurely lock where it is, and prevent it from sliding into place.)
6. Once the knot has been fully seated at the repair site, maintain tension on the post strand. Tighten the "locking loop" by pulling back on the wrapping strand while maintaining pressure on the knot with the knot pusher. The "locking loop" will tighten and secure the knot in place.
7. To complete the knot, place three alternating half-hitches to secure the knot.

Alternating Half-Hitches: A Nonsliding Knot Used to Lock Sliding Knots (Figure 4.5)

1. Tie an overhand half-hitch loop over the post. Push it down into the joint and seat it securely on the sliding knot at the repair site.
2. Tension both suture strands, securing the loop in place. Maintain tension on the post and withdraw the knot pusher.
3. Transfer the knot pusher to the other suture strand, which now becomes the new post for the second half-hitch loop.
4. Tie an underhand half-hitch loop by passing the wrapping strand under the new post. Push it down into the joint, seat it completely, and tension it firmly.
5. Transfer the knot pusher back to the original post suture strand and tie a third half-hitch loop by passing the wrapping strand over the original post. Then tighten the loop.

Revo Knot: A Nonsliding Knot: (Figure 4.6)

1. Wrap an overhand half-hitch loop over the post. Push it down to the tissue and maintain tension on the post to secure this loop in place.
2. Wrap a second identical overhand half-hitch loop around the same post. Push it down on top of the first loop and tension it to secure the first loop.
3. While maintaining tension on the post, tie a third half-hitch loop underhand (in the reverse direction) around the same post. Push it down to the knot and tension it.
4. Withdraw the knot pusher and change it to the opposite suture limb (now the new post).

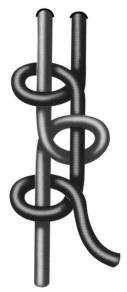

FIGURE 4.5. Alternating half-hitches.

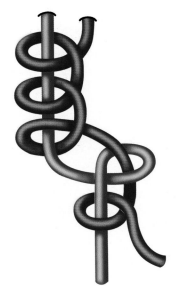

FIGURE 4.6. Revo knot.

5. Wrap an overhand half-hitch loop over the new post and push it down to the knot. Push the knot pusher past the knot (past pointing), tension the loop to tighten it, and secure the first three half-hitches.

6. Withdraw the knot pusher and change it back to the opposite suture limb (the original post suture).

7. Wrap an underhand half-hitch loop around the original post and push it down to the knot. Use past pointing to tighten the loop and complete the knot.

References

1. Bacilla P, Field LD, Savoie FH. Arthroscopic Bankart repair in a high demand population. *Arthroscopy* 1997;13:51–60.

2. Burkhart SS, De Beer JF. Traumatic glenohumeral bone defects and their relationship to failure of arthroscopic Bankart repairs: significance of the inverted-pear glenoid and the engaging Hill–Sachs lesion. *Arthroscopy* 2000;16:677–694.

3. Burkhart SS, Danaceau SM, Pearce CE. Arthroscopic rotator cuff repair: analysis of results by tear size and by repair technique—margin convergence versus direct tendon-to-bone repair. *Arthroscopy* 2001;17:905–912.

4. Gartsman GM, Khan M, Hammerman SM. Arthroscopic repair of full-thickness tears of the rotator cuff. *J Bone Joint Surg Am.* 1998;80(6):832–840.

5. Loutzenheiser TD, Harryman DT II, Ziegler DW, Yung SW. Optimizing arthroscopic knots using braided or monofilament suture. *Arthroscopy* 1998;14:57–65.

6. Loutzenheiser TD, Harryman FT II, Yung SW, France MP, Sidles JA. Optimizing arthroscopic knots. *Arthroscopy* 1995;11:199–206.

7. Chan KC, Burkhart SS, Thiagarajan MB, Goh JCH. Optimization of stacked half-hitch knots for arthroscopic surgery. *Arthroscopy* 2001;17:752–759.

Recommended Reading

Burkhart SS, Fischer SP, Nottage WM, Esch JC, Barber FA, Doctor D, Ferrier J. Tissue fixation security in transosseous rotator cuff repairs: a mechanical comparison of simple versus mattress sutures. *Arthroscopy* 1996;12:704–708.

Burkhart SS, Diaz-Pagan JL, Wirth MA, Athanasiou KA. Cyclic loading of anchor-based rotator cuff repairs: confirmation of the tension overload phenomenon and comparison of suture anchor fixation with transosseous fixation. *Arthroscopy* 1997;13:720–724.

Burkhart SS, Wirth MA, Simonick M, Salem D, Lanctot D, Athanasiou KA. Loop security as a determinant of tissue fixation security. *Arthroscopy* 1998;14:773–776.

Burkhart SS, Wirth MA, Simonick M, Salem D, Lanctot D, Athanasiou KA. Knot security in simple sliding knots and its relationship to rotator cuff repair: how secure must the knot be? *Arthroscopy* 2000;16:202–207.

Chan KC, Burkhart SS. How to switch posts without rethreading when tying half-hitches. *Arthroscopy* 1999;15:444–450.

Gunderson PE. The half-hitch knot: a rational alternative to the square knot. *Am J Surg* 1987;154:538–540.

Kim SH, Ha KI. The SMC knot—a new slip knot with locking mechanism. *Arthroscopy* 2000;16:563–565.

Kim SH, Ha KI, Kim SH, Kim JS. Significance of the internal locking mechanism for loop security enhancement in the arthroscopic knot. *Arthroscopy* 2001;17:850–855.

Shimi SM, Lirici M, Vander Velpen G, Cuschieri A. Comparative study of the holding strength of slipknots using absorbable and nonabsorbable ligature materials. *Surg Endosc* 1994,8:1285–1291.

Trimbos JB. Security of various knots commonly used in surgical practice. *Obstet Gynecol* 1984;64:274–280.

Trimbos JB, Van Rijssel EJC, Klopper PJ. Performance of sliding knots in monofilament suture material. *Obstet Gynecol* 1986;68:425–430.

Trimbos JB, Booster M, Peters AAW. Mechanical knot performance of a new generation polydioxanone suture (PDS-2). *Acta Obstet. Gynecol Scand.* 1991;70:157–159.

SECTION TWO

Glenohumeral Pathology

5

Arthroscopic Treatment of the Arthritic Shoulder

Gregory S. Bauer, Theodore A. Blaine, and Louis U. Bigliani

The value of shoulder arthroscopy in the treatment of glenohumeral arthritis has not been clearly defined. Ogilvie-Harris and Wiley reported the results of arthroscopic debridement for osteoarthritis in 54 patients in 1986.[1] At 3 years followup, successful results were achieved in two-thirds of patients with mild disease, and in one-third of patients with severe degenerative disease. Somewhat earlier, Cofield had described the use of arthroscopy in eight men with glenohumeral arthritis.[2] Although all patients were thought to have benefited from the procedure, four of the patients were scheduled for additional reconstructive procedures based on the arthroscopic findings. These mixed early results, combined with the success of shoulder arthroplasty for the treatment of arthritis, probably explain the paucity of reports on arthroscopic treatment of glenohumeral arthritis.

Arthroscopy in shoulder arthritis has reemerged as a result of recent developments:

- Earlier detection of glenohumeral arthritis due to the increased popularity of shoulder arthroscopy
- Greater understanding of the complications of shoulder arthroplasty and recent research on cartilage regeneration has led to an emphasis on joint-preserving procedures

PATHOPHYSIOLOGY, STAGING, AND TREATMENT

Pathophysiology

A cascade of cellular and biochemical events leads to the breakdown of articular cartilage. Osteoarthritis of the shoulder includes both primary and secondary forms. Primary degenerative osteoarthritis is uncommon, occurring in less than 1% of the general population. Secondary degenerative arthritis can occur as a result of prior fracture, dislocation, instability, osteoneurosis, surgery, or infection (Table 5.1).

The biochemical events that are associated with osteoarthritis include a loss of the collagen matrix, an increase in water content, alterations in proteoglycan composition, and an increase in proteolytic enzymes and cytokines.

A biochemical analysis of the synovial fluid of 96 patients who had surgical procedures (arthroscopy or arthroplasty) for glenohumeral osteoarthritis was reported in 1996.[3] In this study, cartilage breakdown products (sulfated glycosaminoglycan, keratan sulfate, and link protein) were identified and correlated with the severity of osteoarthritis.

Potential benefits of arthroscopic debridement in osteoarthritis include the following:

1. Washout of cytokines and inflammatory mediators that initiate and maintain the process of joint destruction
2. Debridement of inflamed synovium that may contribute to cartilage degradation and pain
3. An improvement in joint mechanics through capsular release and removal of cartilage flaps and debris

Staging

For purposes of uniformity in outcome reporting, osteoarthritis is staged on the basis of radiographic criteria. Weinstein recently published a radiographic staging classification for glenohumeral osteoarthritis[4] (Table 5.2). Stage I has normal radiographs, while stage II has minimal joint space narrowing and a concentric joint. Stage III shows moderate narrowing and inferior osteophytes. Stage IV includes severe joint space loss, osteophyte formation, and loss of concentricity between the humeral head and glenoid. The severity of arthritis can also be assessed by visual inspection at arthroscopy. The Outerbridge classification system,[5] initially developed for chondromalacia patellae, is one of the earliest and most commonly used classification systems for grading osteoarthritis (Table 5.3).[5] Grade I is characterized by softening and swelling of the ar-

TABLE 5.1. Causes of (Noninflammatory) Glenohumeral Arthritis.

Primary osteoarthritis
Posttraumatic
Postinfectious
Postinstability
Postcapsulography
Charcot arthropathy
Osteonecrosis

TABLE 5.3. Arthroscopic Grading Criteria.

Grade	Cartilage
Grade I	Softening and swelling
Grade II	Fragmentation and fissuring < 0.5 in.
Grade III	Fragmentation and Fissuring > 0.5 in.
Grade IV	Exposed subchondral bone

ticular cartilage. Grade II has fragmentation and fissuring in an area less than 0.5 in. in diameter, while Grade III has fissuring in an area greater than 0.5 in. in diameter. An area of exposed bone of any size is considered to be grade IV.

Treatment Indications and Contraindications

Arthroscopic treatment is an accepted treatment alternative for stages I and II osteoarthritis when there is adequate supporting periarticular bone. Management of stage III arthritis has traditionally required prosthetic replacement, but may be considered for arthroscopic treatment depending on patient factors. Stage III arthritis with eccentric glenoid wear has been associated with less favorable results when treated arthroscopically and may constitute a relative contraindication.[1] In stage IV arthritis, there is extensive bony erosion, and most orthopedists consider this stage to be a contraindication to arthroscopic treatment. In each patient, the potential benefits of arthroscopic treatment must be weighed against the risks of delaying prosthetic replacement, including further bone loss and soft tissue compromise. Although the indications for arthroscopic treatment of shoulder arthritis are still being defined, some of the accepted indications are listed in Table 5.4.

Pain that is not responsive to conservative treatment is a relative indication for arthroscopic debridement. Failed conservative treatment consists of a course of nonsteroidal drugs, supervised physical therapy, and up to three intra-articular corticosteroid injections.

Arthroscopy may be indicated for the release of a contracted and stiff capsule associated with arthritis.[6]

Shoulder arthroscopy can be utilized to remove loose bodies or large osteophytes that may restrict motion. Although Neer found little benefit to open debridement of large osteophytes in glenohumeral osteoarthritis,[7] a more limited debridement of smaller osteophytes as seen in stage III arthritis may be warranted. Removal of these loose bodies clearly has the potential to provide improved joint mechanics and alleviate associated pain.

Arthroscopic treatment may provide an alternative, less invasive strategy for some patients in whom a more extensive procedure may be contraindicated.[8] Examples include deltoid dysfunction resulting from neurological or neuromuscular disease, complete rotator cuff dysfunction, the presence of active infection, medical conditions that might prohibit an extensive operative procedure, or other conditions that might prevent active participation in a postoperative rehabilitation program. Shoulder arthroscopy may provide a diagnostic and therapeutic benefit in these difficult situations when all other nonoperative treatment options have failed.

Arthroscopy can be useful diagnostically, identifying pathology not predicted by preoperative clinical or radiograph exam. Ogilvie-Harris and coworkers, for example, found a 9% incidence of significant biceps tendon tears and a 13% incidence of glenoid labral

TABLE 5.2. Radiographic Staging Criteria for Osteoarthritis.

Stage	Radiographs
Stage I	Normal
Stage II	Mild joint space narrowing
	Concentric wear
Stage III	Moderate joint space narrowing
	Early osteophyte formation
Stage IV	Severe joint space narrowing
	Extensive osteophyte formation
	Eccentric wear

TABLE 5.4. Indications for Arthroscopy in Glenohumeral Arthritis.

To confirm diagnosis
To identify and treat additional pathology
To determine prognosis (grade)
To relieve pain
To restore motion
To improve joint mechanics
To remove loose bodies
To slow disease progression
To delay larger definitive procedure

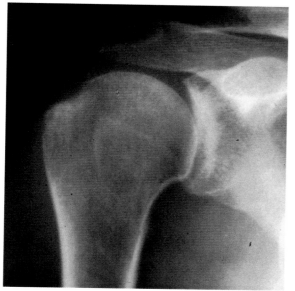 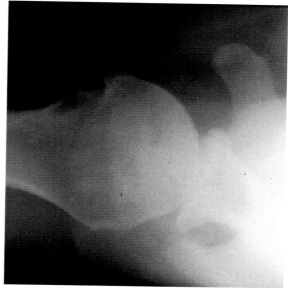

FIGURE 5.1. True AP (A) and axillary (B) radiographs of a patient with stage III osteoarthritis. There is moderate joint space narrowing with early osteophyte formation.

pathology in a group of patients undergoing arthrosocpy for osteoarthritis.[1] Weinstein and coauthors found a 32% incidence of coexisting intra-articular pathology, including labral tears, rotator cuff tears, and lesions involving the biceps anchor.[4]

PREOPERATIVE EVALUATION

Evaluation of the arthritic shoulder begins with a thorough patient history. Important components include systemic and other joint involvement, response to nonoperative treatment, and night or rest pain. The physical exam focuses on localization of pain, active and passive range of motion, and provocative tests. Soft tissue integrity, including rotator cuff and deltoid function, should be assessed. Differentiation of subacromial from intra-articular source of pain can be difficult. Along with impingement signs for subacromial pathology, one test that may be useful in localizing pain to the glenohumeral joint is the compression rotation test described by Ellman.[9] With the patient lying in the lateral decubitus position and the affected shoulder up, compression of the glenohumeral joint by the examiner while the arm is rotated may accentuate pain originating in the glenohumeral joint. An additional test that is both diagnostic and therapeutic is selective injection of the subacromial space and/or glenohumeral joint with a local anesthetic/corticosteroid mixture.

Other diagnostic tests include routine shoulder radiographs, consisting of a true anteroposterior (AP) view in neutral, internal, and external rotation, as well as a scapular lateral and an axillary view. The axillary view is critical in evaluation of the amount and pattern (eccentric or concentric) of glenoid wear (Figure 5.1). Magnetic resonance imaging is not routinely necessary in the evaluation of patients with osteoarthritis unless there is concern about the integrity of the rotator cuff. A CT scan can also be useful to assess glenoid wear patterns if the axillary view is not adequate.

SURGICAL TECHNIQUE

Positioning/Setup

We prefer interscalene regional anesthesia because of the muscular relaxation obtained and the prolonged postoperative pain relief achieved. This may be supplemented with an endotracheal tube or laryngeal airway mask if warranted. While lateral decubitus or beach chair positioning is a matter of surgeon preference, we prefer the beach chair position so that the surgeon may easily convert to an open procedure if necessary.

Instrumentation

An arthroscopic pump that permits independent pressure and flow rate adjustment is utilized. A standard 4.0 mm, 30° arthroscope is used, and a 70° arthroscope should be available. We use a 5.5 mm shaver; however smaller diameter shaver blades (3.5–4.5 mm) may

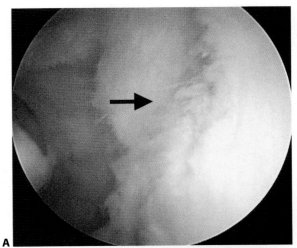

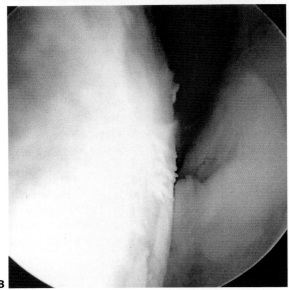

Diagnostic arthroscopy is carried out with the scope first placed in the posterior portal, inspecting the humeral and glenoid articular cartilage (Figure 5.2). The labrum, biceps, and rotator cuff are inspected for pathology. An anterior portal is established in the rotator interval with the aid of an 18-gauge spinal needle, placed just lateral to the tip of the coracoid. This serves as the working portal for debridement of loose cartilage flaps, fibrillation, synovitis, and soft tissue lesions using a combination of motorized resector and electrocautery (Figure 5.3). Surgical treatment should be aimed at removing the mechanical debris (cartilage breakdown products), products of inflammation (cytokines and proteases), and cells that generate inflammatory mediators (synovial and inflammatory cells). Therefore it is important to remove all inflamed synovium in osteoarthritis. A thorough lavage should also be performed with at least 3 L of irrigating solution.

Mechanical causes of pain and limited function should also be addressed. Osteophytes are debrided. Loose bodies are located and removed en bloc with a grasper through an enlarged portal, or piecemeal with the motorized resector (Figure 5.4) If a loose body is removed en bloc, it is important to have good visualization and a portal large enough to ensure that it will not be lost in the soft tissues during extraction. Loose bodies may settle in the subscapularis recess; a 70° arthroscope can aid in visualizing and removing these.

In contrast to patients with adhesive capsulitis, a formal manipulation is not performed in patients with osteoarthritis. Their older age, in combination with disuse osteopenia, presents a significant risk for ia-

FIGURE 5.2. (A) Arthroscopic view from posterior portal (beach chair position, left shoulder) shows grade IV glenoid chondral defect (arrow). (B) Grade III wear on the humeral head (posterior viewing portal, beach chair position, left shoulder).

be required if the joint is tight. A standard set of arthroscopic biters and graspers is useful for loose body removal and capsular release. We use an electrocautery device for tissue ablation and cauterization.

Surgical Technique

An examination under anesthesia is performed to assess stability and range of motion. Landmarks are carefully drawn with a marker. A posterior portal is established in the soft spot, located approximately 2 cm inferior and 2 cm medial to the posterolateral corner of the acromion, and the 30° arthroscope is introduced.

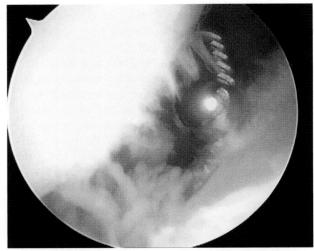

FIGURE 5.3. A motorized shaver is introduced from anterior portal to debride chondral flaps and fibrillation (scope in posterior portal, beach chair position, left shoulder).

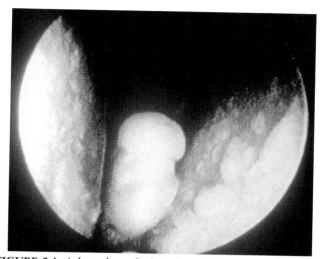

FIGURE 5.4. A large loose body is located between the humeral head and glenoid (scope in posterior portal, beach chair position, left shoulder).

trogenic fracture. Range of motion is increased through a thorough synovectomy and debridement. The shoulder is also placed through a gentle range of motion while under direct visualization. If an arthroscopic release is performed, circumferential release may be necessary. Frequently, however, an anterior release alone is sufficient in the setting of osteoarthritis with accompanying anterior capsular contracture. We perform capsular release by using a combination of motorized shaver, electrocautery, and biters under direct visualization. The anterior capsule is debrided from the anterior edge of the biceps tendon to the superior edge of the subscapularis (Figure 5.5). Care is taken to completely free the biceps and subscapularis while not injuring these tendons. In the pouch, proximity of the axillary nerve to the inferior capsule must always be remembered, and only a gentle synovectomy is performed, as well as debridement of humeral osteophytes. If the patient has a significant loss of internal rotation, a posterior capsular release is performed with the arthroscope in the anterior portal. The motorized shaver or electrocautery is placed in the posterior portal, and the posterior capsule is debrided under direct visualization. It is important to remember that patients with osteoarthritis often develop posterior humeral subluxation and an attenuated posterior capsule. The patient may eventually require an arthroplasty, and an aggressive posterior capsular debridement could compromise future posterior stability.

It is important to address associated pathology in the subacromial space and acromioclavicular (AC) joint. A single lateral portal or two lateral working portals may be utilized, and bursectomy and decompression performed using the combination of electrocautery and motorized shaver. Like synovial debridement in the glenohumeral joint, subacromial decompression should be aimed at thorough debridement of bursal tissue, which can be a source of inflammatory mediators that produce pain. In 1996 Ide et al. demonstrated the presence of substance P, a neural mediator, in bursal tissue in patients with impingement pain.[10] Thorough debridement of fibrous adhesions, which have formed in response to inflammation, is also important. Release of these adhesions can significantly improve shoulder motion in patients with shoulder stiffness.

Distal clavicle excision is appropriate in patients with preoperative evidence of AC joint pain. While it is often helpful to examine preoperative radiographic studies for the presence of degenerative AC arthritis, up to 82% of patients may have radiographic evidence of degenerative disease without any symptoms.[11] Therefore, one should not perform an AC arthroplasty based on radiographic evaluation. We perform arthroscopic AC arthroplasty only on patients with physical evidence of pain localized to the AC joint. A diagnostic injection of lidocaine directly into the AC joint as part of the preoperative workup is helpful if the diagnosis is in question.

The portals are closed with simple absorbable monofilament sutures and covered with steri-Strips and a sterile dressing.

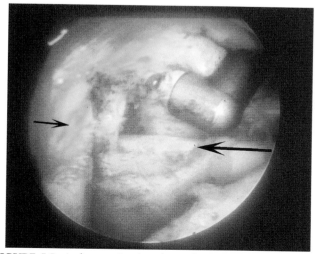

FIGURE 5.5. Arthroscopic view from the posterior portal (beach chair position, right shoulder). The rotator interval capsule is released by using electrocautery above the subscapularis tendon (large arrow). The anterior glenoid labrum is indicated by the small arrow on the left.

POSTOPERATIVE MANAGEMENT

If a significant capsular release has been performed, the patient will be admitted and an additional interscalene block performed the following morning, or the indwelling interscalene catheter reinjected. These patients are usually discharged on postoperative day 2, having received physical therapy twice on each postoperative day. If a debridement has been performed without extensive capsular release, the procedure is performed on an outpatient basis. Patients begin active assisted and passive range-of-motion exercises on the first postoperative day. A sling is generally worn for 3 or 4 days for comfort. Active range-of-motion exercises are initiated approximately 2 weeks postoperatively, after the swelling from the procedure has resolved.

RESULTS

Neer initially reported poor results with open release, debridement, osteophyte removal, and soft tissue balancing for osteoarthritis.[7] Naranja and Iannotti indicated that best results are achieved with arthroscopic debridement when there is near-normal preoperative range of motion.[8] Despite these reports, Ogilvie-Harris and Wiley found that the patients who benefited most from shoulder arthroscopy for osteoarthritis were those who had a concomitant frozen shoulder and underwent release.[1]

Three recent studies support the role for arthroscopic debridement in arthritis of the shoulder. Weinstein and coauthors, in a retrospective study of 25 patients with an average 34-month follow-up, reported good or excellent results in 80% of patients with primary or secondary glenohumeral arthritis.[4] Improvement in both pain and range of motion was demonstrated, with a postoperative average forward elevation of 167° and external rotation at the side of 53°. Initial pain relief lasted an average of 7 months, and only 24% of patients noted deterioration of pain relief over the follow-up period. No significant difference could be demonstrated based on radiographic stage or pathological grade of osteoarthritis.

A consistent finding in 92% of patients in this study was the presence of a thickened subacromial bursa.[4] Debridement of the subacromial inflammation and fibrosis was an important component of the improvement in motion and pain in these patients. These findings are consistent with a recent study presented by Bae and coworkers.[12] In a retrospective study of 36 patients with glenohumeral arthritis who had arthroscopic subacromial decompression, shoulder outcome scores improved from 32 to 77 points with an average

4.5-year follow-up. Results correlated with the extent of degenerative joint disease noted at the time of arthroscopy. Patients with severe degenerative disease as diagnosed by radiographs or arthroscopic exam had less predictable results. The authors concluded that the presence of mild to moderate glenohumeral degenerative disease (grades I–III) did not preclude a satisfactory result.

A third recent study, by Cameron and coworkers, reported on 45 patients at an average of 2 years following arthroscopic debridement of grade IV glenohumeral osteoarthritis, with or without capsular release.[13] Satisfactory results were obtained with significant pain relief in 88% of patients at an average of 28 months after surgery. These results suggest that arthroscopic debridement may be considered even for high-grade arthritis. One related study by Harryman supports the role of capsular release in providing functional improvement.[6] In this prospective study of 30 patients who had been arthroscopically debrided, within 6 months of surgery 88% of patients recovered excellent function, which remained high at an average of 33 months postoperatively. Final motion averaged 93% of the unaffected side.

COMPLICATIONS

Complications of arthroscopic debridement can be intraoperative and postoperative. Intraoperative complications include inadequate debridement or release, overzealous debridement and pain, axillary nerve injury, and iatrogenic fracture from the manipulation. Postoperative complications include pain, infection, portal wound breakdown, and inadequate postoperative therapy. In Harryman's series of 30 patients with arthroscopic capsular release, there was a single axillary neuropraxia that recovered without further treatment.[6]

CONCLUSIONS

Arthoscopic debridement has proven to be an effective strategy for the treatment of some patients with osteoarthritis. Additional studies with long-term follow-up are necessary to prove the durability of this treatment.

References

1. Ogilvie-Harris DJ, Wiley AM. Arthroscopic surgery of the shoulder. A general appraisal. *J Bone Joint Surg Br* 1986;68:201–207.
2. Cofield RH. Arthroscopy of the shoulder. *Mayo Clin Proc* 1983;58:501–508.

3. Ratcliffe A, Flatow EL, Roth N, Saed-Nejad F, Bigliani LU. Biochemical markers in synovial fluid identify early osteoarthritis of the glenohumeral joint. *Clin Orthop* 1996:45–53.

4. Weinstein DM, Bucchieri JS, Pollock RG, Flatow EL, Bigliani LU. Arthroscopic debridement of the shoulder for osteoarthritis. *Arthroscopy* 2000;16:471–476.

5. Outerbridge RE. The etiology of chondromalacia patallae. *J Bone Joint Surg Br* 1961;43:752–757.

6. Harryman DT II, Matsen FA III, Sidles JA. Arthroscopic management of refractory shoulder stiffness. *Arthroscopy* 1997;13:133–147.

7. Neer CS II. Replacement arthroplasty for glenohumeral osteoarthritis. *J Bone Joint Surg Am* 1974;56:1–13.

8. Naranja RJ, Jr, Iannotti JP. Surgical options in the treatment of arthritis of the shoulder: alternatives to prosthetic arthroplasty. *Semin Arthroplasty* 1995; 6:204–213.

9. Ellman H, Harris E, Kay SP. Early degenerative joint disease simulating impingement syndrome: arthroscopic findings. *Arthroscopy* 1992;8:482–487.

10. Ide K, Shirai Y, Ito H. Sensory nerve supply in the human subacromial bursa. *J Shoulder Elbow Surg* 1996;5: 371–382.

11. ShubinStein B, Wiater J, Pfaff C, Bigliani L, Levine W. Detection of acromioclavicular joint pathology in asymptomatic shoulders using magnetic resonance imaging. *J Shoulder Elbow Surg* 2001;10:204–208.

12. Bae H, Guyette T, Warren R, Craig E, Wickiewicz T. Results of subacromial decompression in patients with subacromial impingement and glenohumeral degenerative joint disease. Paper presented at: 67th Meeting of the American Academy of Orthopaedic Surgeons; 2000; Orlando, FL.

13. Cameron B, Galatz L, Williams G, Ramsey M, Iannotti J. Nonprosthetic management of grade 4 osteoarthritis. Paper presented at: 67th meeting of the American Academy of Orthopaedic Surgeons; 2000; Orlando, FL.

Synovectomy for Synovial Disease

John J. Klimkiewicz

Primary synovial disease of the shoulder represents a small proportion of patients presenting with shoulder symptoms. Diagnosis of these entities is often difficult and delayed. While rheumatoid arthritis represents the most common synovial disease, other entities can afflict the shoulder as well, including other types of inflammatory arthritis, metabolic arthritis (gout, pseudogout), synovial chondromatosis, pigmented villonodular synovitis (PVNS), and hemophilia (Table 6.1).

INDICATIONS/CONTRAINDICATIONS

Accurate diagnosis (and treatment) of synovial disease depends upon a combination of history, physical examination, laboratory tests (including synovial fluid analysis), and radiographic imaging. Occasionally, synovial biopsy is necessary for diagnostic confirmation. Arthroscopy of the shoulder can be a useful diagnostic tool in this otherwise difficult clinical setting.

Treatment of most synovial conditions relies upon medical management, including activity modification, physical therapy, anti-inflammatory medications, corticosteroid injections, and systemic drug therapies. Synovectomy is reserved for patients in whom such nonoperative treatment has been ineffective. The clinical benefit of arthroscopic synovectomy has been demonstrated in patients with rheumatoid arthritis, synovial chondromatosis, PVNS, and hemophilia. Long-term treatment efficacy in these cases depends upon thorough synovectomy. An arthroscopic approach allows a more complete inspection of the glenohumeral joint and subacromial space. While most of the literature details open synovectomy for these recalcitrant cases, arthroscopy provides tremendous advantages in terms of morbidity (pain, stiffness) with fewer surgical complications.

PREOPERATIVE PLANNING

In established cases of rheumatoid arthritis, the cervical spine should be imaged prior to the administration of a general anesthetic for arthroscopy, to evaluate for coexistent cervical spine pathology. Patients most appropriate for arthroscopic synovectomy demonstrate minimal glenohumeral joint destruction and good range of motion, and they lack rotator cuff and acromioclavicular pathology. Careful preoperative assessment of the glenohumeral joint, acromioclavicular joint, and subacromial space is helpful in customizing one's surgical approach.

SURGICAL TECHNIQUE

Positioning/Setup

Shoulder arthroscopy can be performed with the patient in either the lateral decubitus or beach chair position; positioning is a matter of surgeon preference. I prefer a general anesthetic. Pharmacological hypotension is often helpful in controlling bleeding during this procedure, and it is especially helpful when the synovium is highly vascular.

Instrumentation

Standard arthroscopic instrumentation includes a standard 4 mm scope with a 5.5 mm cannula, and both 30 and 70° lenses. Mechanical pump assistance, the addition of epinephrine (1:100,000 U/3 L bag of normal saline), and use of a cautery device (Arthrocare, Arthrocare Corp, Sunnnyvale, CA), are necessary to assist in hemostasis. Additional equipment includes disposable cannulas, switching sticks, and motorized shaver blades (4.5–5.5 mm resectors).

TABLE 6.1. Synovial Disorders of the Shoulder.

Inflammatory arthritis
    Rheumatoid arthritis
    Juvenile rheumatoid arthritis
    Psoriatic arthritis
    Ankylosing spondylitis
    Reiter's syndrome
    Systemic lupus erythematosus
Crystalline Disorders
    Gout (uric acid)
    Pseudogout (calcium pyrophospahate)
    Milwaukee shoulder (hydroxyapatite)
Synovial chondromatosis
Pigmented villonodular synovitis (PVNS)
Infection
Systemic disorders
    Hemophilia
    Hemochromatosis

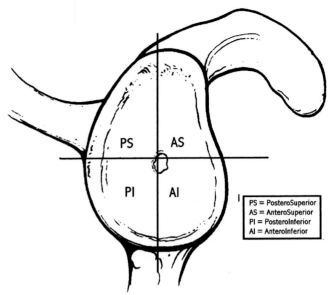

FIGURE 6.1. The glenohumeral joint is divided into quadrants: AS, anterosuperior; AI, anteroinferior; PI, posteroinferior; PS, posterosuperior.

Surgical Technique

Because fluid extravasation can distort orientation once the work has begun, anatomical landmarks should be outlined to assist in portal placement prior to arthroscopy. A traditional posterior portal is established in the anatomic "soft spot" posteriorly (approximately 1–2 cm inferior and 1 cm medial to the posterolateral corner of the acromion). This portal serves as the primary viewing portal to visualize the anterosuperior, anteroinferior, and posteroinferior quadrants of the glenohumeral joint, as well as the subacromial space (Figure 6.1). It can also be utilized as a working portal when one is performing synovectomy of the posterosuperior quadrant.

An "outside-in" anterior portal is then made within the rotator interval (between the subscapularis and biceps tendon) under direct visualization with the assistance of an 18-gauge spinal needle. This will serve as the primary working portal. Synovectomy can be performed through this portal for anteroinferior, anterosuperior, and for most of the posteroinferior glenohumeral joint. In addition, this portal can be helpful in visualizing the posterosuperior quadrant of the glenohumeral joint as well as the subscapular recess. A 70° scope permits an increased field of view through either portal.

A posteroinferior ancillary portal can be useful during arthroscopic glenohumeral synovectomy. This portal is made 1 to 2 cm inferior and slightly lateral to the initial scope placement (Figure 6.2). Care should be taken to establish this portal a few centimeters away to avoid instrument crowding. Conversely, to avoid axillary nerve injury, placement should not be more than 5 cm distal to the acromion. This accessory portal provides excellent access to the pos-

teroinferior quadrant of the joint and the axillary recess.

By using the portals just named, systematic synovectomy can be performed with a full-radius synovial resector shaving blade. Electrocautery is effective in ablating tissue. A holmium–YAG laser also permits effective hemostasis and tissue ablation, and does so in a noncontact "paint brush" manner.

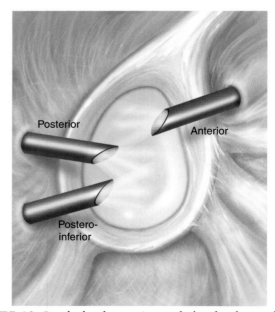

FIGURE 6.2. Standard arthroscopic portals for glenohumeral synovectomy include the standard posterior portal, an anterior portal within the rotator interval, and when necessary, an accessory posterior–inferior portal.

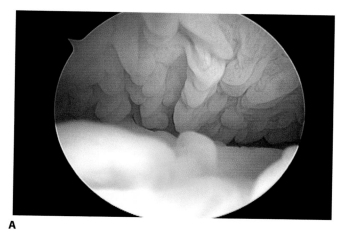

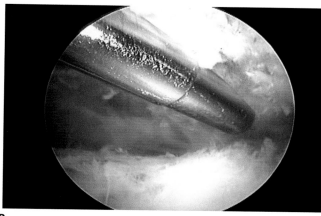

FIGURE 6.3. (A) Synovial hypertrophy typical of that seen in rheumatoid arthritis is arthroscopically visualized throughout the subacromial space in this 42-year-old female with a 4-month history of painful swelling in her left shoulder. (B) The bursa has been debrided with synovectomy and cautery, leaving a more normal appearing subacromial space. (View from posterior scope portal, beach chair position.)

Following glenohumeral synovectomy, the arthroscope is withdrawn and redirected through the same posterior portal into the subacromial space. The scope cannula with blunt obturator is directed under the acromion, which is palpable with the tip of the blunt trocar. A second portal is then established laterally under direct visualization using an 18-gauge spinal needle. This portal is usually placed toward the anterior half of the lateral acromion, since this is predominantly the location of the subacromial bursa. The portal should be made approximately 2 cm distal to the lateral edge of the acromion. Synovectomy and visualization of the rotator cuff within this area can usually be performed through these two portals (Figure 6.3). Strict attention to hemostasis, including fluid management, electrocautery, and hypotensive anesthesia, is essential. At the conclusion of the procedure arthroscopic portals are closed with 3.0 nylon suture and sterile dressings are placed. Drains are typically not employed.

POSTOPERATIVE MANAGEMENT

Postoperative treatment management includes an early range-of-motion program to prevent postoperative stiffness. The sling is discontinued within the first postoperative week, and active range of motion is permitted as tolerated. Physical therapy is begun in the first postoperative week.

RESULTS/OUTCOME

Literature results following synovectomy focus primarily on open approaches. Improvement following arthroscopic treatment has been reported in the early stages of rheumatoid arthritis (prior to extensive osseous involvement) in both range of motion and pain relief. Arthroscopy appears to be less successful in more advanced stages. Success has also been reported with arthroscopic synovectomy in case reports for synovial chondromatosis, PVNS, and hemodialysis-related shoulder arthropathy.

COMPLICATIONS

Complications related to arthroscopic shoulder synovectomy include bleeding, formation of fistulae at portal sites, and neurovascular injuries secondary to aberrant portal placement. Use of epinephrine in the saline trigation (HCC 1:1000), hypotensive anesthetic (when safe), and meticulous hemostasis (bipolar, monopolar, or laser) are critical for adequate visualization and satisfactory completion of the procedure. One should be familiar with the anatomical course of the axillary and musculocutaneous nerves, as well as the cephalic vein, since these structures can be at risk, primarily with anterior portal placement. Careful synovectomy of the axillary recess should be performed secondary to the proximity of the axillary nerve within this region.

Recommended Reading

Mahieu X, Chaouat G, Blin JL, Frank A, Hardy, P. Arthroscopic treatment of pigmented villonodular synovitis of the shoulder. *Arthroscopy* 2001;17(1):81–87.

Matthews LS, LaBudde JK. Arthroscopic treatment of synovial diseases of the shoulder. *Orthop Clin N Am* 1993; 24(1):101–109.

Matthews LS, Wolock B, Martin D. Arthroscopic management of inflammatory arthritis and synovitis of the shoulder. *Oper Arthrosc.* 1991;46:573–581.

Richman JD, Rose DJ. The role of arthroscopy in the management of synovial chondromatosis of the shoulder. A case report. *Clin Orthop* 1990;257:91–93.

Wakitani S, Imoto K, Saito M, MurataN, Hirooka A, Yoneda M, Ochi. Evaluation of surgeries for rheumatoid shoulder based on the destruction patterns. *J Rheumatol* 1999;26(1): 41–46.

SLAP and Biceps Lesions

7

Treatment of SLAP Lesions

Jeffrey T. Gittins, Mehrdad Ganjianpour, and Stephen J. Snyder

In 1984 Andrews described tears of the glenoid labrum in 73 overhead athletes.[1] In 1990 Snyder et al. described a pattern of injury to the superior labrum beginning posteriorly and extending anteriorly and introduced the term SLAP (superior labrum anterior and posterior) lesion.[2] The understanding of SLAP injuries has led to the evolution of their treatment.

DEFINITIONS AND INDICATIONS

SLAP Lesions

A SLAP lesion is a tear in the superior labrum, which, when one is viewing the glenoid face, occurs between 10 and 2 o'clock. SLAP lesions always include the area of the biceps tendon anchor complex. The superior labrum in this area serves as the anchor of the biceps tendon to the glenoid, and the labrum in this area is likely to be large, with a meniscoid appearance. A review of the arthroscopic appearance of these lesions resulted in a classification into four basic types of SLAP tears.[2]

A type I SLAP lesion has fraying and a degenerative appearance of the superior labrum. The attachment of the labrum to the glenoid and the biceps tendon anchor is intact. This may represent a normal finding in the older patient (Figure 7.1).

A type II SLAP lesion may have a degenerative appearance similar to a type I lesion. However, in type II lesions, the superior labrum is also detached from its insertion on the superior glenoid, and along with the biceps tendon, it arches away from the underlying glenoid neck (Figure 7.2).

In a type III SLAP lesion, the superior labrum has a bucket handle tear analogous to that seen in the knee's meniscus. The biceps tendon is intact, as is the labral rim attachment of the peripheral portion of the labrum (Figure 7.3).

With type IV SLAP lesions, a bucket handle tear of the superior labrum extends as a split tear of variable degrees up into the biceps tendon. The torn biceps tendon is displaced with the labral flap into the joint (Figure 7.4).

Complex and combined lesions frequently may be observed. The most common is the combination of a type II and a type IV SLAP lesion. Maffett and colleagues described other variations of SLAP lesions that they labeled types V through VII.[3]

Indications/Contraindications

Although the definitive diagnosis of a SLAP tear can be made only by arthroscopy, a good history and physical examination, complemented by imaging studies, can improve the diagnostic yield.

The two most common complaints of patients with SLAP lesions are pain with overhead activities, and mechanical symptoms of catching, locking, popping, or grinding.[2,4–9] Frequently the pain is impossible to differentiate from impingement-type pain. Other complaints include pain when lying on the shoulder, decreased range of motion, pain with activities of daily living, loss of strength, and symptoms compatible with a "dead arm" syndrome.[4,6,9]

Mechanisms of injury most commonly include traction or compression.[4] Traction injury can occur in several ways. It may occur by sudden inferior load, such as when one loses hold of a heavy object and attempts to keep it under control with the affected arm. It may also occur anteriorly (e.g., when someone is water skiing, or experiences a sudden pull), or it may result from an upward pull (e.g., when an individual grabs an overhead object in an attempt to save himself from falling).[10] In the overhead athlete, biceps anchor injuries may result from the eccentric contraction of the biceps during the follow-through phase of throwing. This injury may also be sustained during an overt glenohumeral dislocation. Compression injuries are also common and are frequently the result of a fall onto an outstretched arm positioned in slight forward flexion and abduction.[2] A direct blow to the shoulder was found to be the cause of injury in up to 17% of patients with isolated SLAP lesions.[5] The insidious onset of shoulder pain has been seen in as many as 33% of patients who have a SLAP lesion.[6]

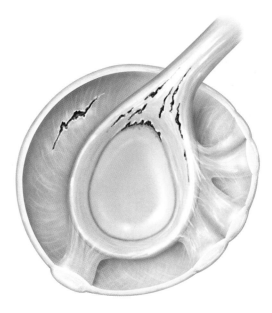

Type I

FIGURE 7.1. Fraying of the superior labrum in a type I SLAP lesion with an intact biceps anchor.

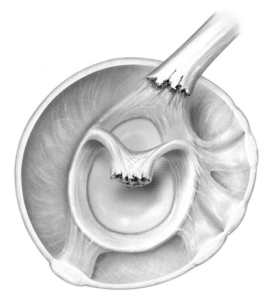

Type III

FIGURE 7.3. A type III SLAP lesion. There is a vertical tear through the labrum resulting in a bucket handle tear, but an intact biceps anchor.

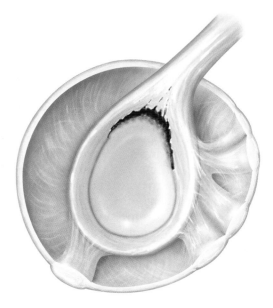

Type II

FIGURE 7.2. A type II SLAP lesion with superior labrum and the biceps anchor torn away from the superior glenoid attachment.

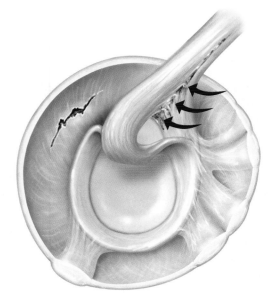

Type IV

FIGURE 7.4. A type IV SLAP lesion with a bucket handle tear of the labrum and extension into the biceps tendon.

PRELIMINARIES AND TREATMENT

Physical Exam

Despite the many physical examination findings suggestive of a superior labral lesion, none have proven very accurate. We therefore rely on a high index of suspicion in the patient with shoulder symptoms and physical findings indicative of a possible SLAP lesion. Making the diagnosis even more difficult, other diagnostic problems often occur in association with superior labral injuries. For example, partial and complete rotator cuff tears are frequently associated lesions in patients with SLAP tears.[2,4,5–9] Crepitation is detected in as many as 43% of patients with isolated SLAP tears in our series.[5] Patients may also have a positive apprehension test. Pain in abduction and external rotation may occur from traction on the torn labrum rather than owing to actual instability. In our experience, 39% of patients had a positive apprehension test; yet only 4% had a positive apprehension suppression test.[5]

Compression–rotation and biceps–tension tests may be positive. Pain with resisted supraspinatus strength testing, pain with resisted external rotation, pain with cross-body adduction, local tenderness, a positive Yergeson sign, and variable instability pattern findings may be present on examination of patients with SLAP lesions.[4–6]

Diagnostic Imaging

Although anterior-posterior (AP), axillary, acromioclavicular (AC), and outlet views should be obtained as part of the diagnostic workup, plain radiographs are not helpful in diagnosing labral tears.

Computerized tomographic (CT) arthrography has improved the detection of labral pathology compared with conventional radiographs. CT arthrography is better, however, for diagnosing bony abnormalities than soft tissue abnormalities, in general.

Magnetic resonance imaging (MRI) is superior to CT for diagnosing labral lesions. It has better soft tissue definition and multiplanar imaging capability than CT or plain films. It is the best noninvasive diagnostic tool for assessing the labrum and rotator cuff in patients with shoulder pain of uncertain origin.[11] However, adequate evaluation of the glenoid labrum and capsule adequately by means of conventional MRI techniques remains difficult. Gadolinium injected into the shoulder joint has been shown to increase the accuracy of the MRI examination.[11–14] In one study, MR arthrography had a sensitivity of 89%, a specificity of 91%, and an accuracy of 90%.[13] In general,

however, MRI remains relatively inaccurate, and frequently "overreads" SLAP lesions.

Owing to the limitations of the history, physical examination, and diagnostic studies in diagnosing labral tears, it is important to maintain a high clinical degree of suspicion regarding these lesions. In patients with persistent shoulder pain whose symptoms do not readily fit into one of the more commonly diagnosed etiologies of shoulder pain, it is important to consider labral pathology. Performing an accurate diagnostic shoulder arthroscopy may be the only way to make the definitive diagnosis of labral pathology.

Surgical Technique

Although MRI may provide useful information for evaluating the glenohumeral joint and labral complex, the diagnosis is generally made during diagnostic arthroscopy.[10] Findings consistent with SLAP lesions of the shoulder include signs of hemorrhage or granulation tissue beneath the biceps tendon and superior labrum, the presence of a space between the articular cartilage margin of the glenoid and the overlying attachment of the labrum and biceps anchor, and arching of the superior labrum mechanism more than 3 to 4 mm away from the glenoid when traction is applied to the biceps tendon.

A normal anatomical variant that may be confused with a SLAP tear is the meniscoid superior labrum. That is, if the superior labrum has a meniscoid appearance, this may be confused with a pathological entity. The labrum commonly attaches below the glenoid articular surface and may be misdiagnosed as a labral tear or avulsion. With acute trauma, the diagnosis is quite evident because of the hemorrhage around the avulsed labral tissue. However, with chronic lesions it may be difficult to diagnose a labral tear because the natural healing process may result in fibrous tissue, which will obscure a pathological detachment that has occurred on the superior neck of the glenoid. The articular cartilage of a normal shoulder extends up to the labral attachment at the superior glenoid. With tension applied to the biceps tendon, the torn superior labrum will be seen to arch away from the underlying bone by approximately 3 to 4 mm. If the labrum has a free margin with normal transition between the labral undersurface and superior glenoid rim, it is not considered to be a SLAP lesion, but a normal variant.

Treatment

Isolated labral tears occurring in otherwise stable shoulders may be treated effectively with debridement of the tear alone. All damaged labral tissue is removed, taking care to preserve the periphery of the labrum and the attachment of the capsule to the glenoid.

Vertical split tears may be resected in a manner similar to a bucket handle tear of the meniscus of the knee, by using basket forceps and shaver blades. When instability is also present with a labral tear, the labrum is debrided to prevent mechanical catching, followed by shoulder stabilization.

SURGICAL TECHNIQUE

Type I

Type I SLAP lesions are treated by debridement of the frayed tissues (Figure 7.5). We prefer to use a 4.0 mm full-radius shaver blade and excise only the torn tissues, avoiding damage to the biceps anchor, the attached anterior superior labrum, or any attached middle glenohumeral ligament. The shaver should be used through the anterior and posterior cannulas while viewing from the opposite side. After shaving, a probe is used to evaluate the labrum.

Type II

At our institutions, type II lesions are repaired by means of a single-anchor double-suture sling (SADS) technique. The 4 mm screw-in anchor is loaded with two strands of strong braided suture and inserted into the superior glenoid just below the biceps tendon. The sutures are then passed through the labrum, one posterior and one anterior to the biceps, forming a sling

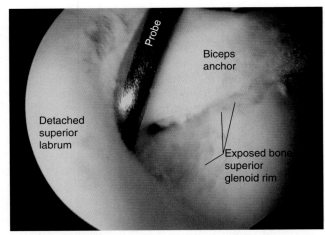

FIGURE 7.6. Type II SLAP: biceps anchor completely detached from the glenoid (posterior portal view, right shoulder, probe from anterior portal, lateral decubitus position).

or harness around the anchor point, affording secure stability for healing. (Figures 7.6, 7.7).

Type III

Type III SLAP lesions must have the unstable bucket handle labral fragment removed before the biceps anchor attachment is inspected (Figure 7.8). Use a motorized shaver first via the posterior cannula to trim the posterior attachment of the fragment. Switch the shaver to the anterior cannula to remove the remaining anterior portion. Very carefully observe the location and attachment site of the middle glenohumeral

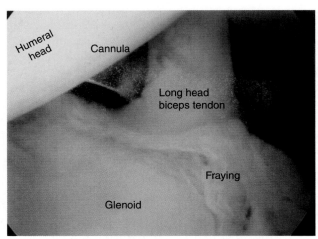

FIGURE 7.5. Type I SLAP lesion (seen from posterior portal, lateral decubitus position, left shoulder).

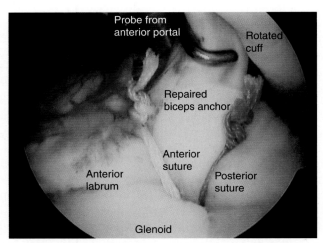

FIGURE 7.7. Double-sling suture anchor repair of type II SLAP lesion (left shoulder, lateral decubitus position; probe palpating repaired SLAP).

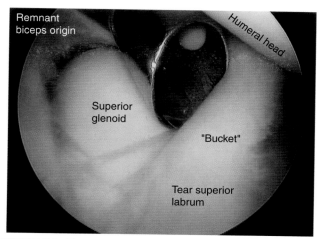

FIGURE 7.8. Type III SLAP lesion. Notice the displaced bucket handle tear of the labrum (right shoulder, lateral decubitus position, viewing from posterior portal; anterior metal cannula palpating and inferiorly displacing bucket).

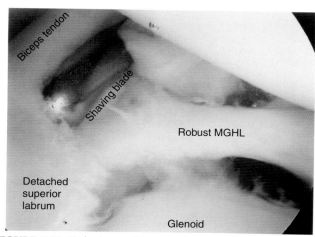

FIGURE 7.10. Buford complex with type II SLAP: a shaver introduced from the anterior portal debrides the undersurface of biceps and labrum, preserving the robust MGHL. (View from posterior portal, right shoulder, lateral decubitus position.)

ligament before completing the anterior resection. On occasion, a significant cordlike middle ligament will attach to the anterior superior labrum, sometimes including the loose portion of the type III or IV SLAP (Figure 7.9). An inadvertent excision of the labral attachment in this situation may lead to a significant anterior instability. If the anchor site of the middle glenohumeral ligament (MGHL) is in doubt, a conservative debridement of the fragment is suggested, leaving a robust tag attached anterior (Figure 7.10). If the anchor seems unstable when traction is applied to

the MGHL with a probe, the tissues can be reattached to the glenoid by using one of two sutures as outlined under SADS repair of type II SLAP (Figure 7.11).

Type IV

Type IV SLAP lesions are treated based on the severity of the biceps tendon split. When more than about 30% of the tendon is included with the displaced labral tear (Figure 7.12), one must consider either repairing the tendon, releasing it and repairing the

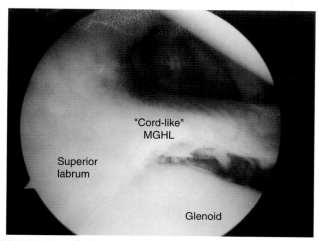

FIGURE 7.9. Buford complex without SLAP lesion (seen from posterior portal, lateral decubitus position, right shoulder).

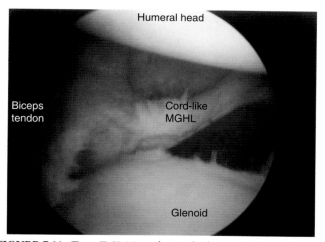

FIGURE 7.11. Type II SLAP with a Buford complex (viewed from posterior portal, lateral decubitus position). Note robust MGHL attached to type II right shoulder, SLAP. The SLAP repair should incorporate an anterosuperior attachment site to secure the MGHL.

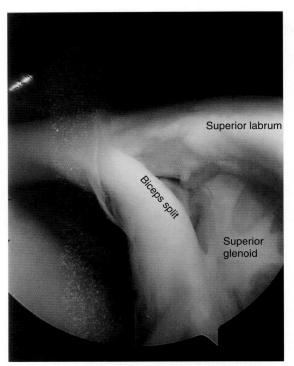

FIGURE 7.12. Type IV SLAP lesion. Notice the tear extending into the biceps tendon (left shoulder, viewed from posterior portal, lateral decubitus position).

labrum (as with a type II SLAP), or performing a biceps tenodesis. The decision depends on the age and activity level of the patient and the condition of the remainder of the biceps tendon. In most cases we prefer to excise the labral fragment along with the attached portion of torn biceps. If the remaining tendon

seems healthy without significant fraying and the anchor site is stable, I will not release or tenodese it. If the tendon appears to be degenerative, it will be released and tenodesed, especially in a young active patient.

STEPS IN THE SADS SLAP REPAIR (FOR TYPE II OR IV)

Labral tears can occur in association with glenohumeral instability. Therefore, shoulder stability should always be evaluated by examination under anesthesia.

1. Begin with the scope in the standard posterior portal and a smooth clear operating cannula in the anterior superior portal (ASP). The key to obtaining proper alignment for inserting the punch or drill bit and the anchor into the superior glenoid tubercle is exact placement of the ASP. It must be precisely in the superior aspect of the rotator interval anterior to the biceps tendon (Figure 7.13). We find it best to create this portal by using an outside-in technique, having first used a spinal needle to locate the ideal spot. Insert the needle into the skin at a point approximately 2 cm from the anterior-lateral corner of the acromion. The path of the needle must approach the superior tubercle under the labrum at an angle of about 45° toward the glenoid (avoid angling parallel to the glenoid "face"). Insert the smooth, clear cannula along the chosen path.

2. Shave the soft tissue off the superior glenoid below the detached labrum and biceps and trim the

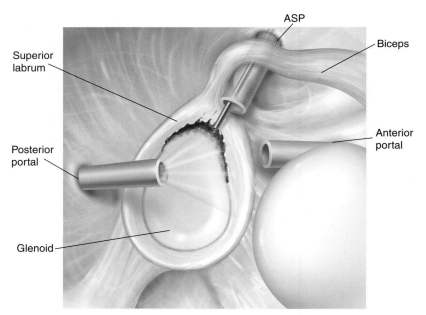

FIGURE 7.13. The anterosuperior (ASP) is carefully established to ensure adequate targeting of the superior glenoid neck.

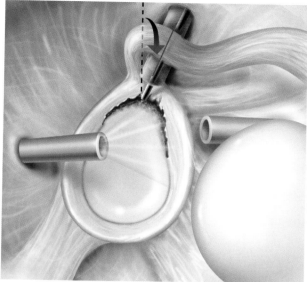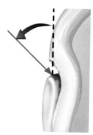

FIGURE 7.14. Suture anchor being placed with a proper angle. Inset shows importance of directing anchor punch medially towards glenoid bone stock.

frayed edge of the labrum. The posterior portion of the lesion and glenoid is best trimmed with the scope anterior and the shaver in the posterior portal. The bone of the superior glenoid is often relatively soft and seldom requires a burr to expose cancellous bone.

3. Insert a 2 mm punch via the ASP and create a pilot hole in the glenoid neck directly below the biceps tendon 2 to 3 mm medial to the articular cartilage. Ensure that the punch does not skive off the bone by carefully observing the progress of the punch. If the anchor skives off the bone, it may fail to support the sutures as well as risk injury to the suprascapular nerve. It is necessary to direct the handle of the punch in a posterior and medial direction, with a little pressure to guide the tip into the bone (Figure 7.14).

4. If one is not already established, create an anterior midglenoid portal (AMGP) with a lipped clear cannula, using outside-in techniques and entering just above the subscapularis tendon.

5. A 4 mm anchor is next loaded with two no. 2 Ethibond sutures in a very specific manner. One of the sutures is white and the other is dark green and, by convention, the white suture is loaded in the deeper side of the eyelet closer to the threads while the green suture is situated more superficially near the top of the eyelet. Half of each suture is marked with a purple surgical marker, both near the eyelet and on the end, to identify it and to aid with suture management. This results in four dissimilar sutures: white, white-purple, green, and green-purple. The sutures are arranged in the anchor so that the purple limb of each suture ex-

its the same side of the eyelet. The anchor is loaded in the driver in a way that allows the purple sutures to exit on the side with the notched vertical orientation line (seen arthroscopically at the driver–implant interface). The screw is then advanced into the bone until the anchor is seated. After the screwdriver has been removed, the sutures are tested for security by gently pulling on them outside the ASP.

Preliminary Step of Arranging the Sutures to Facilitate Passing

6. Change the scope to the AMGP and insert a clear cannula in the posterior portal. Retrieve the all-white suture out the posterior portal by using a crochet hook. (Figure 7.15) For better suture "management," we routinely will then reposition the suture "outside" the portal by inserting a switching stick, removing the cannula, and then reinserting the cannula over the switching stick, leaving the suture "outside" the cannula (Figure 7.16). This is done for both limbs of the white suture. This technique will minimize suture clutter. Return the scope to the posterior portal and the clear cannula to the ASP (Figure 7.15).

7. Retrieve the all-green suture out of the AMGC, using the crochet hook, and store it outside the cannula (Figure 1.16).

8. Retrieve the green-purple suture into the AMGC and store it there by placing a clamp on the end. This is the first suture that will be passed through the labrum posterior to the biceps.

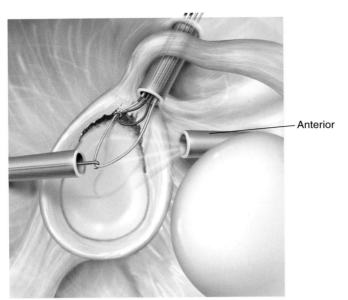

FIGURE 7.15. Using a crochet hook to retrieve the white suture from the posterior portal. This suture is placed outside the cannula by means of a switching rod.

Passing Sutures Through the Labrum

FIRST, POSTERIOR REPAIR

9. Insert the medium-sized crescent hook through the clear cannula via the ASP and position it behind the biceps tendon. Puncture the labrum just posterior to the biceps, and angle the needle to exit just behind the

anchor under the edge of the labrum (Figure 7.17A). Pass 3 cm of the suture shuttle into the joint. Insert an arthroscopic grasping clamp via the AMGP, ensuring that the clamp follows the green-purple suture path exactly (Figure 7.17B). If the clamp passes around one of the other sutures, it will cause the strands to be twisted around each other when the shuttle pulls the suture back through the tissues. Grasp the end of the shuttle, remove the crescent hook, and pull the shuttle out the AMGC (Figure 7.17).

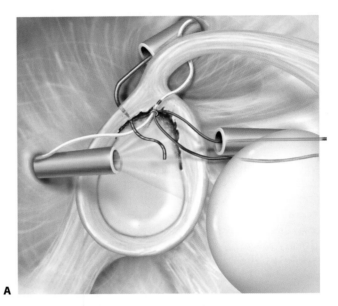

A

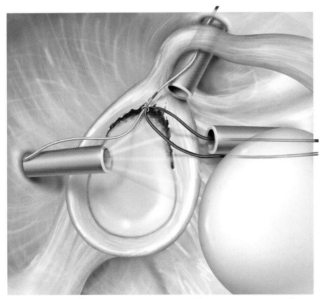

FIGURE 7.16. The sutures are separated into a star pattern for ease of suture management. Note that the white–purple suture has also been stored outside the ASP, using the guide rod technique.

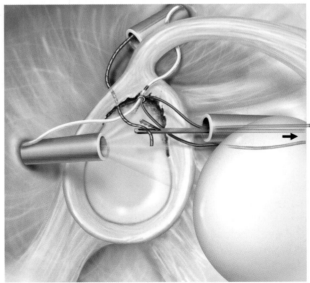

B

FIGURE 7.17. (A) Crescent hook penetrating the labrum. (B) The suture passer is introduced under the labrum posterior to the biceps, and the shuttle is retrieved from the midglenoid portal by means of an arthroscopic grasper.

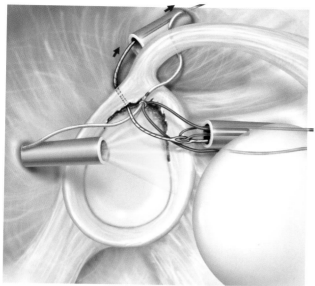

FIGURE 7.18. The purple limb of the green suture is passed through the tissue by means of the shuttle.

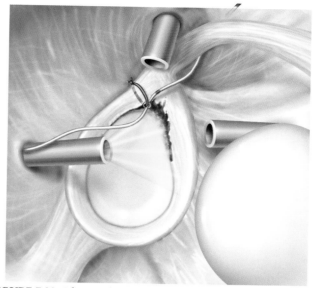

FIGURE 7.20. The purple suture is tied posterior to the biceps tendon.

10. Outside the AMGP portal, load the green-purple suture into the shuttle and pull it back through the tissue and out the ASC (Figure 7.18). Before pulling the suture tight, observe it carefully to ensure that it is not twisted around any other suture.

11. Retrieve the all-green suture out the ASP posterior to the biceps tendon, using the crochet hook (Figure 7.19).

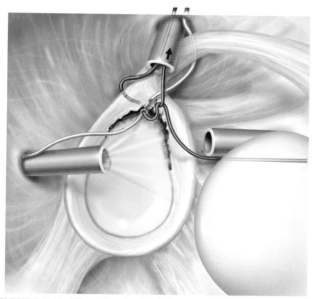

FIGURE 7.19. The other limb of the green suture is retrieved.

12. Tie the suture tails together using a sliding/locking knot. Pull the purple-green suture (the one passing through the labral tissue) to make it the shorter one, and use it as the initial post strand (Figure 7.20).

SECOND, ANTERIOR REPAIR

13. Retrieve the white-purple suture and bring it out the AMGP with a crochet hook.

14. The ASP cannula is repositioned anterior to the biceps tendon. Insert the crescent hook down the ASP and pierce the superior labrum at a point just anterior to the biceps tendon. This point should be in the vicinity of the attachment of the superior glenohumeral ligament and may be at or near the junction of the cordlike middle humeral ligament associated with a Buford complex. Pass the shuttle into the joint and carry it out of the AMGP with an arthroscopic grasping clamp (Figure 7.21).

15. Load the shuttle with the white-purple suture outside the AMGP and carry it back through the joint and labrum tissue and out the ASC (Figure 7.22).

16. Through the ASC, retrieve the all-white suture with the crochet hook from its storage position outside the portal (Figure 7.23).

17. Pull the white-purple suture (the limb that passes through the labral tissue) to make it the shorter limb, and tie the sutures using a sliding/locking knot (Figure 7.24). If the sutures will not slide easily because a twist has been introduced, tie them instead, using a

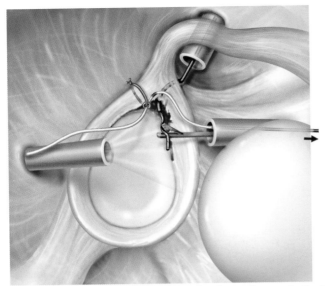

FIGURE 7.21. A switching stick is used to bring the purple limb of the white suture back inside the midglenoid cannula, and the suture passer is introduced under the labrum anterior to the biceps tendon.

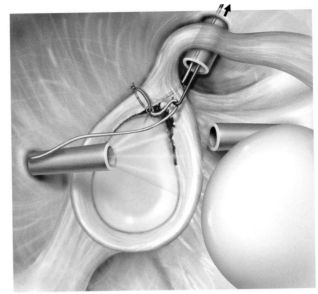

FIGURE 7.23. The other limb of the white suture is retrieved anterior to the biceps tendon from the anterior superior cannula.

nonsliding suture tie technique (such as the multiple half-hitch revo knot: see Chapter 4, Figure 4.6).

19. Test the repair by pulling on the biceps tendon via the AMGC with a probe. The labrum should be firmly attached to the bone, and there should be no gap when tension is applied. In addition, the anterior ligaments should have a stable anchor site with no undue tension upon pulling the biceps (Figure 7.25).

POSTOPERATIVE CARE

The shoulder is protected in a sling for 4 weeks. The patient should begin elbow, wrist, and hand exercises immediately, with gentle pendulum exercises in one week. The shoulder should be protected from excess stress on the biceps tendon for 6 weeks. Progressive resistance exercises are allowed at that point. Vigor-

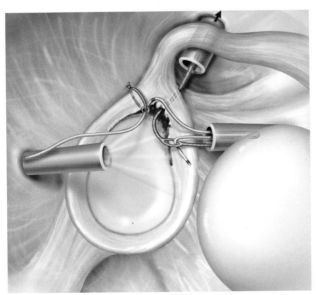

FIGURE 7.22. The purple limb of the white suture is passed through the tissue by means of a shuttle.

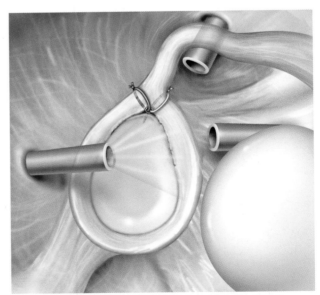

FIGURE 7.24. The white suture is tied, and the double-sling repair of the biceps anchor is completed.

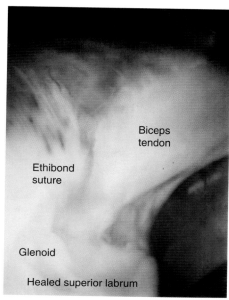

FIGUURE 7.25. Arthroscopic view of healed type II SLAP lesion. Viewing from posteriorly in a right shoulder, lateral decubitus position, notice the biceps anchor completely healed onto the glenoid. A permanent Ethibond suture remains.

ous throwing and strenuous lifting are permitted after 6 months if the patient is asymptomatic and has normal motion.

SUMMARY

Glasgow et al.[15] reported the results of arthroscopic glenoid labral resection in 28 overhead athletes. In patients with stable shoulders, there were 91% good or excellent results at 2-year follow-up. However, these results deteriorated over time, and only 75% of the patients had noteworthy relief. Likewise, Altchek et al.[16] studied 40 athletes following labral debridement. Forty percent of the group had instability on examination at the time of surgery, but 72% of the patients reported considerable pain relief during the first year postoperatively. However, the results deteriorated steadily over time, and only 7% of the patients had noteworthy long-term relief. Both Glasgow and Altchek concluded that labral debridement alone does not generally give satisfactory results in overhead athletes and that treatment in these individuals must focus on the underlying glenohumeral instability.

Payne and Jokl[17] studied 14 patients treated with arthroscopic labral debridement. These patients all had similar shoulder pain with overhead activity but had stable glenohumeral joints on postoperative ex-

amination. Results were initially relatively good, with 93% excellent or good results after 6 months. However, at an average of 2-year follow-up, results had deteriorated to 71% excellent or good. The best results were noted in the superior and anterior inferior labral segments. The authors found that for anterosuperior labral lesions, patients were at risk for delayed development of glenohumeral instability. As a general rule, in the high-level overhead athlete, when labral tears are observed at the time of arthroscopy, glenohumeral instability should be presumed present unless proven otherwise.

Our understanding of SLAP lesions continues to evolve. Despite our concerted efforts in diagnosing labral pathology by history, physical exam, MRI, and MRI arthrography, arthroscopy remains the best tool for the diagnosis of SLAP lesions. In patients who participate in high-level overhead throwing activities, a high index of suspicion should remain for SLAP lesions, particularly in the absence of other identifiable causes. Arthroscopic repair of torn SLAP lesions is effective in the majority of patients. Because these lesions are so frequently associated with other shoulder conditions, one must consider an arthroscopic exam for other pathology, including instability, rotator cuff tears, and paralabral cysts. Improved studies and a constant search for new surgical techniques will help advance our understanding and treatment of superior labral lesions.

References

1. Andrews JR, Carson WG, McLeod WD. The arthroscopic treatment of glenoid labrum tears—the throwing athlete. *Orthop Trans* 1984;8:44.
2. Snyder SJ, Karzel RP, Del Pizzo W, Ferkel RD, Friedman MJ. SLAP lesions of the shoulder. *Arthroscopy* 1990;6:274–279.
3. Maffett MW, Gartsman GM, Moseley B. Superior labrum–biceps tendon complex lesion of the shoulder. *Am J Sports Med* 1995;23(1):93–98.
4. Maffett, MW, Gartsman GM, Moseley B. Superior labrum–biceps tendon complex lesions of the shoulder. *Am J Sports Med* 1995; 22:121–130.
5. Stetson WB, Snyder SJ, Karzel RP, Banas MP, Rahal SE. Long-term clinical follow-up of isolated SLAP lesions of the shoulder. Paper presented at: 64th Annual Meeting of the American Academy of Orthopaedic Surgeons, February 1997.
6. Resch H, Golser K, Thoeni H, Sperner G. Arthroscopic repair of superior glenoid labral detachment (the SLAP lesion). *J Shoulder Elbow Surg* 1993;2:147–155.
7. Snyder SJ, Banas MP, Karzel RP. An analysis of 140 injuries to the superior glenoid labrum. *J Shoulder Elbow Surg* 1995;4:243–248.

8. Field, LD, Savoie FH III. Arthroscopic suture repair of superior labral detachment lesions of the shoulder. *Am J Sports Med* 1993;21:783–790.

9. Yoneda M, Hirooka A, Saito S, Yamamoto T, Ochi T, Shino K. Arthroscopic stapling for detached superior glenoid labrum. *J Bone Joint Surg Br* 1991;73:746–750.

10. Mileski RA, Snyder SJ. Superior labral lesions in the shoulder: pathoanatomy and surgical management. *J Am Acad Orthop Surg* 1998;6:121–131.

11. Tirman PFJ, Applegate GR, Flannigan BD, Stauffer AE, Crues JV III. Magnetic resonance arthrography of the shoulder. *Magn Reson Imaging Clin N Am* 1993;1: 125–142.

12. Chandnani VP, Yeager TD, DeBerardino T, et al. Glenoid labral tears: prospective evaluation with MR imaging, MR arthrography, and CT arthrography. *AJR Am J Roentgenol* 1993;161:1229–1235.

13. Bencardino JT, Beltran J, Rosenberg ZS, et al. Superior labrum anterior-posterior lesions: diagnosis with MR arthrography of the shoulder. *Radiology* 2000;214(1): 1267–271.

14. Karzel RP, Snyder SJ. Magnetic resonance arthrography of the shoulder: a new technique of shoulder imaging. *Clin Sports Med* 1993;1:123–136.

15. Glasgow SG, Bruce RA, Yacobucci GN, Torg JS. Arthroscopic resection of glenoid labral tears in the athlete: a report of 29 cases. *Arthroscopy* 1992;8:48–54.

16. Altchek DW, Warreen RF, Wickiewicz TL, Ortiz G. Arthroscopic labral debridement: a three year follow-up study. *Am J Sports Med* 1992;20:702–706.

17. Payne LZ, Jokle P. The results of arthroscopic debridement of glenoid labral tears based on tear location. *Arthroscopy* 1993;9:560–565.

Recommended Reading

Cooper DE, Arnoczky SP, O'Brien SJ, Warren RF, DiCarlo E, Allen AA. Anatomy, histology, and vascularity of the glenoid labrum: an anatomical study. *J Bone Joint Surg* 1992;74:46–52.

Detrisac DA, Johnson LL. *Arthroscopic Shoulder Anatomy: Pathologic and Surgical Implications.* Thorofare, NJ: Slack; 1986.

Prodromos CC, Ferry JA, Schiller AL, Zarins B. Histological studies of the glenoid labrum from fetal life to old age. *J Bone Joint Surg* 1990;72:1344–1348.

Rodosky, MW, Harner CD, Fu FH. The role of the long head of the biceps muscle and superior glenoid labrum in anterior stability of the shoulder. *Am J Sports Med* 1994;22:121–130.

Snyder SJ, Rames RD, Wolber E. Labral lesions. In: McGinty JB, ed. *Operative Arthroscopy.* New York: Raven Press; 1991:491–499.

Vangsness CT Jr, Jorgenson SS, Watson T, Johsnon DL. The origin of the long head of the biceps from the scapula and glenoid labrum: an anatomical study. *J Bone Joint Surg* 1992;74:46–52.

Williams MM, Snyder SJ, Buford D: The Buford complex—the "cord-like" middle glenohumeral ligament and abscent anterosuperior labrum complex: a normal anatomic capsulolabral variant. *Arthroscopy* 1994;10(3): 241–247.

8

Arthroscopic Biceps Tenodesis

Pascal Boileau, Sumant G. Krishnan, and Gilles Walch

Owing to the multiple possibilities of pathology of the tendon itself and its pulley system, the long head of the biceps is often a cause of shoulder pain. Surgical treatment for disorders of the long head of the biceps is limited to removal of the intra-articular portion of the tendon, with either tenotomy or tenodesis. Biceps tenodesis with or without rotator cuff repair, is a common and well-accepted open surgical procedure. Previous authors have described biceps tenodesis under arthroscopic control, either using isolated sutures (Habermeyer) or sutures with anchors (Snyder, Gartsman). Because of familiarity and success with the technique of interference screw fixation for hamstring anterior cruciate ligament (ACL) reconstruction grafts in a bone tunnel, a similar technique was developed for use in both open and arthroscopic tenodeses of the biceps.

INDICATIONS/CONTRAINDICATIONS

Indications for tenodesis of the biceps (whether open or arthroscopic) include pain associated with significant tenosynovitis, prerupture of the tendon, subluxation, and dislocation. Performing this procedure under arthroscopic control may be beneficial for the patient, regardless of whether the rotator cuff is torn, because decreased morbidity is associated with an all-arthroscopic operation. This procedure can be effectively used in three clinical situations: (1) in association with arthroscopic or mini-open rotator cuff repairs, (2) in cases of isolated pathology of the biceps tendon with an intact cuff, especially in a young athlete, presenting as tendinitis, subluxation, prerupture, or type 4 SLAP lesions with large extension into the biceps anchor; or (3) in cases of massive, degenerative, and irreparable cuff tears with a pathological biceps tendon, where a tenodesis may be preferred to a simple tenotomy, especially in an elderly but active and muscular patient. In this last situation, tenodesis of the biceps may be a preferable alternative to simple tenotomy, avoiding distal retraction and bulging of the muscle at the elbow (which may be a source of painful contracture while working) and slight decrease in supination strength.

A very thin, fragile, almost ruptured biceps tendon may be the technical limit of this arthroscopic technique. In such a situation, the arthroscopic procedure can be easily converted to simple tenotomy alone or to open tenodesis.

PREOPERATIVE PLANNING

Patient history and clinical examination are the hallmarks for diagnosing pathology of the long head of the biceps. Patients often complain of pain in the anterior region of the shoulder, with occasional distal radiation along the anterior aspect of the upper arm. However, these symptoms are often concomitant with impingement symptoms, such as overhead and night pain. Speed's test can be helpful in the preoperative examination. Tenderness with palpation of the bicipital groove (approximately 2 cm distal to the anterolateral acromion with the arm in slight internal rotation) is very often present, with bicipital tenosynovitis, partial rupture, subluxation, and/or dislocation. Tenderness with passive external rotation of the arm, while the examiner palpates the bicipital groove, is also a common sign, as the pathological biceps is "rolled" under the examiner's fingers.

Radiographic examination should include a standard roentgenographic series (anteroposterior x-rays in neutral, internal, and external rotation, an axillary view, and a scapular Y-view/supraspinatus outlet view), to rule in or out any associated abnormalities. Osteophytes around the bicipital groove can also be identified. Specialized imaging studies—for example, magnetic resonance imaging (MRI) with gadolinium, computed tomographic (CT) arthrography, and/or ultrasound imaging—can assist in preoperatively diagnosing pathology of the biceps tendon. In particular, MRI is extremely useful in assessing both the position of the biceps tendon in the groove and the intratendinous pathology that may be present. A subluxation of the biceps, for instance, may not be visible under arthroscopy and should be anticipated with the imaging techniques. These studies can provide significant assistance in the preoperative counseling of a patient with shoulder pain.

SURGICAL TECHNIQUE

Positioning/Setup

Although the lateral decubitus position can be used, the beach chair position allows for easier control of shoulder and elbow flexion and rotation during this procedure. The patient is appropriately padded to protect neurovascular structures, and the head is positioned and secured with the assistance of the anesthesiologist. The procedure may be performed under either general anesthesia or with an interscalene block. The entire scapula and arm are prepped and draped, to allow unrestricted access to the anterior and posterior aspects of the glenohumeral joint.

The shoulder should be placed in approximately 30° of flexion, 10 to 30° of internal rotation, and 30° of abduction ("arthrodesis position"), allowing the anterior part of the subacromial bursa to be adequately filled with irrigation fluid to ensure a clear view of the superior part of the bicipital groove. The elbow is flexed to 90°, to relax tension on the biceps tendon. A classical U-shaped Trillat knee support is used with a Mayo stand to place the shoulder in the desired position. Alternatively, a sterile articulated McConnell arm holder (McConnell Orthopedics, Greenville, TX) may be used to maintain the desired arm position during anterosuperior bursoscopy.

The principle of the operation is to exteriorize the biceps tendon anteriorly, to double it on itself before the biceps tendon is inserted into a humeral socket drilled at the top of the bicipital groove, and to fix the assembly with an absorbable interference screw. The most common technique we use is the transhumeral pin technique because we feel it is easier and faster. However, an alternative technique is sometimes used, in which the biceps tendon long head is pushed, instead of being pulled, in the humeral socket.

[Although this description of the technique involves interference screw fixation, the same technique can be utilized using suture anchor fixation. If this is desired, the appropriate drills and suture anchors must be available. We have found, however, that mechanical fixation is better with an interference screw.]

Technique 1: Transhumeral Pin Technique

INSTRUMENTATION

In addition to the standard arthroscopic instrumentation (4.0 mm arthroscope, 5.5 mm sheath, standard motorized shaver, standard round 4.0 mm arthroscopic burr, arthroscopic probe, arthroscopic locking grasper), another disposable cannula is also necessary for the working instruments. A spinal needle will be required to transfix the biceps tendon after tenotomy, and a vascular clamp is extremely helpful to allow for appropriate exteriorization of the biceps tendon without damaging the tendon itself. A large nonabsorbable suture [no. 5 Ethibond, (Ethicon, of Johnson & Johnson, Norwood, MA) or no. 7 Flexidene (Braun, Germany)], and a smaller absorbable suture (usually no. 0 or 1 Vicryl, from Ethicon) are required. Special equipment also required consists of a guide pin, a cannulated sizer set, a cannulated reamer set, and a Beath (eyelet) passing pin from a standard ACL instrumentation tray. A bioabsorbable interference screw set with matching flexible guide wires and screwdriver for insertion are necessary for final fixation of the tenodesis construct. An electrocautery device with a long tip, such as a meniscal tip Bovie instrument, is helpful to maintain hemostasis. A complete set with all the instruments necessary has been developed, including a guide to make the transhumeral pin passage easier and safer (Shoulder Guide, FMS, Future Medical System, U.S.A.).

Appropriate arthroscopic suturing instruments should be available, in anticipation of encountering a repairable rotator cuff tear. An arthroscopic pump is also very useful during subacromial (especially anterosuperior) bursoscopy, but it should be maintained at a relatively low pressure (approximately 40 mmHg) to prevent excessive fluid extravasations.

SURGICAL TECHNIQUE

Bony landmarks are drawn on the shoulder to identify the spine of the scapula, the acromion, the coracoid process, and the coracoacromial ligament. This procedure requires three arthroscopic portals: the posterior portal is created 1.5 cm inferior and 1.5 cm medial to the posterolateral corner of the acromion, and two anterior portals (anteromedial and anterolateral) are created 1.5 cm on each side of the bicipital groove with the arm in neutral rotation or slight internal rotation. Alternatively, the anterolateral portal is located approximately 2 cm distal to the anterolateral corner of the acromion, along the path of the deltoid fibers. The anteromedial portal corresponds to a low anterior portal just above the intra-articular portion of the subscapularis tendon and lateral to the coracoid process (Figure 8.1). The posterior and anterolateral portals are used for the scope (viewing portals), and the anteromedial portal is used for the instruments (working portal). The surgical technique for arthroscopic biceps tenodesis with interference screw fixation requires six steps.

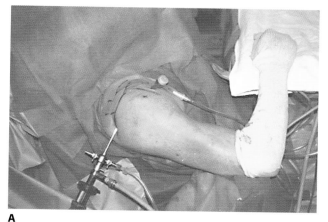

A

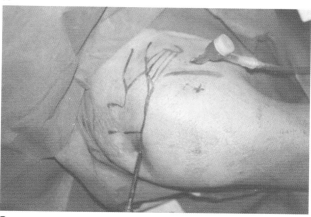

B

FIGURE 8.1. The posterior portal and the two anterior portals: anteromedial and anterolateral, on each side of the bicipital groove. (Reprinted with permission from *Techniques in Shoulder and Elbow Surgery*, Lippincott Williams & Wilkins, Philadelphia.)

STEP 1: GLENOHUMERAL EXPLORATION AND TENOTOMY OF THE LONG HEAD OF THE BICEPS

The glenohumeral joint is first explored with a standard 30° scope through the posterior portal. An anteromedial portal is established with a disposable cannula through the rotator interval, lateral to the coracoid process and the coracoacromial ligament, and just above the subscapularis tendon (Figure 8.1). The rotator cuff is assessed, and pathology of the biceps tendon is confirmed: tenosynovitis, subluxation, dislocation, hypertrophy ("hourglass biceps"), or prerupture. Biceps tendon pathology is very often found in the intertubercular groove portion, and it is important to draw this part of the biceps tendon into the joint with a probe introduced through the anteromedial portal. The long head of the biceps is intra-articularly transfixed with a spinal needle at its entrance into the groove: this will prevent it from retracting into the groove and help to identify its location during subacromial bursoscopy. The tendon is then detached

from its glenoid insertion by using either a knife, a punch, or electrocautery (Figure 8.2).

STEP 2: LOCATION AND OPENING OF THE BICIPITAL GROOVE AFTER ANTEROSUPERIOR BURSECTOMY

The scope, still in the posterior portal, is removed from the joint and reoriented under the acromion, into the subacromial bursa. The same is done for the anteromedial cannula, which is placed into the anterosuperior bursa (directed lateral to the coracoacromial ligament). The bursectomy is begun with a motorized shaver until the spinal needle is located. The anterolateral (third) portal is now created, 3 cm distal to the anterior border of the acromion and 3 cm lateral to the anteromedial portal (Figure 8.1). A space of 3 cm between the anteromedial and anterolateral portals is necessary for triangulation. The arthroscope is removed from the posterior portal and placed in the anterolateral portal. At this point, the anteromedial portal is the working portal and the anterolateral portal is the viewing portal. The remainder of the operation is performed with this configuration. (If visualization is difficult, an outflow cannula can be placed into the subacromial space through the posterior portal.) Instruments are placed in the anteromedial portal to continue the bursectomy and identify the bicipital groove. Shaving of the anterior part of the bursa is essential for visualization and is continued until the groove is located (Figure 8.3A). It is important to maintain elbow flexion during subacromial bursoscopy, to prevent dislodging of the spinal needle from the cut biceps tendon. It is also important to maintain low pump pressure (≤40 mmHg) during bursoscopy, to prevent excessive soft tissue distension.

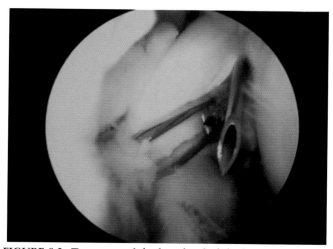

FIGURE 8.2. Tenotomy of the long head of the biceps after transfixion with a spinal needle to prevent distal retraction. (Reprinted with permission from *Techniques in Shoulder and Elbow Surgery*, Lippincott Williams & Wilkins, Philadelphia.)

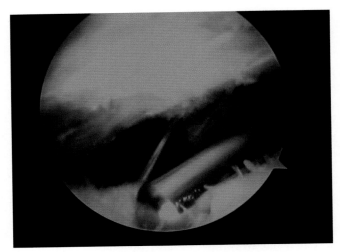

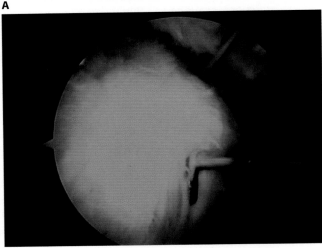

FIGURE 8.3. (A) Anterior bursectomy and location of the spinal needle. (B) Location of the bicipital groove with a probe. (Reprinted with permission from *Techniques in Shoulder and Elbow Surgery*, Lippincott Williams & Wilkins, Philadelphia.)

The rotator cuff is evaluated and, if no tear is found, its insertion into the greater tuberosity is identified. A probe is used to palpate the "soft spot" corresponding to the bicipital groove, which is usually just medial to the lateral part of the greater tuberosity. The probe can be used to feel the "roll" of the biceps tendon in its groove (Figure 8.3B). Of course, this step is facilitated in the presence of a rotator cuff tear. If a rotator cuff tear is encountered, the biceps tenodesis is performed as described, and the cuff is subsequently repaired (either arthroscopically or by a mini-open procedure).

The transverse humeral ligament is now opened in a longitudinal fashion, using an electrocautery because of the leash of vessels on either border of the groove. When the groove is open, the long head of the biceps is probed. At this point, any commercially

available arthroscopic suturing instrument can be used to place a marker suture through the biceps tendon, and the corresponding position of the suture is marked in the bicipital groove with electrocautery, both to locate the future position of the humeral socket and to guide in setting the tension in the tendon during implantation. In our experience, this marking suture is not necessary to appropriately restore biceps myotension once one becomes comfortable with this technique.

The biceps tendon is now lifted out of the groove to free possible adhesions (Figure 8.4). Again, this step is much easier when there is a large cuff tear, with the biceps being uncovered at its entrance in the superior part of the groove. However, this groove can be difficult during one's "learning curve" especially when a small cuff tear or a waterproof cuff is present, and the intra-articular portion of the biceps is covered by the capsule of the rotator interval.

STEP 3: BICEPS EXTERIORIZATION AND PREPARATION
The long head of the biceps is grasped in its groove with a forceps while the spinal needle is removed. The biceps should then be held firmly by its most proximal end with an arthroscopic grasper to facilitate exteriorization. The tendon is exteriorized through the anteromedial portal while the cannula is temporarily removed (Figure 8.5). A vascular clamp is used to grasp the tendon outside the body more distally; this will help to avoid tendon damage and also will allow tendon preparation. About 4 to 5 cm of tendon should be exteriorized, and the tendon is prepared.

A brief tenosynovectomy and trimming of the next proximal 1 cm of the tendon and 2 cm of the tendon

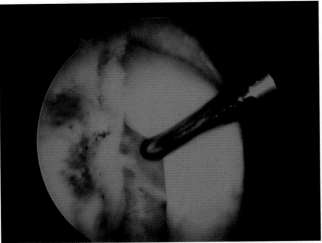

FIGURE 8.4. Lifting the tendon out of the groove to free possible adhesions. (Reprinted with permission from *Techniques in Shoulder and Elbow Surgery*, Lippincott Williams & Wilkins, Philadelphia.)

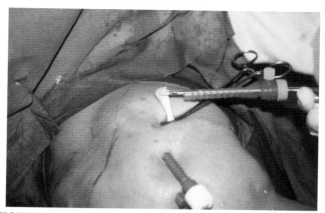

FIGURE 8.5. Tendon exteriorization (outside the arthroscopic cannula). Note the use of the vascular clamp to aid in exteriorizing 5 cm of the tendon. (Reprinted with permission from *Techniques in Shoulder and Elbow Surgery,* Lippincott Williams & Wilkins, Philadelphia.)

is doubled over a no. 5 suture. The tendon is evened, and the end of the tendon whip stitched, using a running baseball stitch with no. 0 or 1 absorbable suture. The tendon should be doubled and sewn to its anterior face for a length of about 2 cm, where a mark is made with a sterile marking pen (Figure 8.6). This mark is used to visualize that the tendon is pulled sufficiently into the humeral socket. By resecting the proximal centimeter, and doubling over a length of 2 cm, appropriate muscular tension is restored with the tenodesis technique—obviating the need for a marker suture (as indicated earlier).

[*NOTE:* If a suture anchor technique is desired, the biceps tendon can be exteriorized or just left in the groove. Two suture anchors are placed in the bicipital groove, at least 1 cm below the most proximal extent of the groove. Both pairs of sutures are also exteriorized through the anteromedial portal next to the biceps tendon. One limb of each suture is placed in the tendon with a locking stitch, at least 4 cm distal to the most proximal end of the tendon and 1 cm apart from each neighboring suture. The proximal 4 cm of the tendon is resected, just above the most superior suture. The free limb of each suture is then tensioned, and (because the sutures slide through the eyelet of the suture anchor), the biceps is delivered to the base of the bicipital groove. Locking sutures are then tied arthroscopically to complete the construct. The authors do not prefer this variation of the technique because patients may feel discomfort from the tenodesis sutures in the anterior part of the shoulder.]

The diameter of the double tendon is measured using the same type of graft sizer used in the knee for ACL reconstruction. The diameter of the double tendon should be 7 or 8 mm. If the tendon is hypertrophic, it must be trimmed by resecting some of the fibers in

a longitudinal fashion with a knife: the goal is to obtain a regular diameter on the 5 cm that has been exteriorized. The size of the double tendon determines the drill diameter needed to drill the humeral socket. The arthroscopic working cannula is reintroduced into the anteromedial portal while the biceps tendon is kept outside the wound and outside the cannula; this is facilitated by placing the no. 5 suture under tension by attaching it to the sterile drapes with a nonpenetrating clamp. To prevent incarceration of muscle fibers from the deltoid when the tendon is pulled into the bone socket, one should ensure that the cannula is introduced in the same canal as the biceps tendon.

STEP 4: DRILLING THE HUMERAL SOCKET

The bicipital groove is cleaned of all fibrous tissue with the shaver or preferably with the VAPR (Mitek, Johnson & Johnson, Norwood, MA). Care must be taken not to shave on the most lateral or medial parts of the groove because the leash of several small vessels will bleed. As with all subacromial arthroscopic work, meticulous hemostasis is essential. The socket placement is assessed with probe measurement: to prevent any anterosuperior impingement with the acromial arch; optimal placement is approximately 10 mm below the top of the groove entrance. The location of the humeral socket is identified and penetrated with a sharp-tipped pick or awl, because the bone within the groove is quite hard; this prevents skivving or sliding of the guide pin along the cortical bone of the groove when drilling.

A guide wire is then placed in the pilot hole and is oriented strictly perpendicular to the humerus and strictly parallel to the lateral border of the acromion (Figure 8.7A–C). The target is the posterior portal. The guide wire is drilled until it just penetrates the pos-

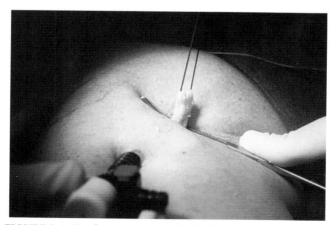

FIGURE 8.6. Tendon preparation: doubled, whip-stitched, marked, and sized. (Reprinted with permission from *Techniques in Shoulder and Elbow Surgery,* Lippincott Williams & Wilkins, Philadelphia.)

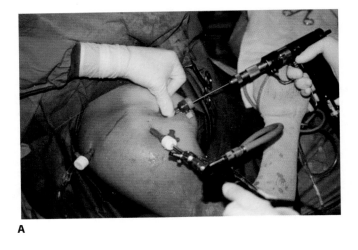

A

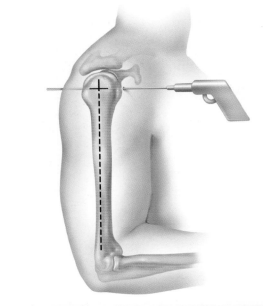

B

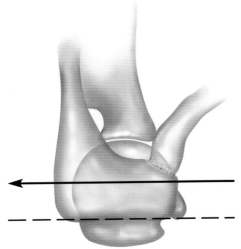

C

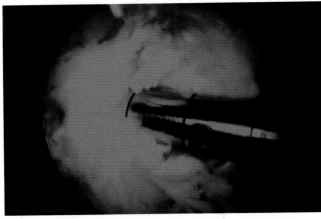

D

FIGURE 8.7. (A) Position for drilling humeral guide pin: strictly perpendicular to humeral shaft, strictly parallel to lateral border of acromion. (B) Humeral guide pin strictly perpendicular to humeral shaft. (C) Humeral guide pin strictly parallel to lateral border of acromion. (D) Reaming the humeral socket. (Reprinted with permission from *Techniques in Shoulder and Elbow Surgery*, Lippincott Williams & Wilkins, Philadelphia.)

terior cortex of the humerus. The humeral guide pin is overdrilled with a 7 or 8 mm cannulated reamer, depending on the size of the double tendon, to a depth of 25 mm (Figure 8.7D). The reamer and the guide pin are then removed. Note that all this work is done through the anteromedial (working) portal. The motorized shaver and an arthroscopic burr are placed through the same portal and into the humeral socket, to clean the socket and chamfer smooth its entrance by removing bone debris and tissues that could contribute to tendon blocking and abrasion. Particular at-

tention should be paid to the inferior part of the humeral socket, where the tendon will enter.

STEP 5: PASSING THE TRANSHUMERAL PIN
A Beath needle pull-through technique is used for tendon placement. This needle has an eyelet on its trailing end and serves as a suture passer. The Beath pin is placed through the anteromedial cannula into the humeral socket. The 7 or 8 mm reamer is used to center the Beath needle in the humeral socket and to keep the direction initially chosen. The direction of the

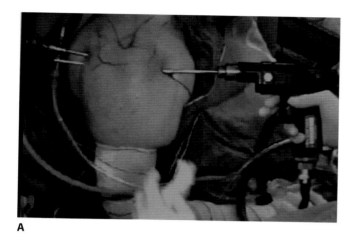

A

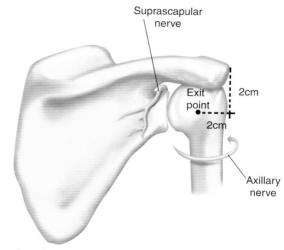

B

FIGURE 8.8. (A) Position of Beath needle: strictly perpendicular to humeral shaft, strictly parallel to lateral border of acromion, and exiting approximately 2 to 3 cm below the posterolateral corner of acromion (and 1 cm below the posterior arthroscopic portal). (B) Po- sition of Beath needle in relation to suprascapular and axillary nerve. (Reprinted with permission from *Techniques in Shoulder and El- bow Surgery,* Lippincott Williams & Wilkins, Philadelphia.)

transhumeral Beath pin is very important: it should be strictly perpendicular to the humerus and strictly parallel to the lateral border of the acromion (Figure 8.8A). The Beath pin is drilled until it exits the skin through the posterior portal (Figure 8.8B). Both ends of the no. 5 suture are threaded through the eyelet of the Beath pin, and the pin/sutures are pulled through the humerus. The suture will be used to pull the bi- ceps tendon into the humeral socket. Before the biceps tendon is pulled into the socket, a flexible guide wire for the interference screw is inserted to prevent screw divergence. To facilitate placement of this guide pin

in the socket, the anteromedial cannula is brought into direct contact with the humeral socket entrance. Once the pin is inside the socket, the biceps tendon is pulled into the humerus. The ink mark at the base of the dou- bled portion of the tendon is visualized to insert com- pletely into the humeral socket (Figure 8.9A).

STEP 6: INTERFERENCE SCREW FIXATION
The tendon is fixed in the hole by means of a bioab- sorbable interference screw, whose dimensions are 8 × 20 mm or 9 × 20 mm (Figure 8.9B). As a general rule, the screw must be 1 mm larger than the humeral

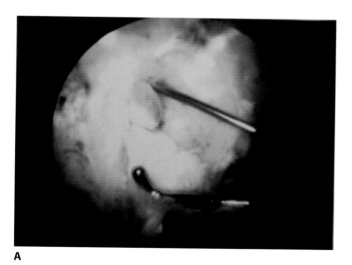

A

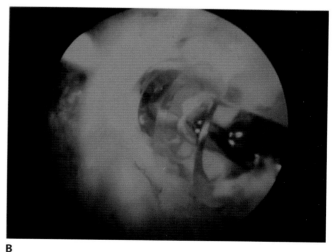

B

FIGURE 8.9. (A) Biceps tendon inserted into socket, with blue mark for depth guide. (B) Inserting the interference screw. (Reprinted with permission from *Techniques in Shoulder and Elbow Surgery,* Lippincott Williams & Wilkins, Philadelphia.)

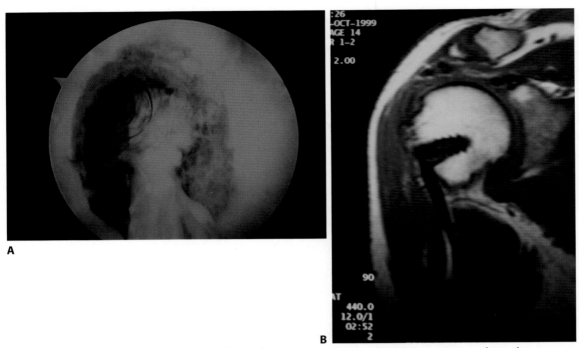

A

B

FIGURE 8.10. (A) Final biceps tenodesis construct with interference screw fixation. (B) MRI appearance of interference screw and final tenodesis. (Reprinted with permission from *Techniques in Shoulder and Elbow Surgery,* Lippincott Williams & Wilkins, Philadelphia.)

socket. An 8 × 20 mm interference screw is used for a 7 mm socket diameter and a 9 × 20 mm interference screw is used for a 8 mm socket diameter. We use a polylactic acid (PLA) screw that was designed specifically for tendon fixation with nonaggressive threads: the Tenoscrew (Physis, Tornier Inc., U.S.A.). The screw is placed on the superior aspect of the tendon while the elbow is still flexed at 90°. When the tip of the screw is engaged between the tendon and the socket wall, the tendon is stabilized by extending the elbow; this prevents twisting and rotation of the tendon during screw placement (Figure 8.10). After complete insertion of the tendon, fixation is checked

by probing the biceps tendon. After flexing and extending of the elbow, fixation of the tendon is rechecked. The transverse humeral ligament may be sutured if desired, using a suture hook, and the rotator cuff is repaired if a tear is present.

TECHNIQUE 2: NON–TRANSHUMERAL PIN TECHNIQUE

An alternative way to place the tendon in the humeral socket is to push the tendon inside the socket (instead of pulling it) by using a Fourk wire (Figure 8.11). (This device is a wire with a slot at the end in order to grasp a suture and to push the tendon in the humeral socket.)

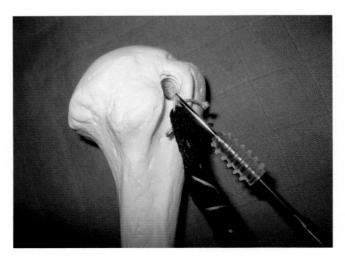

FIGURE 8.11. Alternative way to place the tendon in the humeral socket: the non–transhumeral pin technique.

POSTOPERATIVE MANAGEMENT

Full passive and active elbow flexion, extension, supination, and pronation are allowed the day of surgery, with no immobilization. In the case of isolated biceps tenodesis, complete passive and active motion is allowed for the shoulder as well. In the presence of an associated cuff repair, only passive motion of the shoulder is permitted. Elbow flexion/extension, supination, and pronation activities under stress (i.e., against resistance) are restricted for 6 weeks after the tenodesis.

RESULTS/OUTCOME

This procedure has been performed 43 times since 1997. Minimum clinical follow-up is 2 years. Mean age of the patients was 63 years (range, 25–78). Shoulder function was evaluated by means of the Constant score. The Constant score averaged 43 points (range, 13–60) preoperatively, and averaged 79 points (range, 59–87) at review. No deficit of flexion or extension of the elbow was observed in comparison to the contralateral side. Elbow flexion strength averaged 90% of the other side (range, 80–100%) measured using a spring balance. Two clinical failures of the tenodesis occurred early in the experience with this technique (see Complications section).

This is the only reported series of arthroscopic biceps tenodeses in the published literature. These preliminary (2-year follow-up) results remain encouraging. Advantages of this arthroscopic technique for biceps tenodesis using a bioabsorbable interference screw are multiple. First, after a short learning curve, it is a quick, safe, and reproducible technique. Second, this technique is less traumatic than classical open surgery and avoids violation of an intact rotator cuff if bicipital pathology must be treated in a patient without a cuff tear. Third, this is an "all-arthroscopic" technique. Fourth, interference screw fixation provides secure and strong fixation of the tenodesed biceps, allowing early mobilization of both shoulder and elbow. Fifth, bioabsorbable interference screw fixation does not interfere with MRI evaluation of the shoulder (Figure 8.10B). Finally, if necessary, this tenodesis technique can easily be performed in open surgery as well (the authors have utilized this interference screw technique in open surgery exclusively since 1996).

Doubling the biceps tendon has at least three advantages: (1) it reinforces the strength of the tendon that is not damaged by the interference screw; (2) it prevents a possible sliding of the tendon after screw insertion ("stop-block" effect); and (3) it allows an optimal tensioning of the biceps muscle, whose tension is not changed, as the intra-articular portion of the tendon is placed inside the bone (Figure 8.12).

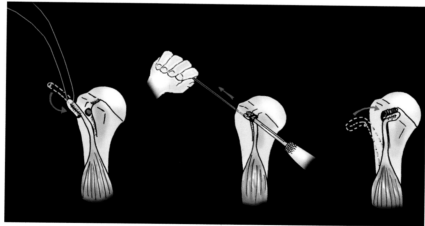

FIGURE 8.12. Advantages of doubling the biceps tendon: *left*, tendon is not damaged by interference screw; *center*, "stop-block" effect, and *right*, optimal tensioning of the biceps muscle, whose tension is not changed.

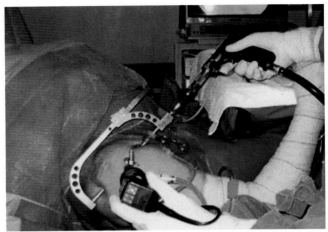

FIGURE 8.13. Shoulder guide (Future Medical Systems, U.S.A.) used to make the passage of the transhumeral pin easier and safer.

COMPLICATIONS

The shape and contour of the biceps muscle was conserved in all but 2 of 43 patients (95%). A failure of the tenodesis in these two cases was observed clinically by distal retraction of the muscle belly. Both failures occurred early in the experience with this technique, owing to technical mistakes. In both cases, the biceps tendon was thin and the interference screw diameter was insufficient (7 mm screw for a 7 mm humeral socket). One technical pitfall can occur if the biceps tendon is passed into the humeral socket without doubling the tendon on itself. If the tendon is very frail, it may tear or slide out of the bone socket. Doubling the biceps tendon reinforces the strength of the tendon and prevents any sliding of the tendon after screw insertion ("stop-block" effect). Another technical mistake is the use of an interference screw of the same diameter as the humeral socket. The screw diameter should be 1 or 2 mm larger than the socket diameter, as a rule. Owing to the habitual size of the biceps tendon, a 7 or 8 mm humeral socket is usually drilled and systematically paired with a 8 or 9 mm interference screw. Not all screws are equal: a PLA screw, with a slow resorption (to avoid inflammatory reactions and pain) should be used. We use the Tenoscrew (Physis-Torin, Inc., USA), specifically designed for this purpose, and have never observed any complications.

No neurological complications were encountered in this series. The axillary nerve is not at risk if the humeral socket is drilled strictly perpendicular to the humeral shaft and parallel to the acromion with the arm at the side. If one follows these guidelines, the transhumeral pin will exit through the posterior portal. Since the axillary nerve has been demonstrated to pass 3 to 5 cm distal to the palpable edge of the acromion, the transhumeral pin stays in the "safe zone" and does not place the nerve in jeopardy. It is important that the arm stay at the side during the transhumeral drilling of the Beath pin because abducting the shoulder to 90° has been shown to decrease the distance of the nerve to the edge of the acromion by nearly 30%. We have designed a guide to make the passage of the transhumeral pin easier and safer (Figure 8.13).

Recommended Reading

Boileau P, Walch G. A new technique for tenodesis of the long head of the biceps using bioabsorbable screw fixation. *J Shoulder Elbow Surg* 1999;8(5):557; abstr 198.

Boileau P, Krishnan SG, Coste JS, Walch G. Arthroscopic biceps tenodesis: a new technique using bioabsorbable interference screw fixation. *Tech Shoulder Elbow Surg* 2001;2(3).

Burkhead WZ, Scheinberg RR, Box G. Surgical anatomy of the axillary nerve. *J Shoulder Elbow Surg* 1992;1(10):31–36.

Constant CR, Murley AHG. A clinical method of functional assessment of the shoulder. *Clin Orthop* 1987;214:160–164.

Gartsman G, Hammerman S. Arthroscopic biceps tenodesis: operative technique. *Arthroscopy* 2000;16(5):550–552.

Goldfarb C, Yamaguchi K. The biceps tendon: dogma and controversies. In: *Sports Medicine and Arthroscopy Review.* Vol 7. Philadelphia: Lippincott Williams & Wilkins; 1999:93–103.

Habermeyer P, Mall U. Arthroscopic tenodesis of the long head of the biceps: technique and results. *J Shoulder Elbow Surg.* 1999;8(5):557; abstr 199.

Snyder SJ. Arthroscope-assisted biceps tendon surgery. In: Snyder SJ, ed. *Shoulder Arthroscopy.* New York: McGraw-Hill; 1994:61–76.

Walch G, Nove-Josserand L, Boileau P, Levigne C. Subluxations and dislocations of the tendon of the long head of the biceps. *J Shoulder Elbow Surg* 1998;7(2):100–108.

Warren RF. Lesions of the long head of the biceps tendon. *Instr Course Lect* 1985;30:204–209.

SECTION FOUR

Instability

9

Using the Suretac Technique for Arthroscopic Treatment of Anterior Instability

Carl W. Nissen and Robert A. Arciero

Arthroscopic repair has become an increasingly recognized option in treating posttraumatic anterior instability. With the development of a bioabsorbable "tack" device in the early 1990s (Suretac, Smith & Nephew Dyonics, Mansfield, MA), an alternative to the use of metallic staples or transglenoid repair became available. This simpler and more effective implant has become a mainstay for arthroscopic repair in the hands of some surgeons.

This bioabsorbable tack, which undergoes hydrolysis and resorption over a 4-week period, is inserted arthroscopically over a guide wire with a small mallet. Initial failure strength has been shown to be equivalent to that of an open suture Bankart repair.[1] Advantages of the bioabsorbable tack include elimination of metal implants in the joint and elimination of arthroscopic knot tying. Given careful patient selection, the use of this tack in arthroscopic Bankart repair can be effective in the majority of patients with unidirectional instability.

INDICATIONS/CONTRAINDICATIONS

We believe that arthroscopic anterior labral reconstruction is indicated in acute, first-time dislocators or in patients with recurrent unidirectional anterior shoulder instability unresponsive to nonoperative measures. Patient selection is critical for successful outcome and may be divided into preoperative and intraoperative criteria (Table 9.1). Contraindications include bidirectional or multidirectional instability (MDI). Although intent to return to contact sports is not an absolute contraindication, the tack should be used for discretion athletes who participate in contact or collision sports.

Further patient selection criteria include diagnostic confirmation of the Bankart lesion with good-quality tissue at the time of surgery. If the capsulo-labral tissues are degenerative or fragmented, the tack should not be used (Figure 9.1). Other contraindications include humeral avulsion of the glenohumeral ligaments (HAGL), obvious gross interstitial glenohumeral ligament damage, and glenoid deficiency. Finally, the tissue must be sufficiently mobile to be able to restore appropriate tension in the anterior ligaments.

PREOPERATIVE PLANNING

Appropriate preoperative planning focuses on careful patient selection through a thorough history, physical, and radiographic exam. History should focus on the event description, arm position, and review of any previous medical records. Physical exam should confirm unidirectional anterior instability and screen out any patients exhibiting additional laxity patterns. X-ray examination includes an axillary or Westpoint view to rule out glenoid deficiency or bony avulsion. Additional tests, such as CT or MRI, are rarely necessary.

SURGICAL TECHNIQUE

Positioning

The procedure may be performed in either the "beach chair" or the lateral decubitus position. We prefer the beach chair position, which we have found provides patient comfort, especially when regional interscalene block anesthesia is used. Patients who are anxious or who desire to be under general anesthesia are encouraged to have both regional and general anesthesia, as we have found the postoperative course to be much smoother when patients are accommodated in this manner.

TABLE 9.1. Indications for Using a Bioabsorbable Tack.
Clinical criteria
Unidirectional instability
Sulcus sign 1+ or absent
Preference for noncontact athlete
Surgeon ability
Equipment availability
Arthroscopic criteria
Presence of a Bankart lesion
Robust labral tissue
Labral repair possible with minimal tension
Ability to eliminate anteroinferior laxity, the "drive-through" sign

Instrumentation

Standard arthroscopic equipment is necessary. Cannulas of appropriate sizes must be available for the Suretac instrumentation set. We have found the use of clear cannulas to be very helpful. To use the beach chair position, an appropriate commercial positioner or table modification is needed to ensure complete access to the posterior shoulder girdle. For the decubitus position, a beanbag with or without kidney rests is necessary, as well as an overhead traction device.

Surgical Technique

After appropriate prepping and draping, which includes setting up the patient in the beach chair position and the placement of appropriate regional anesthesia, diagnostic arthroscopy is performed. The following elements are essential.

1. The diagnostic arthroscopy is begun by using a standard posterior portal.

2. The first of two anterior portals is established as a superior anterior portal through the rotator interval. Externally, this portal is just anterior to the anterior edge of the acromion and can be established by inserting a spinal needle "outside in." Arthroscopically, the portal is seen to enter the joint just below the biceps tendon.

3. A second anterior portal is established immediately above the intra-articular portion of the subscapularis tendon, using an "outside-in" approach with an 18-gauge needle. This needle ensures the proper angle of approach to the glenoid to facilitate subsequent drilling (Figure 9.2).

4. A thorough diagnostic arthroscopy is performed. Specific emphasis is placed on accurately visualizing and understanding the Bankart lesion, Hill–Sachs pathology, and the degree of associated capsular patholaxity. In addition, we examine for a possible HAGL lesion, superior labrum anterior and posterior (SLAP) pathology, and injury to the rotator cuff.

5. The labrum is elevated from the glenoid down to the 6 o'clock position. Visualization of the subscapularis tendon (between the labrum and anterior glenoid neck) confirms satisfactory elevation. This is best seen through the ASP (anterosuperior portal).

6. The inferior glenohumeral ligament is mobilized, ensuring that it can be translated superiorly with either a grasping forceps or a suture through the superior anterior portal.

7. The glenoid neck is debrided down to bleeding bone.

8. The guide wire is placed within the drill bit such that it is about 3 mm proud and is locked into position (Figure 9.3A). The guide wire–drill assembly is

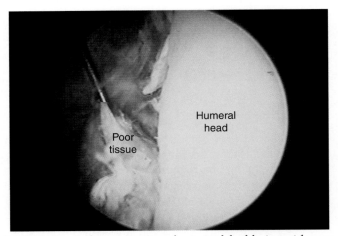

FIGURE 9.1. Arthroscopic view of anterior labral lesion with poor tissue quality. (View from posterior portal, beach chair position, left shoulder.)

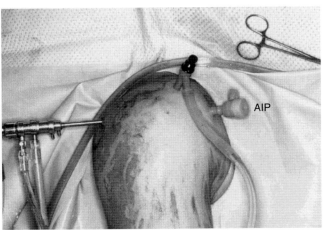

FIGURE 9.2. Patient in the beach chair position with camera and portals in place (right shoulder): AIP, anterior interior portal.

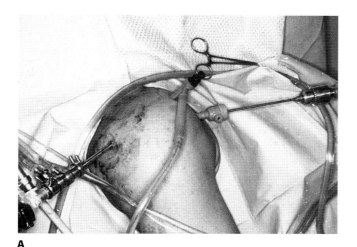

A

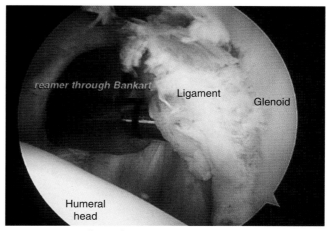

FIGURE 9.4. Drilling of reamer over the guide wire, through the anterior capsular tissue. (View from posterior left shoulder, beach chair position.)

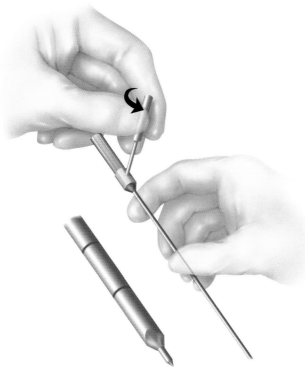

B

FIGURE 9.3. (A) Setup as seen externally with reamer and guide wire assembled for drilling (right shoulder). Initially, piercing of the anterior labral and ligamentous structures should be done with the guide wire extended approximately 3 mm proud of the reamer. (B) Diagramatic representation of guide wire extended 3 mm beyond reamer tip.

sufficient "bite" of labrum has been taken, avoiding inadvertent tissue amputation by the larger diameter drill, and that the drill is properly angled into the glenoid, avoiding "skiving" under the articular cartilage. If the drill is not angled into the glenoid, but is instead parallel to its face, the cartilage may be "burrowed" up off the subchondral bone.

10. Before disengagement from the drill, the guide wire should be tapped to ensure that it is securely engaged in the glenoid. The drill is then removed by hand. Manual pressure on the guide pin externally will prevent inadvertent removal with the drill (Figure 9.5).

11. The bioabsorbable tack is then introduced over the guide wire and impacted by mallet through the labrum

then introduced through the inferior anterior portal and pierces the labrum at the appropriate position for the first drill tack (Figure 9.3B). For a right shoulder, this is about 4 o'clock, in a left, 8 o'clock.

9. The guide wire engages the articular margin and the guide wire–drill assembly is advanced into the glenoid (Figure 9.4). Care must be taken to ensure that a

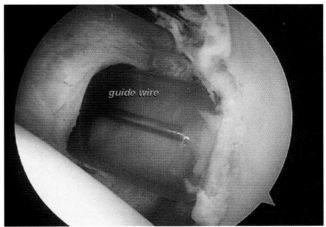

FIGURE 9.5. The reamer is loosened from the guide wire and backed out, leaving the wire in place. (View from posterior, left shoulder, beach chair position.)

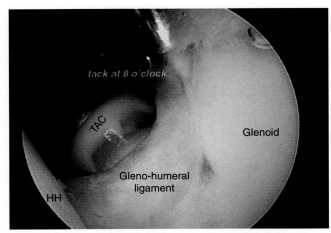

FIGURE 9.6. Tack is impacted over guide wire. (View from posterior, left shoulder, beach chair position.): HH, humeral head.

and into the bone, taking care not to drive the tack through the labral tissue. (Figure 9.6).

12. Additional tacks (usually a total of two or three) at 3 and 2 o'clock (right shoulder) and 9 and 10 o'clock, respectively (left shoulder), are then placed, depending upon ligament/labrum appearance. Placement below the 8 o'clock (left) or 4 o'clock (right) position is usually difficult, even when the inferior anterior portal is used.

POSTOPERATIVE MANAGEMENT

Postoperatively, a shoulder immobilizer is worn for 4 weeks. The device is removed only for personal care and elbow, wrist, and finger range-of-motion exercises. Efforts to restore normal motion begin at 4 weeks with pendulum and active-assistive exercises. Strengthening exercises are initiated at 6 weeks postoperatively. Active overhead motion is permitted at 3 to 4 months, assuming full range of motion and arm control strength have been achieved. Pitching and/or repetitive overhead motion and contact/collision sports are permitted at 6 months after surgery.

RESULTS/OUTCOME

Overall results with the Suretac device have been very good. Our initial review demonstrated 86% good to excellent results, with four of five recurrences occurring after a traumatic episode.[2] Motion was preserved, with only 6% of patients losing more than 10° of external rotation. Athletes involved in contact sports tended to do less well than those in a noncontact sport, but this trend was not statistically significant. A pre-

operative sulcus sign of 1+ or more was associated with a greater chance of postoperative failure as well. These results have remained durable at greater than a 5-year follow-up.[3]

Warner and Warren[4,5] reported a 10% failure rate in a group of 20 patients at 2-year follow-up. Speer et al.[6] reported a 21% redislocation rate in a group of 52 patients at 2- to 5-year follow-up. These data suggest that arthroscopic repair with the bioabsorbable tack is an effective alternative in treating the Bankart lesion. Treating capsular laxity at the time of arthroscopy, either by capsular plication or by thermal modification of the capsule, may be necessary to improve results. A current randomized trial at our institution may help answer this question.

COMPLICATIONS

Complications are infrequent but include nerve injury, motion restriction, synovitis, and failure. Suprascapular nerve injury can occur if the glenoid neck is penetrated posteriorly with the drill or guide wire. Motion problems, especially the loss of external rotation, are relatively uncommon. The difficulty in addressing associated capsular patholaxity with this device, however, may either limit the effectiveness of the technique or require adjunct technology, such as suture or thermal techniques, to address capsular laxity. Excessive tension on the repair construct can also lead to device failure due to "unbuttoning" of the head, which can "pop off" if implant hydrolysis occurs prior to tissue healing.

The most common complication associated with this device is recurrent instability. Although the importance of careful patient selection cannot be overemphasized, causes of such instability are multifactorial: the Suretac device may be placed improperly on the glenoid neck; there may be failure to advance the capsule superiorly; and a bleeding bony bed may not have been created on the glenoid neck. The Suretac, like other fastening systems including suture anchors, can fail to deploy or hold with sufficient strength. This eventuality must be assessed intraoperatively and corrected if necessary. Bioabsorbable implants have been reported to cause inflammatory syndromes,[7,8] although we have not observed this complication. Failure to place the implant inferiorly enough may also jeopardize the success of repair, a limitation in many arthroscopic systems, though perhaps more pronouncedly with the Surtac, given the difficulties in placement of a large enough cannula as inferior as possible relative to the subscapularis tendon.

References:

1. McEleney E, Donovan M, et al. Initial failure strength of open and arthroscopic Bankart repairs. *Arthroscopy* 1995;11(4):426–431.
2. Nissen C, Shea K, et al. Treatment of shoulder instability with a bioabsorbable, arthroscopically placed tack. Paper presented at: Specialty Day of the American Orthopaedic Society for Sports Medicine; Atlanta.
3. Nissen C. Five year follow-up on anteriorly unstable shoulders treated with Suretac device. *Unpublished;* 2000.
4. Warner J, and Warren R. Arthroscopic Bankart repair using a cannulated, absorbable device. *Op Tech Orthop* 1991;1:192–198.
5. Warner J, Pagnani M, et al. Absorbable Bankart repair utilizing a cannulated absorbable fixation device. *Orthop Trans* 1991;15:761.
6. Speer K, Pagnani M, et al. Arthroscopic Bankart with the Suretack device: a 3–5 year follow-up. Paper presented at: Annual Meeting of the American Association of Orthopaedic Surgeons; New Orleans.
7. Edwards D, Hoy G, et al. Adverse reaction to an absorbable shoulder fixation device. *J Shoulder Elbow Surg* 1994;3:230–233.
8. Cheng J, Wolf E, et al. Pigmented villonodular synovitis of the shoulder after anterior capsulolabral reconstruction. *Arthroscopy* 1997;13:257–261.

Recommended Reading

Arciero R, Taylor D, et al. Arthroscopic bioabsorbable tack stabilizations of initial anterior shoulder dislocations: a preliminary report. *Arthroscopy* 1995;11:410–417.

Arciero R, Wheeler J, et al. Arthroscopic Bankart repair versus non-operative treatment for acute, initial, anterior shoulder dislocations. *Am J Sports Med* 1994;22:589–594.

10

Arthroscopic Anterior Capsulolabral Shoulder Stabilization Using the Suture Anchor Technique

Richard G. Levine, Sandra J. Iannotti, and Leslie S. Matthews

Multiple techniques have been proposed for arthroscopic repair of the unstable shoulder, including the use of staples, transglenoid passage of sutures, biodegradable tacks, and suture anchors.[1–8] Reports on the use of staples to reattach the labrum have had poor results, with high recurrence rates, an average loss of 9° of external rotation,[2] staple loosening, migration, and impingement on the articular surface.[9,10] Transglenoid techniques have lower reported redislocation rates but are technically difficult and pose a risk of damaging the suprascapular nerve.[11] The use of biodegradable tacks in arthroscopic instability repair is becoming more common; however, a reabsorption synovitis rate of 6% has been reported.[12] Additional disadvantages caused by single-point fixation include difficulty with poor-quality ligamentous tissue, and ineffectiveness in tightening capsular redundancy.[13]

Suture anchors offer an alternative method for the repair of glenohumeral instability.[14,15] They are commonly used in open shoulder surgery in both rotator cuff repair and biceps tenodesis, and were described for open Bankart reconstruction in 1991.[16] Cadaveric study of suture anchors has demonstrated significantly decreased failure rates compared with transosseous bone tunnels in rotator cuff repairs[17] and a statistically superior load to failure for a suture anchor versus a staple and a bioabsorbable tack.[18] Suture anchor constructs most often fail by suture breakage as opposed to pullout from bone.[18] However, most reports have shown that arthroscopic techniques have had higher redislocation and resubluxation rates[2,12,19–23] than are found following open Bankart repair, with reported recurrent instability of 0 to 5%.[24–26]

INDICATIONS

The suture anchor technique is indicated in patients with symptomatic anterior shoulder instability and a capsulolabral avulsion from the anterior-inferior rim of the glenoid—the Bankart lesion. Ideal candidates (for both open and arthroscopic repair) are patients with an initial traumatic event whose instability is clearly anterior, unidirectional, and involuntary. These patients usually have a discrete Bankart lesion.[27] Patients with atraumatic multidirectional instability are less likely to have a discrete labral injury. Additionally, patients with recurrent instability, especially with a component of posterior or inferior laxity, may have an element of capsular redundancy in addition to the structural labral lesion. This capsular laxity, if present, should be addressed because it may contribute to failed isolated anterior labral repairs.[12,23]

Arthroscopic techniques may be preferred in patients in whom the morbidity of an open repair is undesirable and in patients who wish to preserve the maximal amount of external rotation (especially throwing athletes). Ideal candidates may be noncontact athletes with a discrete Bankart lesion and a substantial labrum that is not degenerative (Figure 10.1). Conversely, patients who regard stability as their highest priority are more likely candidates for open anterior capsulolabral repair. Contraindications to arthroscopic Bankart repair include the absence of the Bankart lesion and surgeon inexperience with arthroscopic techniques. Some surgeons have shown higher failure rates with a degenerated labrum and stretched capsule.[23,28] Contact athletes may benefit from open stabilization. Additionally, concurrent pathology, such as capsular laxity and a large Hill–Sachs lesion,

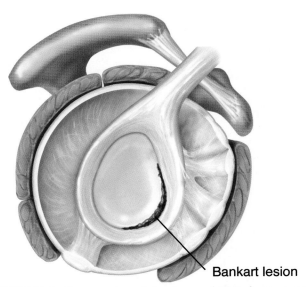

FIGURE 10.1. Cutaway view of glenohumeral joint, demonstrating detachment of anterior inferior glenohumeral ligament–labrum complex from glenoid rim, usually from approximately 3 to 6 o'clock on a clock face.

a bony Bankart lesion, and global ligamentous laxity, may justify open anterior stabilization.

There is increasing consensus that the ideal patient for arthroscopic repair of the anterior-inferior capsulolabral complex is the young active patient with a first-time traumatic anterior dislocation. This patient population has been shown to have an extremely high redislocation rate with conservative treatment, and studies have shown that arthroscopic stabilization following the acute dislocation dramatically reduces the incidence of recurrent instability.[29] Arthroscopic repair following first-time dislocation may be more effective because it prevents the capsular redundancy and labral degeneration associated with repeated instability events, and thus has a better success rate than chronic repair; however, this remains unproven. Additionally, preliminary data show that acute arthroscopic stabilization may afford a better quality of life than conservative treatment.[30]

PREOPERATIVE PLANNING

Although often straightforward, the diagnosis of shoulder instability can be difficult. A careful history is essential, and it must be combined with a thorough physical exam and radiographic evaluation. A search for glenoid fractures and Hill–Sachs lesions with appropriate radiographic views may influence surgical decision making. For labral avulsions, sensitivity to

magnetic resonance imaging is dramatically increased when intra-articular contrast is used.[31]

POSITIONING/SETUP

Prior to patient positioning, an examination under anesthesia for instability is performed, and the results are compared to the unaffected shoulder. The patient is then placed in the lateral decubitus position on a beanbag for support, with care to pad the peroneal nerve and lateral malleolus of the downside extremity. A pillow is placed between the patient's knees and legs for additional padding, and the hips and knees are flexed to assist with patient balance and stability. Foam and adhesive tape are used to hold the affected arm in an overhead shoulder positioner with 7 to 10 lb of skin traction. The tape is cut into small strips and applied noncircumferentially to the arm. Several shoulder positioners are commercially available. The addition of a lateral traction strap can be helpful for visualization of the anterior shoulder structures[32] (Figure 10.2). The arm is held in approximately 70° of abduction and 15° of forward flexion. Internal rotation can be helpful to relax the anterior structures and increase the working space available. The patient is rotated slightly toward his or her back to allow unobstructed use of instruments through the anterior portal. A watertight impervious drape is placed on the upper chest, neck, and back to prevent fluid from leaking onto the patient's head or into the ear during the procedure. The table is then rotated 45° to allow circumferential access to the shoulder, with the anesthesiologist located opposite the operative surgeon at the level of the patient's abdomen. The shoulder is then prepared and draped in a sterile fashion. A fluid collection drape with suction attachments is useful to minimize saline spillage.

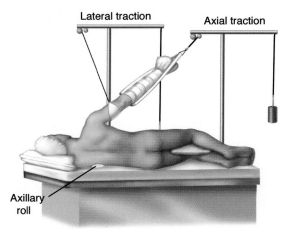

FIGURE 10.2. Schematic illustration of patient in lateral position with use of shoulder holder with lateral traction strap.

INSTRUMENTATION

Standard shoulder arthroscopy equipment is used for this procedure. The following technique utilizes the 30°, 4.0 mm arthroscope for the entire procedure; however the 70° arthroscope can be of assistance in visualization of the anterior structures, and should be available. The use of a fluid pump is helpful to maintain adequate pressure for visualization without causing excessive fluid extravasation. Arthroscopic instrument cannulas 10 mm in diameter are used for anchor placement and suture management. Threaded and lucent cannulas with rubber dams for flow control are essential. Anchors with pullout strengths greater than the suture strength and eyelets that allow for the suture to slide should be chosen. We currently use the 3.5 mm OBL suture anchors, each loaded with two no. 2 braided nonabsorbable sutures (OBL, Smith–Nephew Dyonics). Bioabsorbable anchors that remain functional for greater than 6 months are available, but there have been reports of reactive synovitis with implant failure.[13,33] A variety of commercially available suture passers may be used to transport the sutures through the capsule/labral tissue, though we prefer those made by OBL. Finally, a slotted or closed knot pusher and an arthroscopic periosteal elevator will also be needed.

SURGICAL TECHNIQUE

A diagnostic arthroscopy of the glenohumeral joint is performed through a standard posterior shoulder portal made approximately 3 cm below and 1 cm medial to the posterolateral border of the acromion. Associated pathology is addressed as indicated. Twin anterior portals are then established (Figure 10.3). An anterior superior portal (ASP) is made using an "outside-in" technique, with spinal needle localization midway between the coracoacromial ligament and the base of the coracoid process, entering the joint at the superior end of the biceps tendon to allow space for a second anterior portal to be placed inferiorly. Confirmation and examination of the anterior labral lesion is performed with the use of a probe (Figure 10.4). An anterior inferior portal (AIP) is made lateral to the coracoid, entering the joint just superior to the subscapularis tendon via an "outside-in" technique with spinal needle localization. Several authors prefer to perform this step using an "inside out" technique with a Wissinger rod. Either method is acceptable. It is important to assess the ability of the spinal needle to reach the 5:30 position on the glenoid rim prior to making this portal (Figure 10.5A). Attention must be placed on ensuring a sufficiently lateral AIP placement to facilitate glenoid targeting (Figure 10.5B). With the

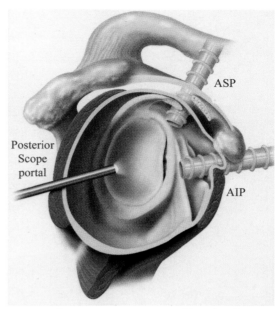

FIGURE 10.3. The anterior superior portal (ASP) and anterior inferior portal (AIP) used during anterior arthroscopic stabilization. The scope is in the posterior portal.

use of a switching stick the arthroscope is then placed in the anterior superior portal for visualization of the inferior glenoid. Care must be taken to ensure that the anterior portals are sufficiently separated externally to avoid "instrument crowding."

With the arthroscope in the posterior scope portal and 7 to 10 lb of traction applied through the lateral traction strap, the anterior labrum is freed from its scarred position on the glenoid neck or rim with a periosteal elevator through the ASP (Figure 10.6). The glenoid rim is then abraded with a burr, an aggressive shaver, or a rasp. Anchors are placed through the AIP

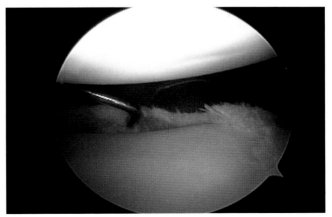

FIGURE 10.4. Arthroscopic photograph (right shoulder, lateral decubitus position, viewing from posterior portal) of a probe from the ASP palpating the detached anterior inferior glenohumeral ligament (Bankart lesion).

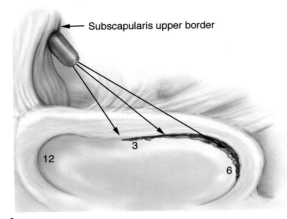

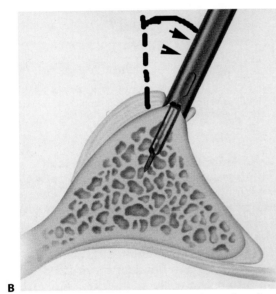

FIGURE 10.5. The AIP must be positioned as inferiorly as possible, immediately above the subscapularis tendon's upper border, to permit inferior targeting of the glenoid's 5 o'clock position (A). Failure to place the portal sufficiently inferiorly can lead to difficulty placing anchors below 4 o'clock. (B) The portal must also be positioned sufficiently laterally such that it has appropriate "angle of attack" to avoid "skiving" off the glenoid.

cannula using standard technique with pre-drilling. Optimal anchor location is on the glenoid rim at the edge of the articular surface. The holes must be made at the anterior border of the cartilaginous surface, not medially on the scapular neck, to allow the repaired inferior glenohumeral ligament labral complex to function as a buttress anteriorly (Figure 10.7). To avoid damaging the articular surface, the position of the drill bit should angle approximately 15 to 20° medially to the plane of the glenoid. Three anchors in total are usually adequate for repair and should be evenly distributed from about the 5:30 to the 3:00 position (right shoulder), with the most inferior anchor placed first. Each anchor is placed, tensioned, passed through tissue and then tied.

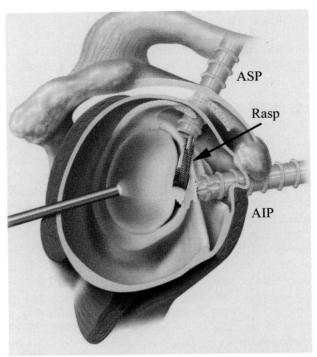

FIGURE 10.6. With 7 to 10 lb of traction applied through the lateral traction strap, the anterior labrum is freed from its scarred position on the glenoid neck or rim with a periosteal elevator introduced through the ASP: ASP, anterior superior portal; AIP, anterior inferior portal.

After each anchor placement, confirmation of anchor stability is obtained by pulling firmly on the corresponding sutures. It is important to assess the ability of the suture to slide through the anchor eyelet to permit the use of a sliding knot technique. The surgeon must be familiar with the anchor used, so that it is op-

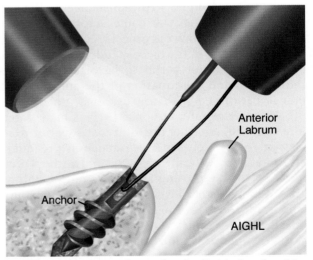

FIGURE 10.7. The first anchor is placed at 5 o'clock and positioned on the articular margin: AIGHL, anterior inferior glenohumeral ligament.

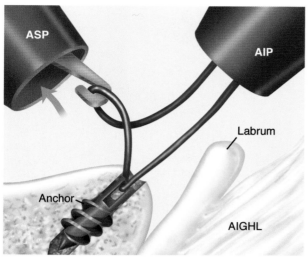

FIGURE 10.8. Following anchor placement, the suture limb to be passed through the labrum is retrieved from the ASP. AIGHL, anterior inferior glenohumeral ligament: ASP, anterior superior portal; AIP, anterior inferior portal.

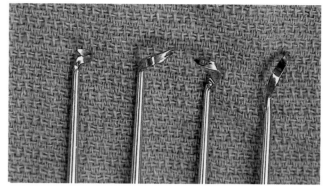

FIGURE 10.10. The OBL suturing device.

timally oriented in line with the intended direction of the suture pull. After anchor placement, the arthroscope is then switched back to the posterior portal.

Alternatively, one can insert anchors while visualizing from the posterior portal. The suture limb to be passed through the capsule and labrum is then retrieved through the ASP (Figure 10.8). When retrieving this suture, care must be taken to avoid anchor "unloading" by viewing the suture at the level of the anchor eyelet.

The second limb of the suture remains clamped outside the AIP. Next, the limb passed out the ASP is shuttled retrograde back through the capsule and labrum. The suturing device should exit near the location of the anchor. The volume and position of the anterior capsule and inferior glenohumoral ligament grasped with the suture should be dictated by the degree of laxity noted in the anterior structures. This maneuver determines the amount of capsular shift performed.

A variety of instruments are available for soft tissue arthroscopic suturing. We prefer to use the DBL suture passer (Figures 10.9, 10.10). This two-step approach can be simplified to a one-step process if using a device which penetrates the labrum capsule and grasps the suture limb. Such an approach is occasionally easier. However, in general, suture passage independent of the anchor suture limb is less technically demanding and causes less disturbance to the capsu-

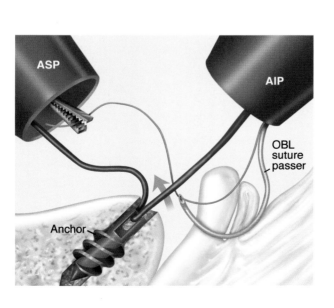

FIGURE 10.9. The suture-passing device has been placed through the AIP and a suture shuttle passed through the labrum. A grasping instrument is used to retrieve the suture shuttle through the ASP, which then permits retrograde shuttling of the anchor suture limb back through the labrum and out the AIP. ASP, anterior superior portal; AIP, anterior inferior portal.

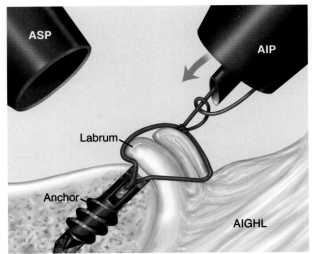

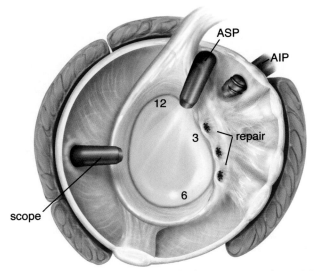

FIGURE 10.11. Both limbs are brought out the AIP, and a sliding knot technique is used to tie the sutures. Note the restoration of the normal labrum–AIGHL buttress against the glenoid margin: ASP, anterior superior portal; AIP, anterior inferior portal; AIGHL, anterior inferior glenohumeral ligament.

FIGURE 10.12. The final repair, with three suture anchors: ASP, anterior superior portal; AIP, anterior inferior portal.

lolabral tissues. Both suture ends are then retrieved through a single anterior cannula, and a knot is tied (Figure 10.11). To remove any twists in the sutures, the knot pusher should be passed down the cannula over the sutures before tying. The suture strand fur-

thest away from the articular margin should be used as the post for knot tying to avoid knot interposition between the tissue and glenoid surface.[34] Many techniques have been reported for tying knots, most of which are acceptable. We prefer the Duncan loop

TABLE 10.1. Results/Outcome Summary of Arthroscopic Suture Anchor Stabilization.

Study	Patients	Patient Age (mean years), average [range]	Mean follow-up (months) [range]	Recurrence rate (%)	Loss of external rotation (°)	Comments
Field et al. (1999)[a]	50	—	33 [24–40]	8	None	Comparison to open with recurrence 0%
Bacilla et al. (1997)[b]	40	18 [16–27]	30 [18–36]	7.5	—	High-risk athletes; 29 of 32 returned to organized sports
Koss et al. (1997)[c]	27	29 [17–44]	40 [26–64]	30	1	90% failures from traumatic events–authors recommend against arthroscopic stabilization in contact athletes; higher failures with > 5 preop dislocations
Hoffman and Reif (2000)[d]	30	26 [16–51]	24 [12–36]	12	5° in 19%; 10° in 30%	Worse results with > 10 preop dislocations
Belzer and Snyder (1995)[e]	37	—	22 [—]	11	5° avg (0–30°)	Additional 13% with mild apprehension
Weber (1996)[f]	40	—	24 minimum	8	"Better than open"	Comparison study to open; arthroscopic repair 3 times more likely to return to throwing sports

[a]Ref. 25.

[b]Ref. 1.

[c]Ref. 22.

[d]Hoffman F, Reif G. Arthroscopic shoulder stabilization using Mitek anchors. *Knee Surg Sports Traumatol Arthrosc* 1995;11:50–54.

[e]Ref. 20.

[f]Weber SC. Arthroscopic suture anchor repair versus open Bankart repair in the management of traumatic anterior glenohumeral instability [abstract]. *Arthroscopy* 1996;12(3):382.

method, which allows for a sliding knot to ensure knot security. Posterior pressure placed on the humeral head by an assistant may be helpful while securing the knot.[5] The preceding steps are then repeated for the remaining two anchors, proceeding from inferiorly to superiorly (Figure 10.12).

POSTOPERATIVE MANAGEMENT

Patients are discharged home in a shoulder immobilizer on the day of the operation. They are instructed to remove the dressings and apply bandaids after 48 h. The immobilizer is worn at all times for the first 10 days except when removed to permit elbow and wrist motion several times a day. At 10 days postoperatively they are seen in the clinic for suture removal and wound check. They are started on gentle pendulum exercises. At this visit we counsel patients on the importance of activity restriction. Patients are often relatively pain free and may inadvertently risk the healing anterior structures if overly active. Physical therapy with active assisted range of motion is started at 6 weeks postoperatively, progressing to a strengthening program by 3 months. Contact activities and heavy lifting are allowed at 6 months postoperatively.

RESULTS/OUTCOME

Table 10.1 shows the results and outcome summary of arthroscopic suture anchor stabilization.

COMPLICATIONS

Issues of migration and loosening make the use of metallic implants a concern, and we currently use absorbable implants. Intraoperative complications inherent with all suture anchors include suture breakage, suture pullout from the anchor, knot tying difficulties, knot abrasion of the articular surface, and knot interposition between the labrum and the glenoid.

References

1. Bacilla R, Field LD, Savoie FH. Arthroscopic Bankart repair in a high demand patient population. *Arthroscopy* 1997;13(1):51–60.
2. Matthews LS, Vetter WL, Oweida SJ, Spearman J, Helfet DL. Arthroscopic staple capsulorrhaphy for recurrent anterior shoulder instability. *Arthroscopy* 1988;4(2): 106–111.
3. McIntyre LF, Caspari RB, Savoie FH. The arthroscopic treatment of anterior and multidirectional shoulder instability. *Instr Course Lect* 1996;45:46–56.
4. Rose DJ. Arthroscopic transglenoid suture capsulorrhaphy for anterior shoulder instability. *Inst Course Lect.* 1996;45:57–64.
5. Higgins LD, Warner JJP. Arthroscopic Bankart repair. Operative technique and surgical pitfalls. *Clin Sports Med* 2000;19(1):49–62.
6. Grana WA, Buckley PD, Yates CK. Arthroscopic Bankart suture repair. *Am J Sports Med* 1993;21(3):348–353.
7. Nelson BJ, Arciero RA. Arthroscopic management of glenohumeral instability. *Am J Sports Med* 2000;28(4): 602–614.
8. Warner JJP, Warren RF Arthroscopic Bankart repair using a cannulated, absorbable, fixation device. *Oper Tech Orthop* 1991;1:192–198.
9. Karr TC, Schenck RC Jr, Wirth MA, Rockwood CA. Complications of metallic suture anchors in shoulder surgery: A report of 8 cases. *Arthroscopy* 2001;17(1):31–37.
10. Zuckerman JD, Matsen FA. Complications about the glenohumeral joint related to the use of screws and staples. *J Bone Joint Surg Am* 1984;66:175–180.
12. Cole BJ, Warner JJP. Arthroscopic versus open Bankart repair for traumatic anterior shoulder instability. *Clin Sports Med* 2000;19(1):19–48.
13. Edwards DJ, Hoy G, Saies A, et al. Adverse reactions to an absorbable shoulder fixation device. *J Shoulder Elbow Surg* 1994;3:230–33.
14. Wolf E. Arthroscopic capsulolabral repair using suture anchors. *Orthop Clin North Am* 1993;24:59–69.
15. Wolf EM, Wilk RM, Richmond JR. Arthroscopic Bankart repair using suture anchors. *Oper Tech Orthop* 1991;1(2):184–191.
16. Richmond JC, Donaldson WR, Fu F, Harner CD. Modification of the Bankart reconstruction with a suture anchor. Report of a new technique. *Am J Sports Med* 1991;19(4):343–346.
17. Burkhart SS, Diaz Pagan JL, Wirth MA, Athanasiou KA. Cyclic loading of anchor-based rotator cuff repairs: confirmation of the tension overload phenomenon and comparison of suture anchor fixation with transosseous fixation. *Arthroscopy* 1997;13(6):720–724.
18. Shall LM, Cawley PW. Soft tissue reconstruction in the shoulder: comparison of suture anchors, absorbable staples, and absorbable tacks. *Am J Sports Med* 1994;22(5): 715–718.
19. Sperber A, Hamberg P, Karlsson J, Sward L, Wredmark T. Comparison of an arthroscopic and an open procedure for posttraumatic instability of the shoulder: a prospective, randomized multicenter study. *J Shoulder Elbow Surg* 2001;10(2):105–108.
20. Belzer JP, Snyder SJ. Arthroscopic capsulorrhaphy for traumatic anterior shoulder instability using suture anchors and nonabsorbable suture [abstract]. *Arthroscopy* 1995;11:359.
21. Guanche C, Quick D, Sodergren K, et al. Arthroscopic versus open reconstruction of the shoulder with isolated Bankart lesions. *Am J Sports Med* 1996;24:144–148.

22. Koss S, Richmond JR, Woodward JS. Two-to five-year followup of arthroscopic Bankart reconstruction using a suture anchor technique. *Am J Sports Med* 1997;25(6): 809–812.

23. Horms HJ, Laprell HG. Developments in Bankart repair for treatment of anterior instability of the shoulder. *Knee Surg Sports Traumatol Arthrosc* 1996;12:228–231.

24. Rowe CR, Patel D, Southmayd WW. The Bankart procedure: a long-term end-result study. *J Bone Joint Surg Am* 1978;60:1–16.

25. Field LD, Savoie FH, Griffith P. A comparison of open and arthroscopic Bankart repair [abstract]. *J Shoulder Elbow Surg* 1999;8:195.

26. Hoveluis L, Thorling J, Fredin H. Recurrent anterior dislocation of the shoulder: results after the Bankart and Putti–Platt operations. *J Bone Joint Surg Am* 1979;61: 566–569.

27. Rowe CR. Acute and recurrent anterior dislocations of the shoulder. *Orthop Clin North Am* 1980;11:253–270.

28. Kandziora F, Jager A, Bischof F, Herresthal J, Starker M, Mittlmeier T. Arthroscopic labrum refixation for post traumatic anterior shoulder instability: suture anchor versus transglenoid fixation technique. *Arthroscopy* 2000;16(4):359–366.

29. Arciero RA, Wheeler JH, Ryan JB, and McBride JT. Arthroscopic Bankart repair versus nonoperative treatment for acute, initial anterior shoulder dislocations. *Am J Sports Med* 1994;22(5):591–594.

30. Kirkley A, Griffin S, Richards C, Miniaci A, Mohtadi N. Prospective randomized clinical trial comparing the effectiveness of immediate arthroscopic stabilization versus immobilization and rehabilitation in first traumatic anterior dislocations of the shoulder. *Arthroscopy* 1999;15(5):507–514.

31. Iannotti J, Zlatkin M, Esterhai J, et al. Magnetic resonance imaging of the shoulder. Sensitivity, specificity, and predictive value. *J Bone Joint Surg Am* 1991;73:17–29.

32. Snyder SJ, Banas MP, Belzer JP. Arthroscopic treatment of anterior shoulder instability using threaded suture anchors and nonabsorbable suture. *Instr Course Lect* 1996;45:71–81.

33. Bukhart A, Imhoff AB, Roscher E. Foreign-body reaction to the bioabsorbable Suretac device. *Arthroscopy* 2000;16(1):19–25.

34. De Beer JF. Arthroscopic Bankart repair: some aspects of suture and knot management. *Arthroscopy* 1999; 15(6):660–662.

Recommended Reading

Barber FA, Click SD, Weideman CA. Arthroscopic or open Bankart procedures: what are the costs? *Arthroscopy* 1998;14(7):671–674.

Cole BJ, Warner JJP. Arthroscopic versus open Bankart repair for traumatic anterior shoulder instability. *Clin Sports Med* 2000;19(1):19–48.

Instructional Course Lectures, Vol. 45: Sec II (Shoulder); 1996.

Arthroscopic Treatment of Posterior Instability

Jeffrey S. Abrams

Posterior glenohumeral instability is a relatively uncommon problem in comparison to anterior instability. Yet it remains an important condition that is arthroscopically treatable. Posterior instability can be unidirectional, or it may be the predominant symptomatic direction of multidirectional instability. Unidirectional posterior instability is more often the result of trauma. Conversely, multidirectional instability may include a posterior and inferior component and is more often due to repetitive overuse, such as in repetitive overhead athletics, or associated with generalized laxity.

Arthroscopic reconstruction not only offers the opportunity to repair the posterior labral and capsular pathology but also addresses anterior, inferior, or superior pathology.

INDICATIONS/CONTRAINDICATIONS

Patients considered for surgery should have completed an organized rehabilitative program. Included in the nonoperative approach are scapular stabilization and external rotator cuff strengthening.

Involuntary subluxators who fail nonoperative treatment are candidates for arthroscopic repair. There are two groups here: (1) those who can demonstrate posterior instability by positioning their extremity in forward flexion and internal rotation, and (2) those who cannot demonstrate subluxation but have symptoms reproduced through provocative testing.

Ideal indications include traumatic onset, labral detachment from the posterior glenoid, and satisfactory capsular ligaments. Additional findings that may be addressed include anterior labral tears or separation, superior labral tears, and an enlarged rotator interval (interval between the middle and superior glenohumeral ligaments). Rotator cuff pathology can coexist, although most commonly these are partial-thickness articular side tears.

Patients with capsular insufficiency or significant bone loss may not be appropriate for this procedure.

PREOPERATIVE PLANNING

Preoperative evaluation should include a careful history, with physical and radiographic examinations. During the physical examination, the patient should be asked to demonstrate the subluxation if possible or to place his or her arm in the painful position. Evaluation of instability should be done in comparison with the opposite side. The patient should be examined for the presence of generalized laxity. A load-and-shift test can demonstrate asymmetry in posterior translation in a relaxed patient. A sulcus sign can demonstrate excessive inferior translation. If a patient has excessive winging of the scapula, an electromyographic study of the serratus anterior may be helpful. Neurologic studies are usually normal, and winging may be the result of involuntary, abnormal posturing of the scapula.

Plain radiographic evaluation includes a true anteroposterior view of the glenohumeral joint, transscapular Y view, and an axillary view. In chronic cases, posterior glenoid wear may be present. Magnetic resonance imaging provides sensitive, though not always accurate, indications of posterior labral pathology.

SURGICAL TECHNIQUE

Positioning/Setup

The arthroscopic repair can be accomplished in the lateral decubitus position or in the beach chair position. In either instance, access to the posterior and anterior glenoid should be unimpeded.

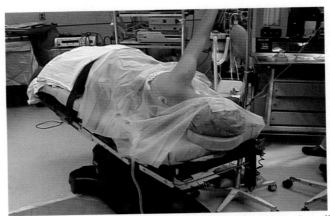

FIGURE 11.1. Patient is in lateral decubitus position, with downside well padded.

With the patient in the lateral decubitus position, traction can be minimal, the glenoid is oriented parallel to the floor or table, and the arm can be positioned in slight abduction, allowing easy access to the inferior pouch. The surgeon's arms can be maintained at the side, reducing fatigue, and allowing assistants and the anesthesiologist to be uncrowded and able to see the monitor. The torso can be secured with a beanbag, with additional tape to prevent movement. The arm is abducted 25° with minimal flexion, and balanced suspension is utilized, rather than traction (Figure 11.1). An axillary roll supports the chest wall, protecting the axillary contents.

Instrumentation

Arthroscopic instruments including a 30°, 4 mm scope, spinal needles, shaver, and switching sticks are standard. In addition, an 8 mm diameter disposable clear cannula is needed to permit passage of larger surgical instruments.

Special instrumentation includes suture anchors and suture-passing devices for labral repair. Suture hooks from the Spectrum Repair Set (Linvatec, Largo, FL) can be used to pass or retrieve sutures through the labrum and/or capsule (Figure 11.2). The Spectrum repair system relies on use of either a shuttling device or a monofilament suture to retrieve braided sutures.

Because knot tying is an important part of this procedure, appropriate instruments such as knot pusher and cutter are also required.

Surgical Technique

An examination under anesthesia is performed on both shoulders in the supine position. This examination should focus on range-of-motion assessment as well as laxity testing.

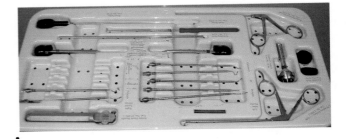

A

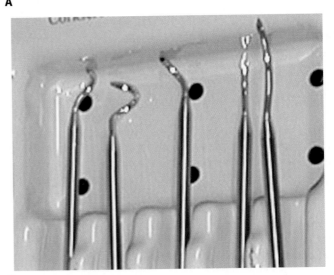

B

FIGURE 11.2. (A) Spectrum repair set (Linvatec) includes a thumbwheel and (B) various angle tips for suture passage.

A posterior portal is established after joint inflation with saline via an 18-gauge spinal needle. Begin viewing with the arthroscope posteriorly. Joint inspection should include the entire labrum, posterior capsule, and articular surfaces. Upon pulling back on the scope and focusing inferiorly, a complete assessment of the full length of the posterior capsule can be made. An anterior portal is established by using an "outside-in" technique, with a spinal needle entering between the acromion and the lateral margin of the coracoid process. The scope is then placed anteriorly and the joint inspection is repeated. Visualize and probe the anterior labrum, inferior glenohumeral ligament, and posterior labrum (Figure 11.3). Visualize your posterior portal entry. Confirm that the position is lateral to the glenoid, or reestablish the position to ensure satisfactory suture anchor placement. Using a switching stick, replace the posterior cannula with an 8 mm clear disposable cannula.

With the scope anteriorly, the posterior capsule is abraded with a motorized shaver, beginning inferiorly in the pouch at 6 o'clock. This will facilitate a healing response.

In the cases of labral detachment, a drill and drill guide are used to establish holes for the anchors along the glenoid rim. Anchor drill holes are placed along the articular edge, directing the drill into the glenoid (Figure 11.4). Be careful not to skive on the articular surface or delaminate the cartilage from the bone. Extra care is needed to make sure drill entry is into solid bone. If the angle of drilling and anchor insertion are inadequate, readjust or reestablish a more laterally positioned cannula.

The first (most inferior) suture anchor is placed, taking care to ensure proper seating and tensioning. The posterior cannula can be used, or an accessory to

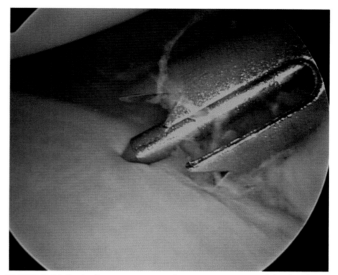

FIGURE 11.4. Arthroscopic view from anterior portal (right shoulder, lateral decubitus position). Note that the drill guide introduced through the posterior portal allows precise drill hole and suture anchor placement along the articular margin, angled into the glenoid bone.

2 cm more inferior portal established. The braided suture limbs are retrieved and brought out through an accessory inferior posterior portal, established 1 to 2 cm distal to the posterior working portal.

Next, curved suture hooks are introduced through the primary posterior portal (Figure 11.5A). The Spectrum tray (Linvatec) provides variably angled and curved tips that can penetrate the capsule and deliver a monofilament suture toward the glenoid (Figure 11.2). Beginning inferiorly in the pouch, the posterior capsule is penetrated and the monofilament suture advanced with the thumb wheel. To use the Spectrum repair set, a monofilament suture must be at least 30 in. long. In cases of capsular laxity, this "bite" inferiorly must be generous enough to sufficiently advance (and thereby reduce) a large inferior pouch. After the Spectrum tool has been removed, the monofilament limb emerging closest to the glenoid is grasped and pulled out through the accessory cannula (containing the braided suture limbs). A knot is then made in the monofilament suture and used to "shuttle" one limb of that anchor's braided suture through the labrum and/or capsule. The braided suture can now be tied as a "simple slider" knot (Figure 11.5B). A knot pusher is used to slide the knot down the cannula. After the knot has been seated, apply additional traction on the nonpost stitch and past point, locking the knot. Additional half-hitches are added, preventing any subsequent loosening.

If a mattress construct is desired, the repair needle can be passed a second time through the labrum or capsule adjacent to the first. The second arm of the braided suture is shuttled and a secure sliding knot is

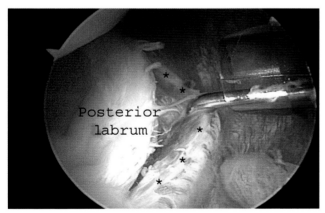

FIGURE 11.3. Viewing from an anterior superior portal, a probe displaces the posterior labral detachment, seen here from the 10 o'clock position (right shoulder, lateral decubitus perspective).

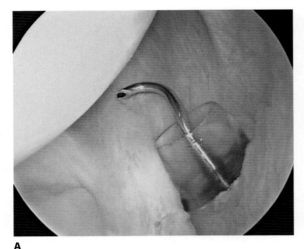

A

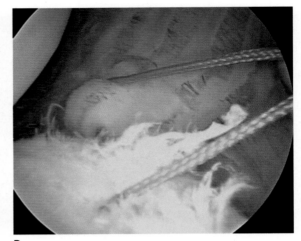

B

FIGURE 11.5. Arthroscopic photos (scope anterior, right shoulder, lateral decubitus position). (A) Curved suture hook poised to penetrate and reduce the posterior inferior pouch. (B) One limb of an

Ethibond suture successfully shuttled through posterior inferior capsule, other limb emerging from glenoid rim at site of anchor.

placed. These steps are repeated until the labrum has been completely repaired (Figure 11.6). In cases of posterior instability without labral detachment, in which posterior capsular laxity is the cause of the instability, suture anchors may not be necessary. Instead, after posterior capsular abrasion, capsular advancement is performed by means of the Spectrum hooks, beginning inferiorly and progressing superiorly. Each capsular bite is advanced superiorly, and the labrum is used as an anchoring structure for capsular plication. This often requires a two-step maneuver after the capsule has been penetrated. The needle tip is advanced and a second bite including the labrum is taken. Anchors can be used to facilitate this plication, in cases

of labral insufficiency. Sutures are tied as they are placed.

These steps are repeated as the posterior labrum is repaired and the capsule is advanced. As we approach the primary posterior cannula, the reversed, curved suture hooks can apply 0-PDS monofilament suture to further plicate or close the cannula hole.[1]

At this time, the camera is returned to the posterior portal and any other identified pathology is addressed; assessment of the rotator above the cannula interval (between the biceps and the subscapularis) is included in this sequence. If the interval is thought to contribute to the instability pattern, the 8 mm cannula is placed anteriorly (Figure 11.7A). An interval-

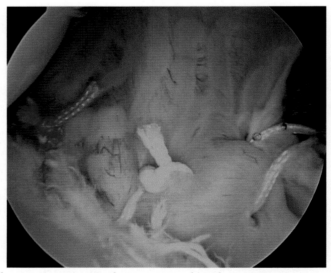

FIGURE 11.6. Arthroscopic view showing suture repair along posterior glenoid rim. Remaining superior suture has been placed to pleat and further tighten superior posterior capsule at site of working portal (scope anterior, right shoulder, lateral decubitus position).

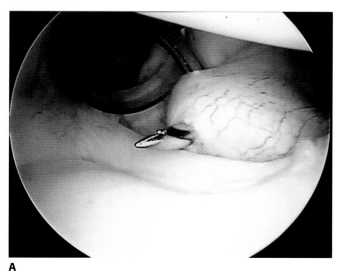

A

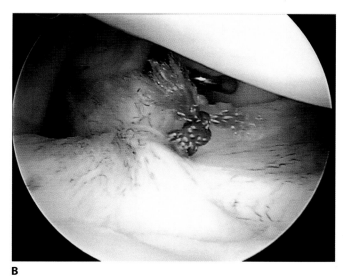

B

FIGURE 11.7. (A) With scope in posterior portal (left shoulder, lateral decubitus position), the rotator capsular interval is now addressed if suspected of contributing to posterior instability. Note the placement of a large working clean cannula with suture hook placed to pierce the superior bind of the middle glenohumeral ligament. (B) Final view of rotator capsular interval between the middle and superior ligaments, which has been closed with multiple sutures (posterior scope portal, left shoulder, lateral decubitus position).

closing stitch is placed by using a curved suture hook to grasp the superior portion of the middle glenohumeral ligament and advancing this up to the superior glenohumeral ligament. Reduction or closure of the interval can be completed by placing multiple sutures beginning medially at the glenoid, and working laterally to the cannula (Figure 11.7B). It is not necessary to grasp either the subscapularis or supraspinatus tendinous structures. Absorbable 0 PDS or no. 2 braided sutures can be used, depending on the clinical situation. In cases of atraumatic multidirectional instability, permanent braided sutures are recommended. For treatment of traumatic unidirectional instability, absorbable sutures are usually selected. The scope portals are closed with simple sutures, and a sterile dressing is applied. The final appearance can be seen in Figure 11.8.

POSTOPERATIVE MANAGEMENT

An Ultrasling (DonJoy, Carlsbad, CA) is worn for 4 to 6 weeks (Figure 11.9). The timing of sling removal is based on the degree of inferior laxity. Traumatic unidirectional posterior instability is immobilized for 4 weeks, and atraumatic posteroinferior multidirectional instability is immobilized for 6 weeks. During this period, patients are allowed external rotation to 30° while holding the injured arm at the side. Forward flexion and internal rotation are avoided. Shrugs and scapular exercises are started early.

After sling removal, patients begin active-assisted forward flexion. While a patient is lying supine (to control the scapula), the good arm actively assists elevation of the surgical shoulder. The hand is permitted to reach the back pocket, but maximal internal rotation and extension are avoided during the first 3 months.

At 8 weeks, upright forward flexion is continued. Proper neuromuscular control and scapular rotator strengthening and movement are emphasized. External rotation strengthening using Theraband tubing

FIGURE 11.8. Note the final appearance of the rotator interval that has been closed with absorbable monofilament sutures (arrows). (B, biceps long head; HH, humeral head.) (scope posterior, right shoulder, lateral decubitus perspective.)

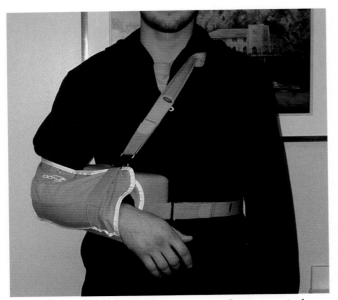

FIGURE 11.9. Ultrasling (DonJoy) is used postoperatively.

and rowing exercises with light resistance are started. Wall pushups with a neutral grip are begun as well. Motion in elevation and external rotation is usually normal by 10 weeks.

Return to activities is between 4 and 6 months, depending on the preoperative laxity, security of the repair, motion, protective strength, and anticipated sport. Many sport-specific rehabilitation programs begin at 3 months and continue until the player has successfully returned to the sport.

RESULTS/OUTCOME

Posterior arthroscopic stabilization is successful in approximately 90% of patients. There have been several reports on arthroscopic posterior capsule plication. Wolf and Eakin reported on 14 patients with unidirectional recurrent posterior subluxation.[1] Eight patients required suture anchors, and two patients needed repair of additional anterior labral tears. There were 93% stabilized and 86% good and excellent results. Antoniou, Duckworth, and Harryman reported on 41 patients with posteroinferior instability.[2] This included 9 revision surgeries, 10 patients with multidirectional instability, and 19 patients receiving workers' compensation. Thirty-five patients (85%) had improved stability after surgery, and 68% of the patients had perceived stiffness. Review of these studies and others suggests that elite throwers, patients who have had revision instability surgery, and patients on workers' compensation may have inferior results.

In my personal series, 39 patients have been followed for 2 to 5 years. These include patients with traumatic unidirectional posterior instability, as well as patients with overuse posteroinferior instability, who could demonstrate subluxation with forward elevation. None of these patients had symptomatic inferior laxity.

Arthroscopic findings included an enlarged posterior pouch (39), posterior labral tear (20), anterior labral tear (11), SLAP lesion (3), rotator cuff tear (3), and loose bodies (2). Repairs included suture anchor repairs of the posterior labrum, posterior capsule plication, anchor repair of anterior or superior labral detachment, and closure of the rotator capsular interval. Successful stabilization occurred in 92%, with one recurrence, and two shoulders that were painful. Ninety percent of the athletes returned to their sport, including nine high-level baseball and tennis players. Six of eight patients who had experienced on-the-job injuries (workers' compensation) returned to full active duty. Four of five patients who had had revision surgery returned to their former activities and had successful stabilization.

COMPLICATIONS

Complications can be classified based on technical error, recurrent instability, stiffness, and pain.

Technical error is most concerning because of the use of articular suture anchors. There are challenges in placing anchors into the posterior glenoid. This may be due to less familiarity with glenoid angulation, as well as to the orientation of the posterior portals, the presence of posterior labral tears without true separation, and bone changes making it easy to slide under articular cartilage and delaminate it. A drill guide can facilitate the placement of suture anchors. Careful orientation to the glenoid is necessary to make proper bone penetration. If the bone is hard and screw-in anchors are to be used, consider a tap. Regardless of the anchor choice, make sure the anchor is well seated below the articular surface.

Recurrent instability due to subsequent trauma or long-term capsular remodeling is probably the most common "complication." Emphasis on scapular control can limit symptoms and may allow some athletes to continue their activity despite mild postoperative instability symptoms.

Stiffness can occur for a number of reasons. A significant reduction in capsular volume is achieved with both anterior and posterior repairs. Many shoulders will gradually loosen with stretching over time. If gains have plateaued after 6 months, one may consider arthroscopic capsulotomy and lysis of adhesions. This is seldom necessary.

Patients with ongoing pain after a "successful" posterior stabilization need further evaluation. Look to the scapular mechanics for a possible clue. Abnormal scapulothoracic rhythm during elevation and abduction may suggest problems extrinsic to the glenohumeral joint. Posterior capsular reduction can theoretically contribute to subacromial and coracoid impingement symptoms. Only one patient has needed a subacromial decompression owing to recurrent shoulder pain.

References

1. Wolf EM, Eakin CL. Arthroscopic capsular plication for posterior shoulder instability. *Arthroscopy* 1998;14: 153–163.
2. Antoniou J, Duckworth DT, Harryman DT II. Capsulolabral augmentation for the management of posteroinferior instability of the shoulder. *J Bone Joint Surg Am* 2000;82:1220–1230.

Recommended Reading

Bell RH, Noble JS. An appreciation of posterior instability of the shoulder. *Clin Sports Med* 1991;10:887–900.

Bigliani LU, Pollock RG, McIlveen SJ, Endrizzi DP, Flatow EL. Shift of the posteroinferior aspect of the capsule for recurrent posterior glenohumeral instability. *J Bone Joint Surg Am* 1995;77:1011–1020.

Harryman DT, Sidles JA, Harris SL, Matsen FA III. Role of the rotator interval capsule in passive motion and stability of the shoulder. *J Bone Joint Surg Am* 1992;74:53–66.

Hawkins RJ, Koppert G, Johnson G. Recurrent posterior instability of the shoulder. *J Bone Joint Surg Am* 1984;66: 169–174.

Nobuhara K, Ikeda H. Rotator interval lesion. *Clin Orthop* 1987;223:44–50.

Pagnani MJ, Deng XH, Warren RF, Torzilli PA, Altchek DW. Effect of lesions of the superior portion of the glenoid labrum on glenohumeral translation. *J Bone Joint Surg Am* 1995;77:1003–1010.

Tibone JE, Bradley JP. The treatment of posterior subluxation in athletes. *Clin Orthop* 1993;291:124–137.

Warner JD, Deng XH, Warren RF, Torzilli PA. Static capsuloligamentous restraints to superior–inferior translation of the glenohumeral joint. *Am J Sports Med* 1992;20:675–685.

Weber SC, Caspari RB. A biomechanical evaluation of the restraints to posterior shoulder dislocation. *Arthroscopy* 1989;5:115–121.

12

Multidirectional Instability: Suture Plication Technique

Felix H. Savoie III

Multidirectional shoulder instability (MDI), first described by Neer and Foster in 1980, is due to the presence of inferior instability in combination with anterior and/or posterior instability. Although Matsen has characterized MDI as atraumatic in etiology, others have noted an association between MDI and repetitive trauma. Recent attention on the rotator interval has suggested its possible role in MDI as well.

Open management of MDI was first described by Neer with his glenoid-based open inferior capsular shift. Altchek and Warren modified his technique to address associated labral pathology. Open shifts for MDI using a variety of modifications of Neer's original procedure have led to 80 to 90% good-to-excellent results.

Arthroscopic management of MDI was pioneered by Caspari, initially using a transglenoid technique. Technical developments have facilitated the evolution of arthroscopic techniques. The time-honored approach upon which our technique is based is that of capsular plication, in which sutures are used to eliminate capsular patholaxity. The alternative approach, thermal modification of the capsule, has been described by many authors, met with early initial success, but has shown deterioration with longer follow-up (see Chapter 13). This chapter presents the current technique for suture plication in the management of multidirectional instability of the shoulder.

INDICATIONS AND CONTRAINDICATIONS

Surgical management of multidirectional instability is indicted for patients with pain, functional impairment, and a failure of rehabilitation. The most difficult part of managing MDI is often making the di-

agnosis. Multiple exam techniques have been described, but the authors primarily rely on the "sulcus" sign with the arm positioned in adduction, which persists despite external rotation or abduction. Anterior and posterior load and shift testing (in adduction and various degrees of abduction) is also helpful. A shift of the humeral head past the rim of the glenoid suggests abnormal laxity and is considered a positive test.

Upon establishment of the diagnosis, initial management focuses on rehabilitation. Kibler, who has noted the association of scapular winging with instability, described a comprehensive rehabilitation program. In essence, patients with capsular laxity depend on the functional integrity of the rotator cuff and periscapular muscles to maintain the congruous relationship between the humeral head and the glenoid. Instability becomes symptomatic when the delicate balance of these muscles is lost, resulting in uncontrolled shifting of the humeral head on the glenoid. In attempting to control the instability, the rotator cuff can overwork and become irritated, producing the symptoms of secondary impingement so often associated (especially in overhead athletes) with this disorder. Failure to successfully resolve the tendinitis then results in "protective" winging of the scapula, with further loss of rotator cuff function and ultimately a loss of normal shoulder proprioception.

Rehabilitation centers on stabilizing the scapula by strengthening the lower trap and serratus anterior, followed by standard rotator cuff exercises and the addition of complex movement patterns until normal function is achieved. The first round of management may be limited to pain control and elimination of the inflammation in the rotator cuff muscles and tendons. Therapy then continues as the pain and functional level of the shoulder allows. A minimum of 6 months of therapy, including a home program, should be followed before surgical intervention is considered.

The indications for surgery are continued pain and functional impairment despite an adequate rehabilitation program.

Contraindications to surgical management of MDI include the absence of the foregoing indications, a lack of adequate experience in the management of disorders of the shoulder, and a lack of equipment necessary for arthroscopic reconstruction.

PREOPERATIVE PLANNING

Positioning/Setup

Arthroscopic reconstruction is best accomplished in the lateral decubitus position. Although the beach chair position is favored by many surgeons, we have found that access to the inferior capsule is more easily accomplished in the lateral position. A standard arm holder, video equipment, and an anesthetist familiar with hypotensive anesthesia are also necessary. A second arm holder to distract the shoulder (lift the humeral head away from the glenoid) is used by some surgeons and should be available if desired.

Instrumentation

Surgical management of multidirectional instability requires specialized equipment. In addition to the usual arthroscopy equipment such as 30 and 70° arthroscopes, shavers, and various hand instru-

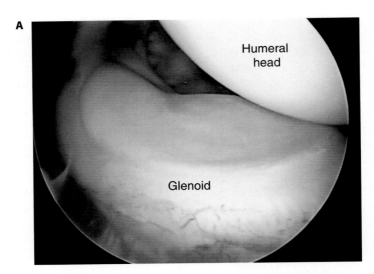

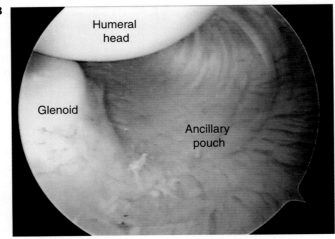

FIGURE 12.1. (A) With the arthroscope positioned in the posterior portal (right shoulder, lateral decubitus position), note the "stadium view" afforded with near 360° visualization in this patient with marked capsular laxity. (B) With the arthroscope directed inferiorly, note the capacious axillary pouch, a consistent finding in patients with multidirectional instability.

ments, a hand rasp, a thermal device of some type, and multiple methods of suture passage and placement should be available. We favor the use of the Spectrum tissue repair set (Linvatec, Largo, FL) and various angled suture retrievers (Mitek, Johnson & Johnson, Norwood, MA). A 2-0 prolene suture (48 in. long) or a suture shuttle (Linvatek) is also helpful in passing 2-0 Ethibond sutures. Disposable cannulas whose inner diameters permit instrument passage are standard.

One additional requirement for this procedure is the familiarity with and surgical ability in arthroscopic knot-tying techniques (see Chapter 4), and the ability to place and retrieve sutures through cannulas.

SURGICAL TECHNIQUE

After adequate induction of general anesthesia, the patient is positioned in the lateral decubitus position and rolled posteriorly 30°. The arm is placed in the arm holder with 5 to 10 lb of "suspension" traction, abducted 30 to 45° and in 90° external rotation. A second suspension system to distract the humeral head from the glenoid may be used, but the authors favor simple manual pressure used only to avoid potential injury to the brachial plexus.

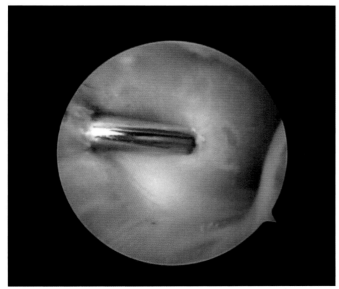

FIGURE 12.2. Viewing from the posterior scope portal (right shoulder, lateral decubitus position), a shaver from the anterior portal is used to roughen the anterior–inferior capsule prior to plication.

A posterior portal is established in line with the equator of the joint in the raphe of the infraspinatus. A diagnostic arthroscopy is performed, and the diagnosis of capsular laxity is confirmed (Figure 12.1). Management of associated and labral tears, capsular splits, and rotator cuff pathology is discussed elsewhere in this text. An anterior portal is then placed: an "outside-in" technique is used, with optimal portal placement determined by means of a spinal needle. Although the external portal position may vary between patients, it should always enter the shoulder through the "soft spot" in the interval. If the use of a suture shuttle is contemplated, an anterior superior portal is also placed along the anterior lateral corner of the acromion, entering the joint at the anterior margin of the supraspinatus.

The rasp or shaver is then used to roughen or freshen the capsule to be plicated. A minimum of one centimeter of capsule from the glenoid labrum laterally should be treated to form a bleeding surface. Resection is not necessary, but a healing area must be created (Figure 12.2). By keeping the suction turned off during the shaving, an abrasion-type healing response, rather than tissue removal, is facilitated. Care is taken to ensure adequate capsular preparation along the anterior–inferior capsule, including the rotator interval.

Alternatively, a thermal device of some kind may be used to treat the capsule in this area in preparation for suture placement. The area treated should remain within the planned area of suture placement, however.

The first stitch should be placed at the 6 o'clock position. This is best accomplished by utilizing the angled suture hook to grasp the capsule lateral to (on the humeral side) the previously treated capsule, whereupon the needle tip is delivered through this nontreated tissue. The hook is then pulled superiorly and medially, and is then placed through the labrum—actually, between the labrum and the glenoid (Figure 12.3). Next the suture is wheeled into the joint until it is completely within the instrument. In most cases the suture placed though the hook is a doubled 2-0 prolene or a suture shuttle.

Alternatively, a suture shuttle can be used. Once the retriever has been removed, the two free ends of the suture are pulled out the same canula. A no. 2 Ethibond suture is then placed through the looped end of the prolene (in the lower anterior cannula) and shuttled through the capsule. A self-locking knot is then tied and used to plicate the capsule, shifting the capsule superiorly and eliminating the inferior redundancy (Figure 12.4). Maintaining the arm in 90° of ex-

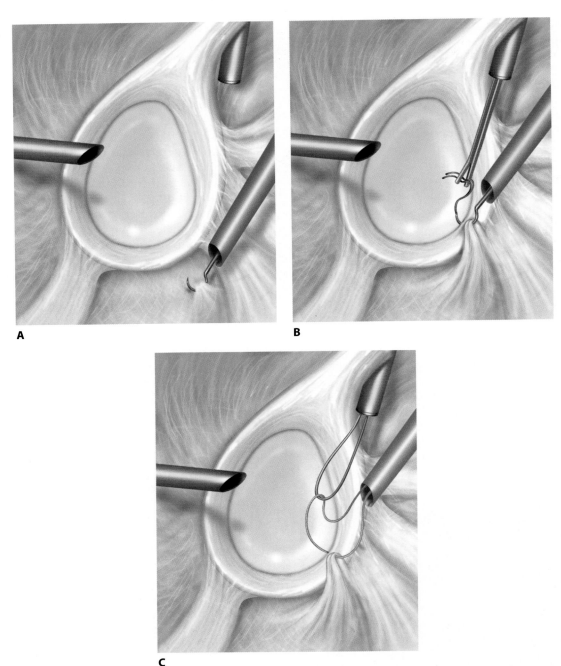

FIGURE 12.3. (A) Side view of the shoulder with the capsular hook shifting tissue superiorly and medially. (B) Suture hook passing the suture between the glenoid and labrum. (C) Suture in place for capsule plication.

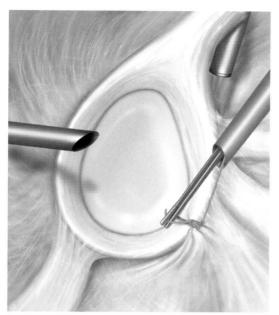

FIGURE 12.4. An arthroscopic knot is tied through the anterior portal, eliminating capsular redundancy.

ternal rotation during the placement of the suture prevents overtightening. A second stitch is placed near the 5 o'clock position, followed by additional sutures at the 3 and 1 o'clock positions (Figure 12.5).

The arthroscope is then placed in the anterior portal and the posterior capsule evaluated. The posterior capsule is prepared with a synovial shaver or rasp to generate a healing reponse. Additional sutures can be placed in a fashion similar to the anterior sutures (Figure 12.5). These are placed at the 7 and 9 o'clock positions. When the capsule is too thin, an alternative method may be used to accommodate suture fixation. A large-lumened 18-gauge spinal needle is placed percutaneously through the infraspinatus tendon and lateral portion of the capsule (Figure 12.6A). A no. 2 Ethibond suture is placed through the needle, "fed" into the joint, and retrieved through the medial capsule and out the posterior canula utilizing an angled (15 or 30°) suture retriever (Figure 12.6B). The posterior canula is then redirected into the subacromial area, and a crochet hook is used to retrieve the lateral limb of the suture from the same posterior canula. A modified Roeder knot is tied to plicate both capsule and infraspinatus tendon, creating a thickened band in the posterior capsule and tendon (Figure 12.7).

As with the anterior capsular plication, three sutures are placed to stabilize the posterior capsule. The arthroscope is then placed in the posterior portal and the rotator interval plicated.

Arthroscopically, pathology may be noted as a "bulging out" appearance to the interval; widening,—

noted primarily by experience; failure of the widened interval to contract with external rotation; and visible perforations. Unfortunately, there is a wide variety to the normal anatomy in this area. Experience in looking at this area is the best guide to understanding and differentiating true interval pathology from normal anatomy.

The technique for rotator interval closure (Figure 12.8) has been described by Treacy and utilizes the same spinal needle-retriever technique described for the posterior capsule. A large lumen 18-gauge needle is inserted through the superior aspect of the interval 1-cm medial to its humeral insertion at the anterior edge of the supraspinatus. A #2 Ethibond suture is placed through the needle and into the joint. Through the anterior canula, a retrograde retriever is then placed through the layers of the interval anterior and posterior to the subscapularis and passed superior to the biceps. The suture is then grasped and pulled out the cannula. A hemostat is placed on this limb of the suture. A switching stick is then placed into the cannula and redirected into the subacromial bursa. The superior limb of the suture is then grasped in the bursa using a crochet hook and pulled out this same canula while keeping the arthroscope in the joint. The arm is held in 45° of abduction and 90° external rotation while the suture is tightened. Once tied, inferior subluxation should be eliminated. If inferior subluxation persists, additional sutures are placed until completely eliminated. Up to three sutures may be required to effect interval closure.

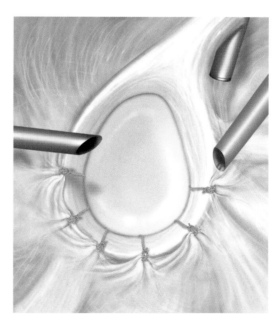

FIGURE 12.5. Sequential stitches may then be placed as needed to eliminate capsular redundancy. Note that plication sutures have been placed along both the anterior and posterior glenoid rim.

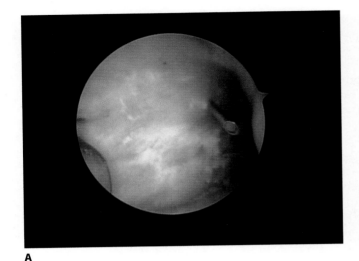

A

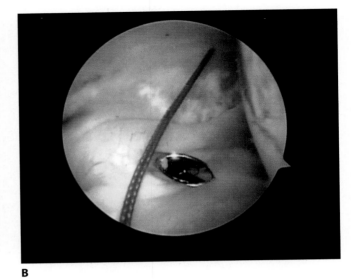

B

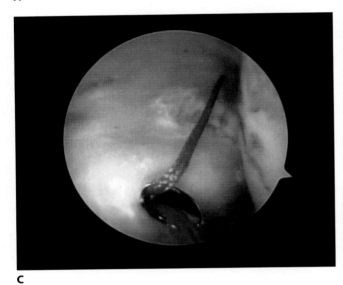

C

FIGURE 12.6. View from the anterior portal (left shoulder, lateral decubitus position). (A) Large spinal needle placed percutaneously through the infraspinatus tendon and lateral capsule. (B) Suture retriever placed between the posterior labrum and glenoid prior to grasping the Ethibond suture. (C) Note the roughened capsule in the area between the stitches. The posterior cannula (through which the suture was placed) has been pulled back just outside the joint.

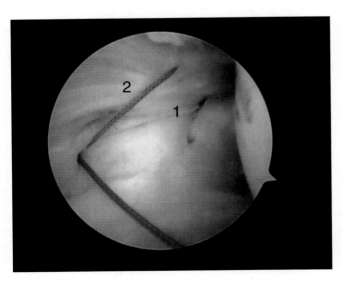

FIGURE 12.7. The first suture (1) has been tied outside the capsule. A second stitch (2) has been placed and partially retrieved, but not yet been tied. (1, first stitch tied; 2, second stitch being pulled out of capsule [arrow], not yet tied.) (View from anterior portal, left shoulder, lateral decubitus posterior.)

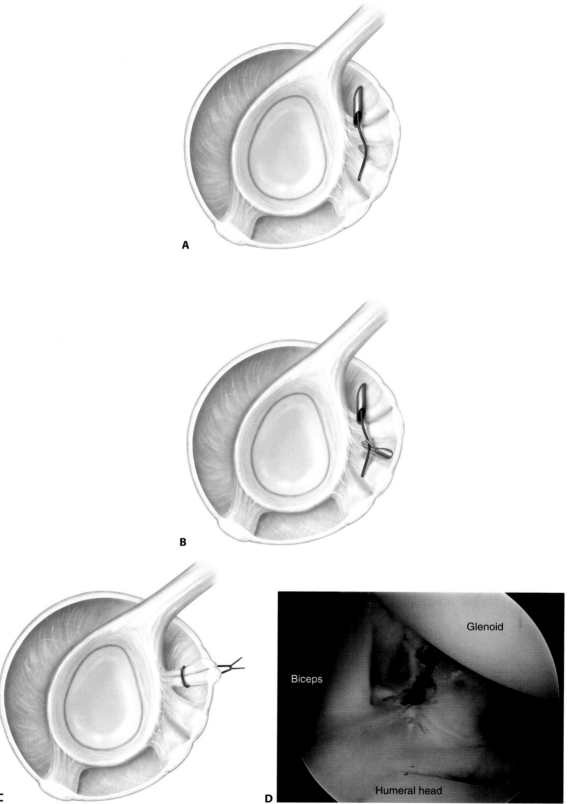

FIGURE 12.8. Diagrams and arthroscopic views of plication of the rotator interval. (A) A large diameter (to permit easy introduction of braided ethibond suture) spinal needle is placed percutaneously beside the anterior margin of the supraspinatus tendon through the superior portion of the rotator interval capsule. A suture is then advanced through the spinal needle into the glenohumeral joint. (B) A retriever is passed through the anterior and posterior layers of the rotator interval inferiorly (via the anterior cannula). (C) The stitch is retrieved through the anterior portal and tied with a modified Roeder knot in the anterior subdeltoid subacromial space. Up to three sutures may be necessary to close the interval. (D) Arthroscopic view from posterior portal, right shoulder, lateral decubitus perspective.

TABLE 12.1. Results of Suture Plication for MDI.

Year	Author	Number of patients	Diagnosis	Average follow-up	Good to excellent (%)	Motion (% normal)
1993	Duncan and Savoie[1]	10	MDI	12 months	100	99
1999	Treacy et al.[2]	25	MDI	60 months	88	99
1997	McIntyre et al.[3]	19	MDI	25 months	95	95
1997	Wichman and Snyder[4]	24	MDI		79	
2001	Gartsman et al.[5]	47	MDI	35 months	94	99
1997	Treacy et al.[6]	50	Inferior	Short	"Very encouraging"	
2001	Lyons et al.[7]	26	MDI	24 months	96	
1998	Wolf and Eakin[8]	14	Posterior	33 months	86	100

POSTOPERATIVE MANAGEMENT

The patient is placed either in a small abduction sling or in a gunslinger brace (for patients with a predominant posterior instability component) in slight abduction and neutral rotation. It is important to support the humeral head and prevent inferior subluxation and excessive tension on the repaired rotator interval and the inferior capsule.

Immobilization is continued for 3 to 6 weeks, depending on the quality of the repair and the patient's healing response. When the repair seems to be maturing, a home movement program is initiated, keeping within guidelines set at the time of surgery—usually external rotation to 15 or 30° in adduction, flexion to 90° in neutral rotation, and scapular rotation. The patient is also started on scapular retraction exercises. The pillow sling is removed for these movements twice a day.

Approximately 4 to 6 weeks postfixation, the patient begins waist-level rotator cuff exercises, as well as lower trapezius and serratus anterior exercises, and is allowed to remove the immobilization device. Physical therapy begins 2 weeks later, with an emphasis on scapular position during all exercises. The patient is allowed unrestricted active stretching and exercises as long as the scapula remains in a retracted position; stretching by the therapist, however, is delayed until a minimum of 3 months except in unusual circumstances. True multidirectional instability patients will regain motion without requiring aggressive stretching.

A progressive exercise program including proprioceptive neuromuscular facilitation exercises, plyometrics, and Kibler integrated rehabilitation is initiated at 12 weeks after surgery and advanced as tolerated by the patient. Sport-specific conditioning and fast-paced exercises follow. Both the therapist and the patient must understand the importance of maintaining proper scapular position throughout the rehabilitation program. The most common error during

this time is to attempt to progress through the exercises too rapidly, with resultant scapular winging and secondary cuff tendinitis.

The majority of patients will resume normal function by 6 months postsurgery.

RESULTS/OUTCOME

Results following arthroscopic management of MDI have been mixed. The current technique seems to be producing satisfactory results, but follow-up in the 5-year range is lacking for this particular method. However, since the initial report by Duncan and Savoie of 10 patients with 100% satisfactory results at short term follow-up, a number of other authors suggest consistently good outcomes (Table 12.1).[1–8] Treacy has reported 88% good-to-excellent results with a 5-year follow-up. McIntyre reported on 19 patients with 95% good-to-excellent results at a 3-year follow-up. Gartsman reported a 94% success rate in 47 patients.

COMPLICATIONS

Fortunately, reports of complications during arthroscopic suture management of MDI have been rare. Complications may be grouped into preoperative, intraoperative, and postoperative. Preoperative complications including diagnostic error and inadequate preoperative rehabilitation are probably the most common. Distinguishing congenital MDI from instability due to repetitive stress or multiple traumatic injuries is often difficult even for experienced clinicians. Patients with true collagen disorders (Marfan's syndrome, Ehlers–Danlos type 2, etc) or psychiatric problems also present a subset doomed to failure if operative intervention is utilized.

Reported intraoperative problems are rare. Failure to recognize coexisting labral or cuff tears may compromise outcome. The potential for injury to the axillary nerve has been noted in cases of thermal capsular management, but no such damage has been reported with the suture plication technique. Risk of making the shoulder "too tight" is real, though this result is rarely reported.

Postoperative complications are influenced predominantly by rehabilitation. It is important to remember that a true congenitally lax MDI patient will regain normal motion without aggressive stretching. MDI due to repetitive stress or trauma, however, may require more aggressive therapy to achieve normal motion. Frequent postoperative assessment and communication with the therapist are imperative.

References

1. Duncan R, Savoie FH. Arthroscopic inferior capsular shift for multidirectional instability of the shoulder: a preliminary report. *Arthroscopy* 1993;9:24–27.
2. Treacy SH, Savoie FH, Field LD. Arthroscopic treatment of multidirectional instability. *J Shoulder Elbow Surg* 1999;8:345–350.
3. McIntyre LF, Caspari RB, Savoie FH. The arthroscopic treatment of multidirectional shoulder instability: two-year results of a multiple suture technique. *Arthroscopy* 1997;13(4):418–425.
4. Wichman MT, Snyder SJ. Arthroscopic capsular plication for multidirectional instability of the shoulder. *Oper Tech Sports Med* 1997;5:238–243.
5. Gartsman GM, Roddey TS, Hammerman SM. Arthroscopic treatment of multidirectional glenohumeral instability: 2 to 5 year follow-up. *Arthroscopy* 2001;17(3):236–243.
6. Treacy SH, Field LD, Savoie FH. Rotator interval capsule closure: an arthroscopic technique. *Arthroscopy* 1997;13(1):103–106.
7. Lyons TR, Griffith PL, Savoie FH. Laser-assisted capsulorrhaphy for multidirectional instability of the shoulder. *Arthroscopy* 2001;17(1):25–30.
8. Wolf EM, Eakin CL. Arthroscopic capsular plication for posterior shoulder instability. *Arthroscopy* 1998;14:153–163.

Recommended Reading

Altchek DW, Warren R. T-plasty modification of the Bankart procedure for multidirectional instability of the anterior inferior type. *J Bone Joint Surg Am* 1990;73:105–112.

Savoie FH, Caspari RB. Instability of the shoulder: superior, posterior, and multidirectional. In: McGinty JB, Caspari RB, Jackson RW, et al., eds. *Operative Arthroscopy*. New York: Raven Press, 1991:709–723.

Harryman DT II, Sidles JA, Harris SL, et al. The role of the rotator interval capsule in passive motion and stability of the shoulder. *J Bone Joint Surg Am* 1992;74:53–66.

Matsen FA III, Thomas SC, Rockwood CA Jr. Anterior glenohumeral instability. In: Rockwood CA Jr, Matsen FA III, eds. *The Shoulder*. Philadelphia: WB Saunders; 1990:526–622.

Neer CS II, Foster CR. Inferior capsular shift for involuntary inferior and multidirectional instability of the shoulder: a preliminary report. *J Bone Joint Surg Am* 1980;62:897–908.

Snyder SJ, Stafford BB. Arthroscopic management of instability of the shoulder. *Orthopedics* 1993;16:513–517.

13

Arthroscopic Treatment of Multidirectional Instability: Thermal Technique

James P. Bradley, Jon K. Sekiya, Bernard C. Ong, and Kenneth R. Thompson

Multidirectional instability of the shoulder can be a difficult management problem. It usually presents in adolescents and young adults with hyperlaxity of several joints. Initial management of multidirectional instability is directed at a supervised exercise program consisting of rotator cuff, deltoid, and periscapular strengthening exercises. While conservative therapy is the mainstay of treatment and often successful, a subset of patients fails to improve, and surgical intervention is necessary to effectively restore shoulder stability.

The use of thermal energy has become increasingly popular in arthroscopic surgical procedures, in part because of its ease of use. While thermal capsulorrhaphy is a useful tool in the arthroscopic management of shoulder instability, basic science studies have shown that there are limits to the amount of capsular tissue that can be shortened before collagen is significantly weakened and denatured, to a point that is detrimental to healing.

Therefore, in the following clinical application, we describe the use of thermal capsulorrhaphy as an adjunct to other arthroscopic interventions in the treatment of multidirectional shoulder instability. Thermal capsulorrhaphy enhances and augments other arthroscopically performed stabilization procedures, further improving the results that could be obtained with either procedure alone.

INDICATIONS/CONTRAINDICATIONS

An open inferior capsular shift procedure with rotator interval closure has been successful in treating multidirectional shoulder instability and is considered to be the gold standard of operative intervention.[1–3]

Recent reports of arthroscopic thermal capsulorrhaphy procedures to treat multidirectional instability have shown promise, with good success rates.[4,5] The best results may come from a combined arthroscopic approach, first performing suture capsulorrhaphy with rotator interval closure and suture capsular plication in the areas of greatest instability (anterior and/or posterior as determined by the examination under anesthesia), followed by thermal augmentation to further address any residual laxity.

Contraindications to the arthroscopic treatment of multidirectional instability enhanced with thermal capsulorrhaphy include (1) revision surgery, (2) bony abnormalities such as glenoid hypoplasia, glenoid deficiency (bony Bankart lesions, or inverted-pear glenoid), and/or humeral head deficiencies (engaging Hill–Sachs lesions), and (3) thin or inadequate capsular tissue.

We believe that in the absence of these contraindications and when long-term follow-up becomes available, arthroscopic anterior and posterior capsular plication augmented with thermal capsulorrhaphy and rotator interval closure for multidirectional shoulder instability will yield results comparable to those from open procedures, hopefully with less perioperative morbidity.

PREOPERATIVE PLANNING

Preoperative planning depends upon a comprehensive history and physical examination, documenting the frequency and predominant direction of dislocation (if any), the mechanism of injury (traumatic or nontraumatic, voluntary or involuntary), history of any systemic medical diseases such as Ehlers–Danlos syndrome, whether the patient has global laxity including the unaffected shoulder, and if inferior sulcus testing improves with external rotation.

In addition, standard plain radiographs, including anteroposterior internal and external rotation of the shoulder, axillary lateral, West Point, and Stryker notch views, are essential to evaluate for bony abnormalities. We also routinely use gadolineum-enhanced (intra-articular) magnetic resonance imaging (MRI) to obtain an arthrogram to evaluate for labral injuries and/or other associated pathology such as humeral avulsions of the glenohumeral ligament (HAGL lesion), which may modify our management plan.

SURGICAL TECHNIQUE

Positioning/Setup

The procedure can be performed in either the beach chair or the lateral decubitus position. We prefer the lateral decubitus position with a beanbag, utilizing a traction setup (Figure 13.1). The downside should be well padded, including use of an axillary roll and pillows to pad the peroneal nerve and bony prominences.

Instrumentation

In addition to standard instrumentation for performing arthroscopic stabilization procedures, a thermal energy system is required. Thermal energy can be delivered arthroscopically using either laser or radiofre-quency energy. More recently, radiofrequency energy has gained increased popularity in orthopedic surgery. These delivery systems pass a high-frequency, alternating current from an electrical generator from the probe into the tissue. The current passes between the probe tip and the grounding pad in monopolar applications (Oratec Interventions, Menlo Park, CA) or between two points on the probe tip in bipolar systems (Arthrocare, Arthrocare Corp., Sunnyvale, CA; Mitek, Johnson & Johnson, Norwood, MA). We use the Oratec monopolar radiofrequency probe with the system set at 75°C and 40 W of power.

Surgical Technique

An examination under anesthesia is performed to document the degree and direction of the shoulder instability. We inject the glenohumeral joint with 1% lidocaine with epinephrine before beginning a standard posterior-portal-based arthroscopy. If a posterior capsulorrhaphy is anticipated, our initial posterior portal is made a little "high" and closer to the acromion, to make room for a possible "low" portal. Inspection of the joint is performed to evaluate the global capsular laxity (Figures 13.2, 13.3). If labral tears are identified, they are repaired by using suture anchors. Other intra-articular pathology is definitively addressed and/or ruled out.

The direction of predominant instability is addressed first. For anterior instability, two anterior portals are made, one anterior superior portal (high portal) and one anterior inferior portal (low portal). This high anterior portal should be placed lateral to the coracoid process just inferior to the biceps tendon and

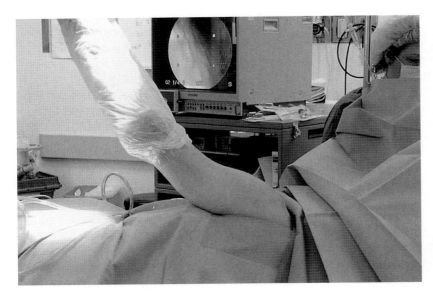

FIGURE 13.1. The patient is placed in the lateral decubitus position with the left shoulder suspended by 10 lb of traction. All bony prominences and neurovascular structures are well padded and protected.

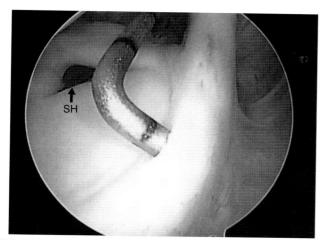

FIGURE 13.2. Intra-articular structures of a left shoulder viewed from the posterior portal (lateral decubitus). Notice the capsular laxity and increased volume of the posterior superior structures. Incidentally, there is a normal sublabral hole (SH) anteriorly.

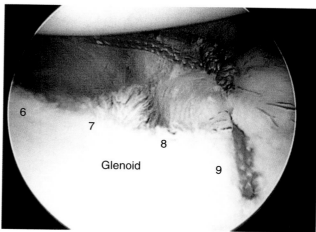

FIGURE 13.4. An anterior capsular plication suture tightens the middle glenohumeral ligament to the glenoid rim in a left shoulder at the 9 o'clock position (lateral decubitus). Notice the remaining capsular laxity inferior to this between 6 and 8 o'clock positions.

is used to place arthroscopic capsular plication sutures at a position between 8 and 10 o'clock in a left shoulder (Figure 13.4). The low anterior portal is also placed lateral to the coracoid process, inferior to the biceps tendon and just superior to the edge of the subscapu-

laris tendon. With this portal placed right on the edge of the subscapularis tendon, capsular plication sutures can be placed along the anterior band of the inferior glenohumeral ligament and the anterior inferior capsule (Figure 13.5).

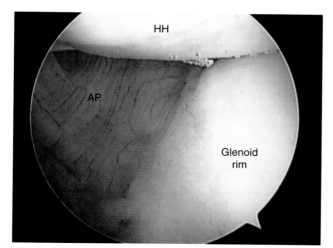

FIGURE 13.3. Intra-articular view of a left shoulder from the posterior portal (lateral decubitus). Notice the laxity and increased volume of the posterior inferior capsular structures and axillary recess: HH, humeral head; AP, axillary pouch.

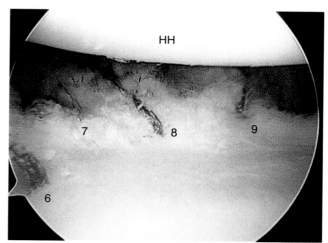

FIGURE 13.5. In this left shoulder viewing from the posterior portal, (lateral decubitus position), anterior plication sutures have tightened up the anterior inferior capsule between 6 and 8 o'clock: HH, humeral head.

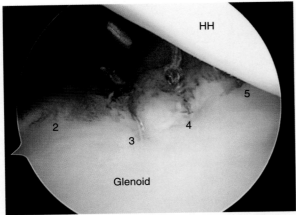

FIGURE 13.6. In this arthroscopic view from anterior portal of a left shoulder (lateral decubitus position) two posterior capsular plication sutures have been placed at about 3 and 4 o'clock: HH, humeral head.

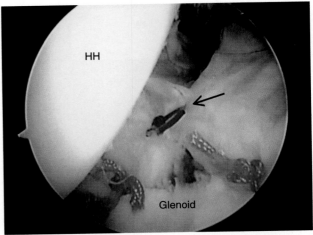

FIGURE 13.8. With the arthroscope looking anteriorly from the "high" posterior viewing portal (left shoulder, lateral decubitus position), the rotator interval is then closed arthroscopically (arrow): HH, humeral head.

If the predominant direction of instability is posterior, or if there is a significant posterior component to the patient's instability pattern, the arthroscope is placed through the high anterior portal looking posteriorly. A second posterior portal is created inferior to the first portal, with care not to be greater than 3 cm inferior to the posterior edge of the acromion (to avoid risk to the axillary nerve). A posterior capsular plication is then performed arthroscopically, beginning with the low portal to place capsular plication sutures in the posterior band of the inferior glenohumeral ligament. As the posterior inferior ligament and capsular tension are restored, plication sutures are continued superiorly, utilizing the high posterior portal (Figure

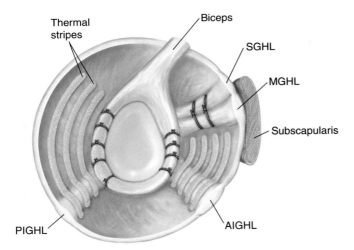

FIGURE 13.7. Schematic drawing of a right shoulder depicting anterior and posterior plication sutures. To further restore adequate capsular tension and volume, thermal stripes are applied as shown, following placement of the plication sutures. Finally, the rotator capsular interval is closed with arthroscopically placed sutures: SGHL, superior glenohumeral ligament; MGHL, middle glenohumeral ligament; AIGHL, anterior inferior glenohumeral ligament; PIGHL, posterior inferior glenohumeral ligament.

13.6). Thermal capsulorrhaphy is then performed to further tighten any residual laxity not corrected by the capsular plication. The radiofrequency device is then used to further tighten any residual laxity not corrected by the anterior capsular plication. It is imperative to use the radiofrequency probe in a striped fashion, leaving untouched segments of capsule between areas of shrinkage to allow for revascularization and healing (Figure 13.7). To avoid potential neurological injury, it is also important to avoid treating areas between the 5 and 7 o'clock positions on the glenoid. Thermal striping is performed at the most inferior area, working anteriorly and superiorly as the capsular tension is restored. It is very important not to press down on the probe and not to leave the probe in any one area for too long, especially when the inferior aspects of the capsule are being treated. Begin with the low anterior portal (and/or low posterior portal) when treating the inferior areas and then switch to the high anterior portal.

Following the anterior and posterior capsular plication and thermal capsulorrhaphy, intra-articular sutures are placed to close the low anterior and low posterior portals arthroscopically. The shoulder is then reexamined, and if residual instability is present, the rotator interval is closed with arthroscopically placed intra-articular sutures (Figure 13.8).

POSTOPERATIVE MANAGEMENT

Following arthroscopic anterior and/or posterior capsular plication, rotator interval closure, and augmentation with thermal capsulorrhaphy, a sling is worn for 6 to 8 weeks to protect the repair. Active and passive range-of-motion exercises of the neck, elbow, wrist, and hand are begun on the first postoperative day. We restrict any abduction, forward elevation, or external rotation past neutral for 4 weeks.

At 4 weeks following surgery, the patient may come out of the sling three times a day for passive pendulum exercises and active assisted range-of-motion exercises. Gentle strengthening exercises are also begun, incorporating the muscles of the shoulder girdle and periscapular area. The limits of shoulder motion are increased to 90° of abduction and forward flexion, 45° of external rotation, and extension to 20°. At 6 to 8 weeks, the sling is discontinued and motion is slowly increased to full range, with the exception of external rotation, which is limited to −15° compared with the other shoulder.

At 12 weeks following surgery, exercises are continued until full pain-free motion and strength have been achieved. At this point, a graduated interval sports program is initiated. By 20 to 24 weeks, a gradual return to unrestricted activities is begun. Shoulder and scapular range of motion and strengthening exercises are continued on their own indefinitely.

RESULTS/OUTCOME

Published results following thermal capsulorrhaphy for multidirectional shoulder instability are limited. Savoie and field prospectively compared 32 shoulders treated with arthroscopic thermal capsulorrhaphy with 25 shoulders managed with an arthroscopic suture capsular shift for multidirectional instability.[4] In the nonthermal group, 10% of patients had recurrent instability, all requiring revision surgery (average follow-up of 52 months). Of the 11 high school or college athletes, 82% were able to return to their previous level of athletic participation. In the thermal group, only 1 of the 32 patients (3%) had recurrent instability requiring revision surgery (average follow-up of 27 months). Of the 17 athletes in the thermal group, 88% returned to their previous levels of participation postoperatively.

Lyons et al. retrospectively evaluated the use of laser-assisted capsulorrhaphy (holmium:YAG laser) in 27 multidirectional instability shoulders with a minimum follow-up of 2 years.[5] All but one of 27 shoulders remained stable (96%); the other patient had recurrent instability. Twelve of the 14 athletes in the study returned to their previous level of athletic activity. Eighty-eight percent of the patients in the study had a satisfactory outcome according to the criteria of Neer and Foster.

There are several unpublished studies on thermal capsulorrhaphy for multidirectional instability. Bradley et al (Bradley JP, D'Allesandro DF, Connor PM,

unpublished data, American Orthopedic Society for Sports Medicine, Annual Meeting, Orlando, FL, March 2000) evaluated 35 shoulders with multidirectional instability following monopolar radiofrequency thermal capsulorrhaphy. With an average follow-up of 12 months, 37% were rated as excellent, 34% rated as satisfactory, and 29% had unsatisfactory outcomes according to the American Shoulder and Elbow Surgeons Shoulder Assessment form. Eight of the 35 patients had recurrent instability symptoms (23%), prompting the authors to increase their postoperative sling immobilization from 2 to 4 weeks to 6 to 8 weeks.

In a continuing study, we have since followed these patients now with 53 shoulders treated with thermal capsulorrhaphy (D'Alessandro DF, Bradley JP, Connor PM, personal communication, 2001). Using the same rating system, 38% of patients had an excellent result, 22% had a satisfactory result, and 40% had an unsatisfactory result (average follow-up of 37 months, minimum 2 years). This high failure rate has prompted the senior author to consider thermal capsulorrhaphy only as an adjunct to an arthroscopic suture capsular plication procedure.

Ciullo (Ciullo JV, unpublished data, American Shoulder and Elbow Surgeons, Annual Meeting, Miami Beach, FL, May 2000) reported his results in 294 patients treated with thermal capsulorrhaphy. The majority of patients had multidirectional instability (93%), with 5% having posterior subluxation and 2% having anterior instability. He reported a 99% success rate with a minimum follow-up of 2 years.

Fanton reported his results with monopolar radiofrequency thermal capsulorrhaphy in 16 patients with multidirectional instability. He reported initial results of nearly 90% good or excellent scores at 1 year, which subsequently deteriorated to 75% at 2 years because several patients developed increased laxity and recurrent instability symptoms.

Karas et al. (Karas S, Noonan T, Horan M, unpublished data, American Orthopedic Society for Sports Medicine Annual Meeting, Sun Valley, ID, 2000) evaluated 10 patients with multidirectional instability following arthroscopic stabilization (5 with associated Bankart lesions) combined with thermal capsulorrhaphy. Seven of 12 shoulders (58%) had successful outcomes at a minimum follow-up of 2 years.

Hawkins (Hawkins RJ, unpublished data, American Association of Nurse Anesthetists, Fall Course, San Diego, CA, November 1999) presented his results in 8 patients with multidirectional instability following combined arthroscopic repair and thermal capsulorrhaphy. There was a single recurrence (13%), and the average American Shoulder and Elbow Surgeons Shoulder Assessment form score was 89, with a minimum follow-up of 1 year.

Williams et al. (Williams GR, Wong K, Ramsey ML, Iannotti JP, unpublished data, American Shoulder and Elbow Surgeons, Annual Meeting, Miami Beach, FL, May 2000) followed seven patients whose recurrent multidirectional instability had been treated with monopolar radiofrequency thermal capsulorrhaphy. Five of seven patients (71%) were satisfied with their results at a minimum follow-up of 2 years.

Basamania (Basamania, unpublished data, International Society of Arthroscopy, Knee Surgery, and Orthopedic Sports Medicine, Washington, DC, June 1999) reported a 92% success with thermal capsulorrhaphy in 52 patients with multidirectional instability. The entire anterior and posterior capsule was treated, and patients were strictly immobilized for 4 weeks following surgery. No length of follow-up was given.

Koh et al. (Koh JL, Wells J, Warren RF, Wickiewicz T, O'Brien SJ, Craig E, Rodeo S, unpublished data, International Society of Arthroscopy, Knee Surgery, and Orthopedic Sports Medicine, Washington, DC, June 1999) evaluated 42 patients following thermal capsulorrhaphy with or without a concomitant arthroscopic stabilization procedure (79%). Of the 42 patients in the study, 27 had multidirectional instability of the shoulder. Three of the 42 patients (7%) had recurrent instability and 2 patients had persistent postoperative pain, for a failure rate of 12% at latest follow-up (no time period given).

COMPLICATIONS

Complications following thermal capsulorrhaphy for multidirectional instability of the shoulder include recurrent instability, neurological injury, capsular necrosis, and adhesive capsulitis.[6] Risk factors for recurrent instability following thermal capsulorraphy include a history of multiple dislocations, revision surgery, involvement with contact sports, or inadequate postoperative immobilization.

Axillary neuritis following thermal capsulorrhaphy has been described in the literature and is usually transient.[7,8] Gryler et al. evaluated the temperatures in the axillary nerve in cadaver shoulders during monopolar radiofrequency thermal capsulorrhaphy and found that during anterior inferior capsular treatment, temperatures in the axillary nerve were as high as 52°C.[9] These elevated temperature readings in the axillary nerve are concerning, and care should be taken when these anterior inferior areas of the capsule are treated. We avoid treating the capsule between 5 and 7 o'clock when we are using thermal techniques.

Another potential complication following thermal capsulorrhaphy is capsular necrosis, with loss of capsular and glenohumeral ligament integrity.[7,10] This problem has been associated with thin capsules, performing the capsular shrinkage in a contiguous paintbrush fashion (rather than leaving untouched areas between treated areas), excessive capsular shrinkage beyond 15 to 20%, and inadequate periods of postoperative immobilization.

Another serious complication following thermal capsulorrhaphy is adhesive capsulitis.[7,10,11] One proposed explanation for this occurrence is that an intensified fibroblast response stimulates global capsulitis, leading to adhesions. Methods of avoiding the problem include avoiding excessive capsular shrinkage, as well as instituting a graduated and progressive exercise program monitored by a physical therapist, following an appropriate period of immobilization.

References

1. Neer CR, Foster CR. Inferior capsular shift for involuntary inferior and multidirectional instability of the shoulder: a preliminary report. *J Bone J Surg Am* 1980;62:897–908.
2. Pollock RG, Owens JM, Flatow EL, et al. Operative results of the inferior capsular shift procedure for multidirectional instability of the shoulder. *J Bone J Surg Am* 2000;82:919–928.
3. Wirth MA, Groh GI, Rockwood CA. Capsulorrhaphy through an anterior approach for the treatment of atraumatic posterior glenohumeral instability with multidirectional laxity of the shoulder. *J Bone J Surg Am* 1998;80:1570–1578.
4. Savoie FH, Field LD. Thermal versus suture treatment of symptomatic capsular laxity. *Clin Sports Med* 2000;19:64–75.
5. Lyons TR, Griffith PL, Savoie FH, et al. Laser-assisted capsulorrhaphy for multidirectional instability of the shoulder. *Arthroscopy* 2001;17:25–30.
6. Sperling JW, Anderson K, McCarty EC, et al. Complications of thermal capsulorrhaphy. *AAOS Instr Course Lect* 2001;50:37–41.
7. Abrams JS. Thermal capsulorrhaphy for instability of the shoulder: concerns and applications of the heat probe. *AAOS Instr Course Lect* 2001;50:29–36.
8. Fanton GS. Monopolar electrothermal arthroscopy for treatment of shoulder instability in the athlete. *Oper Tech Sports Med* 2000;8:242–249.
9. Gryler EC, Greis PE, Burks RT, et al. Axillary nerve temperatures during radiofrequency capsulorrhaphy of the shoulder. *Arthroscopy* 2001;17:567–572.
10. Shaffer, BS. Tibone, JE: Arthroscopic shoulder instability surgical complications. *Clin Sports Med* 1999;18:737–767.
11. Fanton GS. Arthroscopic electrothermal surgery of the shoulder. *Oper Tech Sports Med* 1998;6:139–146.

Recommended Readings

Anderson K, McCarty EC, Warren RF. Thermal capsulorrhaphy: where are we today? *Sports Med Arthrosc Rev* 1999;7:117–127.

Brillhart AT. Complications of thermal energy. *Oper Tech Sports Med* 1998;6:182–184.

Foster TE, Elman M. Arthroscopic delivery systems used for thermally induced shoulder capsulorraphy. *Oper Tech Sports Med* 1998;6:126–130.

Hayashi K, Thabit G, Massa KL, et al. The effect of thermal heating on the length and histologic properties of the glenohumeral joint capsule. *Am J Sports Med* 1997;25:107–112.

Hayashi K, Hecht P, Thabit G, et al. The biologic response to laser thermal modification in an in vitro sheep model. *Clin Orthop* 2000;373:265–276.

Hecht P, Hayashi K, Cooley AJ, et al. The thermal effect of monopolar radiofrequency energy on the properties of joint capsule: an in vivo histologic study using a sheep model. *Am J Sports Med* 1998;26:808–814.

Lopez MJ, Hayashi K, Vanderby R, et al. Effects of monopolar radiofrequency energy on ovine joint capsular mechanical properties. *Clin Orthop* 2000;374:286–297.

Lu Y, Hayashi K, Edwards RB, et al. The effect of monopolar radiofrequency treatment pattern on joint capsular healing: in vitro and in vivo studies using an ovine model. *Am J Sports Med* 2000;28:711–719.

Nath S, DiMarco JP, Haines DE. Basic aspects of radiofrequency catheter ablation. *J Cardiovasc Electrophysiol* 1994;5:863–876.

Obrzut SL, Hecht P, Hayashi K, et al. The effect of radiofrequency energy on the length and temperature properties of the glenohumeral joint capsule. *Arthroscopy* 1998;14:395–400.

Pullin JG, Collier MA, Johnson LL, et al. Holmium:YAG laser-assisted capsular shift in a canine model: intraarticular pressure and histologic observations. *J Shoulder Elbow Surg* 1997;6:272–285.

Schaefer SL, Ciarelli MJ, Arnoczky SP, et al. Tissue shrinkage with the holmium:yttrium aluminum garnet laser: a postoperative assessment of tissue length, stiffness, and structure. *Am J Sports Med* 1997;25:841–848.

Schulz MM, Lee TQ, Sandusky MD, et al. The healing effects on the biomechanical properties of joint capsular tissue treated with Ho:YAG laser: an in vivo rabbit study. *Arthroscopy* 2001;17:342–347.

Thabit G. Therapeutic heat: a historical perspective. *Oper Tech Sports Med* 1998;6:118–119.

Wall MS, Deng XH, Torzilli PA, et al. Thermal modification of collagen. *J Shoulder Elbow Surg* 1999;8:339–344.

14

Arthroscopic Anterior Shoulder Stabilization Using Knotless Suture Anchors

Raymond Thal

Arthroscopic Bankart repair procedures have been developed in an effort to restore stability to the shoulder, while avoiding some of the morbidity associated with open repair. Most current procedures involve the use of suture anchors and arthroscopic knot tying. However, the quality, consistency, and technical challenges associated with arthroscopic knots are concerning. Satisfactory knot tying requires significant practice and use of special knot-tying devices. Mastering this process can be difficult and time-consuming.

The technical challenges associated with arthroscopic suture anchor repair have led to the development of an alternative method of fixation, the Mitek Knotless Suture Anchor. The metallic Knotless Suture Anchor was released by Mitek Products, Inc. (Norwood, MA) in 1998, with a newer bioabsorbable version, the BioKnotless Suture Anchor, released in 2001.

INDICATIONS

Patients with instability in whom nonoperative intervention has been ineffective are candidates for arthroscopic shoulder stabilization using the knotless anchors. Although this chapter focuses on arthroscopic repair of anterior instability, the technique is useful for posterior and multidirectional instability repairs as well. A contraindication for use of this technique is inadequate capsular tissue to perform an arthroscopic repair, which is uncommon.

PREOPERATIVE PLANNING

Standard preoperative x-ray films should be obtained, including a scapular Y and axillary view. An axillary

view should be included to evaluate the glenoid lip for a large bony Bankart lesion or glenoid rim fracture. A history of documented recurrent dislocations precludes the need for other diagnostic studies unless associated rotator cuff pathology is suspected. When subtle instability or subluxation is suspected, a computed tomographic (CT) arthrogram, magnetic resonance (MR) scan, or gadolinium-enhanced MR scan may be useful in evaluating the glenoid labrum, capsule, and biceps tendon, as well as the rotator cuff.

DESCRIPTION OF THE KNOTLESS AND BIOKNOTLESS SUTURE ANCHORS

The Knotless Suture Anchor (Figure 14.1) consists of a titanium body with two nitenol arcs. The arcs have a memory property that creates resistance to anchor pullout after insertion into a small drill hole. The Knotless Suture Anchor differs structurally from conventional anchors in several ways. A channel or slot is located at the tip of the knotless anchor. A short loop of green, no. 1 Ethibond suture, called the *anchor* loop, is attached to the tail end of the anchor. A second, longer loop of white 2-0 Ethibond suture, called the *utility* loop, is linked to the anchor loop and serves as a passing suture.

The BioKnotless Suture Anchor (Figure 14.2) looks like the Mitek Panalok anchor. The BioKnotless Anchor has a wedge-shaped polylactic acid anchor body with a slot located at the tip. White no. 1 Panacryl suture is used for the anchor loop, and green 2-0 Ethibond suture is used for the utility loop.

With either anchor, the *utility* loop is used to pull the *anchor* loop through the soft tissue to be repaired. The anchor loop is then captured in the channel at the tip of the anchor prior to insertion of the anchor

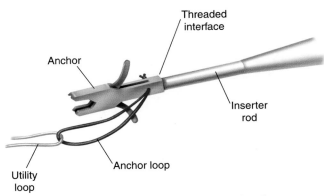

FIGURE 14.1. The Knotless Suture Anchor design.

into bone. The sides of the anchor are flat, to create space for the captured suture loop to pass without abrading the suture.

SURGICAL TECHNIQUE

Patient Setup

Stabilization with Knotless Suture Anchors can be performed with the patient in either the lateral decubitus position or the beach chair position. The author prefers the lateral decubitus position. The shoulder is examined with the patient under anesthesia, testing for instability in 90° of abduction with the application of anterior pressure.

Instrumentation

A standard 4.0 mm arthroscope with 5.5 mm sheath is used for this procedure. An 18-gauge spinal needle is used to initially target the appropriate location for anterior portal placement. Two 5.0 mm disposable cannulas with inflow side ports are used to establish dual anterior portals for ligament and glenoid rim preparation. The anterior-inferior cannula will be replaced with an 8 mm disposable cannula to permit

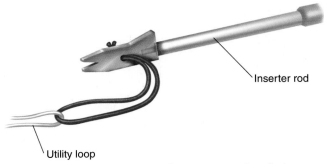

FIGURE 14.2. The BioKnotless Suture Anchor design.

suture passing, and anchor drilling and insertion. Gravity inflow is sufficient and minimizes fluid extravasation, although an arthroscopic pump can be used.

An electrocautery device, a curved 4.5 mm soft tissue suction shaver, and a 5.2 mm suction punch are used for ligament preparation. A high-speed 4.5 mm round burr is used for glenoid rim preparation. A 2.9 mm depth-controlled drill bit (Mitek) is designed for use with the Knotless and BioKnotless Suture anchors. A 3.4 mm suction punch is used for marking the drill hole before anchor insertion.

A variety of instruments are available for arthroscopic suture passage and can be successfully used in passing the utility loop. The author's preferred technique for arthroscopic passage of the utility loop is a suture loop shuttle technique. This technique utilizes the Shutt suture punch (Linvatec, Largo, FL) or the Spectrum suture hooks (Linvatec), and a 2-0 Prolene (Ethicon, Inc. Somerville, NJ) suture loop, 48 in. long, passed through the suture punch. The Prolene suture loop serves as a suture shuttle and is used to pull the utility loop through the anterior inferior glenohumeral ligament. Finally, a small, lightweight mallet is necessary for anchor insertion.

Surgical Technique

Initial arthroscopic visualization is achieved via a standard posterior portal. Dual anterior portals are established for instrumentation. The anterior-inferior portal is placed as close as possible to the superior edge of the subscapularis tendon to allow access to the anterior and inferior aspect of the glenoid rim. The anterior-superior portal is placed in the rotator cuff interval just anterior to the biceps tendon. Inflow is brought through the anterior-superior portal. A thorough arthroscopic evaluation is done, with examination of the articular surfaces, labrum, biceps tendon, rotator cuff, and glenohumeral ligaments.

PREPARATION OF THE ANTERIOR INFERIOR GLENOHUMERAL LIGAMENT AND ANTERIOR GLENOID RIM

Preparation depends upon the pathological lesion that is encountered. Instrumentation is via the anterior-inferior and anterior-superior portals. The exposed labral edge of the Bankart lesion is debrided with a motorized shaver to promote healing. Care is taken to adequately release and mobilize the anterior inferior glenohumeral ligament from the glenoid and underlying subscapularis tendon. When an anterior labroligamentous periosteal sleeve avulsion (ALPSA) lesion is the cause of instability, the periosteum should be incised with an electrocautery device to release the anterior-inferior glenohumeral ligament from the glenoid. This essentially converts an ALPSA lesion to a Bankart lesion.

Associated capsular stretch can be managed in several ways. Complete capsular mobilization, as described earlier, allows for a superior capsular shift that often corrects associated capsular stretch. A variety of capsular plication techniques have been described as well. In the author's experience, capsular plication is rarely needed when the capsule is mobilized adequately and shifted superiorly. When satisfactory tissue quality is present, then a small section of the edge of the detached anterior inferior glenohumeral ligament can be resected using a suction punch to shorten the ligament. The proper amount of anterior inferior glenohumeral ligament to resect is determined by pulling the torn anterior inferior glenohumeral ligament into proximity to the glenoid with an arthroscopic grasper while assessing capsular tension. This is a critical step in the procedure that greatly affects the final outcome and allows for management of capsular stretch by working within the Bankart lesion.

A motorized burr is used to decorticate the anterior glenoid neck from the edge of the articular cartilage medially 1 to 2 cm.

The anterior-inferior cannula then is replaced by a larger 8 mm cannula to accommodate the drill guide, suture passer, and Knotless or BioKnotless Suture Anchors. Three drill holes are created in the anterior glenoid rim, using the Mitek drill guide and the Mitek 2.9 mm arthroscopic superdrill (Figure 14.3). These drill holes are spaced as far apart as possible (1, 3, and 5 o'clock positions on a right shoulder) and at the edge of the articular cartilage. To avoid damage to the articular surface, it is important to direct the drill bit medially, away from the articular surface of the glenoid, by at least a 15° angle. The drill holes are marked with a basket forceps, suction punch, or electrocautery to ease later hole identification for anchor insertion.

KNOTLESS SUTURE ANCHOR REPAIR PROCEDURE

The Mitek Knotless Suture Anchor (Figure 14.1) or BioKnotless Suture Anchor (Figure 14.2) is used to repair the anterior inferior glenohumeral ligament to the glenoid rim. A superior shift of the anterior inferior glenohumeral ligament is also performed.

Prior to implant placement, the utility loop of the knotless suture anchor assembly is passed through the anterior inferior glenohumeral ligament at a selected site via the anterior-inferior portal. This can be achieved by using various arthroscopic suture passing instruments and techniques.

The location of passage of the utility loop and anchor loop through the anterior inferior glenohumeral

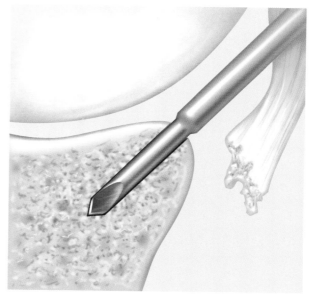

FIGURE 14.3. Three 2.9 mm drill holes are created in the anterior glenoid rim.

ligament is very important. It should be located inferiorly with respect to the glenoid drill hole so that a superior shift of the anterior inferior glenohumeral ligament is achieved when the anchor is inserted into the drill hole. The anchors are inserted in the most inferior site first, progressing to the more superior sites.

SUTURE LOOP SHUTTLE TECHNIQUE FOR ARTHROSCOPIC PASSAGE OF UTILITY LOOP

The author's preferred technique for arthroscopic passage of the utility loop is a suture loop shuttle technique. The use of this technique to pass the utility loop through the ligament at a precise location allows for proper capsule shift. To determine the location for suture loop placement, one grasps the ligament with the suture punch and pulls it superiorly to the drill hole site, while assessing ligament tension (Figure 14.4). A 2-0 Prolene suture loop 48 in. long then is passed through the ligament, using the suture punch. The Prolene suture loop serves as a suture shuttle and is used to pull the utility loop into the anterior-inferior portal, through the anterior inferior glenohumeral ligament, and then out the anterior-superior portal (Figure 14.5).

For the inferior two anchors, pass the utility loop from the intra-articular side of the ligament to the extra-articular side to ease capture of the anchor loop. Pull the utility loop out through the anterior–superior portal to orient the anchor loop at a better angle with

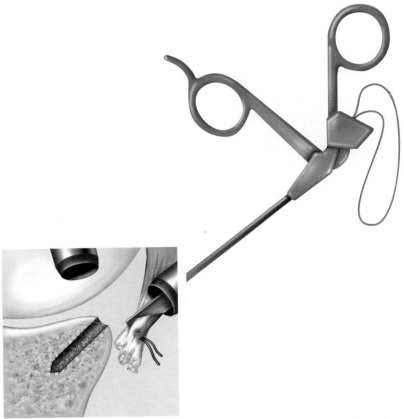

FIGURE 14.4. A suture punch is used to pass a 2-0 Prolene suture loop (purple), 48 in. long, through the ligament.

respect to the anchor and ease loop capture (Figure 14.6).

The utility loop is then used to pull the anchor loop through the anterior inferior glenohumeral ligament. As the utility loop pulls the anchor loop through the anterior inferior glenohumeral ligament, the attached anchor is passed down the anterior-inferior cannula while being controlled on the threaded inserter rod.

Once the anchor loop has passed through the anterior inferior glenohumeral ligament, one strand of the anchor loop is captured or snagged in the channel at the tip of the anchor (Figure 14.7). The anchor then

is inserted and tapped into the glenoid drill hole to the desired depth to achieve appropriate tissue tension (Figure 14.8). This process pulls the anterior inferior glenohumeral ligament to the appropriate position. The anterior inferior glenohumeral ligament shifts superiorly and securely approximates to the glenoid rim. The anchor should not bottom out in the drill hole. The depth of anchor insertion is determined by observing the ligament approximation to the glenoid and by intermittently pulling the utility loop to test the tension of the anchor loop during insertion. Overtensioning can cause the anchor loop to tear through the ligament.

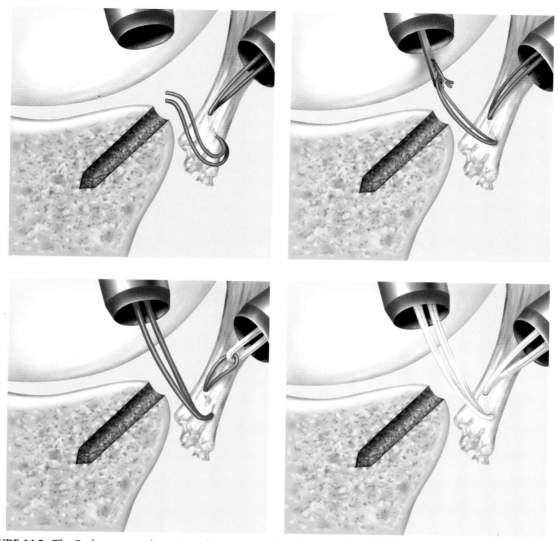

FIGURE 14.5. The Prolene suture loop is used as a suture shuttle to pull the utility loop (white) through the ligament.

The utility loop and inserter rod are removed when repair security is satisfactory. A secure, low-profile repair is achieved, with a superior shift of the anterior inferior glenohumeral ligament (Figure 14.9).

Special attention must be given to the arcs on the *metallic* Knotless Suture Anchor to avoid inadvertent cutting of the anchor loop (Figure 14.10). The anchor is rotated so that the arc that is positioned inside the anchor loop rotates toward the utility loop (Figure 14.11). The utility loop is used to pull the anchor loop over one of the anchor arcs and hold the anchor loop safely away from the arcs during the first stages of anchor insertion. Tension on the anchor loop is relaxed once the arcs have entered the bone.

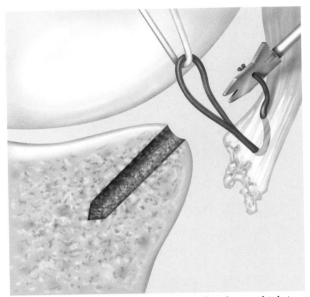

FIGURE 14.6. Tension is applied to the utility loop, which in turn is used to pull the anchor loop through the anterior inferior glenohumeral ligament.

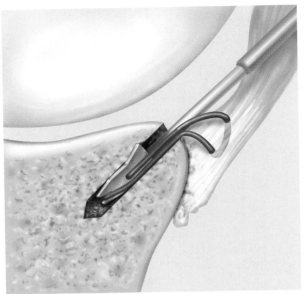

FIGURE 14.8. The anchor is inserted and tapped into the glenoid drill hole to the desired depth to achieve appropriate tissue tension.

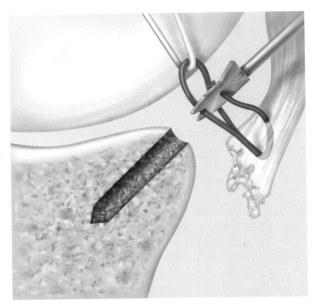

FIGURE 14.7. One suture strand of the anchor loop is captured or snagged in the channel at the tip of the anchor.

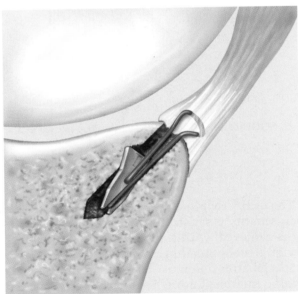

FIGURE 14.9. The utility loop and inserter rod are removed after a secure, low-profile repair has been achieved.

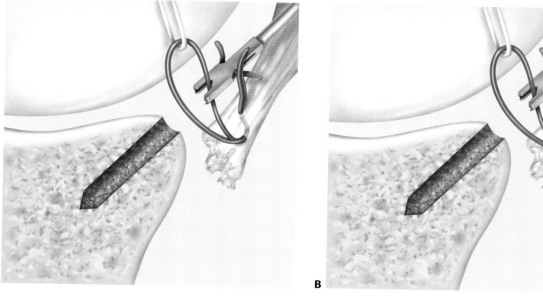

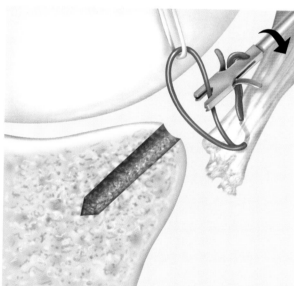

FIGURE 14.10. (A) One anchor arc has not been passed through the anchor loop and will cut the anchor loop when the anchor is inserted into bone. (B,C) The anchor loop is incorrectly wrapped around the anchor.

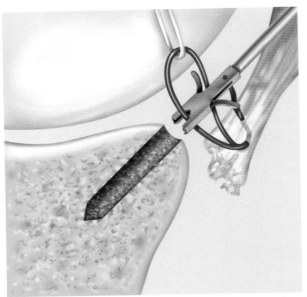

FIGURE 14.11. The anchor has been properly rotated so that the arc that is positioned inside the anchor loop rotates toward the utility loop.

POSTOPERATIVE MANAGEMENT

A sling is used for comfort and protection for the first 4 weeks. During that time, pendulum exercises, passive range-of-motion exercises of the shoulder and elbow, and isometric exercises of the forearm are performed. Active forward flexion with internal rotation is permitted to the forehead level. External rotation is limited to neutral. At 4 weeks postoperatively, progressive active and passive range-of-motion exercises are allowed. External rotation is limited to 45°. In addition, isometric exercises of the deltoid and periscapular muscles are begun. At 6 weeks postoperatively, progression to a full active range of motion is allowed. This program continues until 8 weeks postoperatively, at which time most patients regain normal mobility of the shoulder. At 8 weeks, resistive training with the use of isotonic and isokinetic exercises is performed in a progressive manner. Participation in contact and overhead sports is not allowed until 5 months postoperatively.

RESULTS/OUTCOME

In a prospective evaluation of the first 27 consecutive patients with traumatic anterior instability of the shoulder treated with arthroscopic Bankart repair using the Mitek Knotless Suture Anchor, results at an average 29 months follow-up (range, 24–39 months) were studied.

The study population consisted of 24 males and 3 females with an average age of 28 years (range, 17–59 years). Twelve of the patients were 22 years of age or younger. The dominant shoulder was involved in 18 of the patients (16 right shoulders, 11 left shoulders). The average duration of preoperative symptoms was 66 months (range, 3–192 months). All patients had had an initial traumatic event. All patients had had recurrent instability. Twenty-one patients had had preoperative dislocations (average four dislocations), and six patients had had recurrent subluxations. Five patients underwent repair of a SLAP (superior labrum, anterior and posterior) lesion repair at the time of the Bankart repair.

All the patients reported satisfaction with the surgery. All patients remained stable at the time of follow-up, without feelings of apprehension or episodes of subluxation or dislocation. Twenty patients (74%) regained full range of motion postoperatively. Twenty-five patients (93%) had less than 5° loss of external rotation at 90° of abduction. Two patients had a 10° loss of external rotation at 90° of abduction. The average loss of external rotation was 2°. Average Rowe score was 36 preoperatively and 96 postoperatively. Average score on the American Shoulder and Elbow Surgeons (ASES) form was 62 preoperatively and 94 postoperatively.

One patient (3.8%) experienced a traumatic redislocation 1 year after repair. He was asymptomatic until he fell skiing and dislocated his shoulder. He remains stable after revision arthroscopic Bankart repair using knotless suture anchors.

Previous reports of arthroscopic treatment of anterior inferior glenohumeral instability suggest the need to address capsular laxity with ligament plication or thermal modification in addition to Bankart repair. The success achieved with the current technique suggests that persistent capsular laxity, when present, can be corrected by working within the Bankart lesion. Adequate ligament mobilization and proper ligament repositioning on the glenoid rim are critical. The Knotless Suture Anchor has been shown to provide increased superior capsular shift, compared with a standard suture anchor, as the Knotless Anchor pulls the ligament into the drill hole. This action can address and correct any residual capsular laxity.

Several factors are thought to contribute to the success of the described technique for arthroscopic Bankart repair. Meticulous attention was given to ligament preparation and repositioning of the ligament on the glenoid rim. Secure, consistent suture anchor fixation is achieved arthroscopically using the Knotless Suture Anchor. Increased superior capsular shift can be achieved to address capsular stretch. The procedure is simplified by the elimination of arthroscopic knot tying. The Knotless Suture Anchor fixation eliminates the potential weakness associated with the arthroscopic knots required with the use of standard suture anchors.

COMPLICATIONS

Several anchor loop configurations should be avoided when the metallic Knotless Suture Anchor is used because they can lead to anchor loop breakage. One arc must be passed through the anchor loop before anchor insertion. If this is not done, the anchor loop will be cut on insertion into bone (Figure 14.10A). The anchor loop must pass directly from the base of the anchor into the ligament. If, instead, the anchor loop is allowed to wrap around the body of the anchor, then the anchor loop will be at risk of being cut by the closing anchor arc as the anchor is inserted into bone (Figure 14.10B,C).

From 1998 to 2000, the author inserted 367 Knotless Suture Anchors in 129 patients for various soft tissue-to-bone repairs, including the insertion of 196 anchors in 61 Bankart repairs. Three anchor loops were broken during this time. Two of these three broken anchor loops occurred in the first three Bankart repairs performed, before the importance of proper anchor loop position was recognized. Review of the videotape of these broken anchor loops revealed that the anchor loop was allowed to wrap around the base of the anchor and was cut by the closing anchor arc on insertion into the bone. Repair was successfully achieved by stacking another Knotless Anchor into the same drill hole in each case. Subsequent anchor loop breakage was prevented by attention to proper anchor loop position.

At the time of publication, anchor loop breakage has not occurred in the author's initial experience with the BioKnotless Suture Anchor after insertion of 266 anchors in 94 patients.

Recommended Reading

Benedetto KP, Glotzer W. Arthroscopic Bankart procedure by suture technique: indications, technique, and results. *Arthroscopy* 1992;8:111–115.

Neviaser TJ. The anterior labroligmentous periosteal sleeve avulsion lesion: a cause of anterior instability of the shoulder. *Arthroscopy* 1993;9:17–21.

Thal R. A Knotless Suture Anchor: technique for use in arthroscopic Bankart repair. *Arthroscopy* 2001;17(2):213–218.

Thal R. Knotless Suture Anchor. Arthroscopic Bankart repair without tying knots. *Clin Orthop* 2001;390:42–51.

Thal R. A Knotless Suture Anchor: design, function, and biomechanical testing. *Am J Sports Med* 2001;29(5):646–649.

Thal R. Arthroscopic anterior stabilization of the shoulder with a Knotless Suture anchor: technique and results. *Am J Sports Med* In Press

SECTION FIVE

Stiffness

15

Arthroscopic Treatment of the Stiff or Frozen Shoulder

Kevin L. Smith

Stiff or frozen shoulders are a relatively common problem in the general orthopedic practice. Unfortunately, they can pose a considerably frustrating condition for both the patient and the treating physician. Although reported to be self-limiting, frozen shoulders may take several years to "thaw." Posttraumatic or postsurgical stiff shoulders may pose an even greater therapeutic challenge.

The stiff or frozen shoulder is classified into one of four etiologies: idiopathic frozen shoulder, diabetic frozen shoulder, posttraumatic stiff shoulder, or postsurgical stiff shoulder. Full motion of the shoulder depends upon the scapulothoracic articulation, intracapsular structures, and extracapsular structures. In managing a stiff shoulder, therefore, it is important to consider all the affected areas. Primarily this involves the capsuloligamentous structures and intra-articular scarring; but extra-articular adhesions in the subacromial or humeroscapular motion interface, often seen in the posttraumatic and postsurgical stiff shoulders, must be considered, as well.

Surgery is best reserved for the most severe and recalcitrant cases. Arthroscopic release offers the considerable advantage of restoring motion without violating muscle or tendon origins, usually necessary in open releases. It is, however, a technically demanding procedure and requires substantial experience in arthroscopic shoulder surgery.

INDICATIONS/CONTRAINDICATIONS

The mainstay of treatment for the stiff or frozen shoulder is conservative and includes nonsteroidal anti-inflammatory drugs, physical therapy, intra-articular corticosteroid injections, and alternative modalities. If these fail to restore sufficient comfort, motion, and function within a reasonable period of time, manipulation under anesthesia and arthroscopic or open release of the shoulder may be considered.

Perhaps the only absolute contraindication is an active reflex sympathetic dystrophy or some other type of pain syndrome that might be worsened by surgical intervention. (Degenerative arthritis may be worsened following capsular release and is a relative contraindication.)

PREOPERATIVE PLANNING

In the patient with frozen shoulder, preoperative studies other than x-rays are rarely necessary. The postinjury or postoperative shoulder may require more complex imaging studies, including additional x-ray views or CT scan.

Perhaps the most important component of the preoperative exam is motion assessment. Active and passive motion must be assessed for both shoulders. Range is evaluated in forward flexion, elevation (plane of the scapula), abduction (coronal plane), external rotation (at the side and in abduction), internal rotation (spinal level) and cross-body adduction (distance from antecubital fossa to coracoid process). This critical assessment is repeated under anesthetic before and after manipulation and will help determine which structures require surgical attention. For example, restriction in external rotation usually reflects anterior soft tissue tightness, specifically in the rotator internal and anterior capsule. Abduction limitation is usually due to axillary pouch pathology. Restriction in cross-body adduction and internal rotation reflects posterior capsular tightness.

SURGICAL TECHNIQUE

Positioning/Setup

The procedure can be accomplished in either the beach chair or the lateral decubitus position. The author prefers beach chair positioning, with its familiar anatomical setting and relatively easy conversion to open approaches if necessary. Patients are placed on the operating table and are adequately secured and

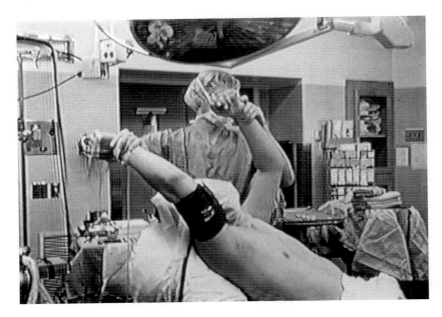

FIGURE 15.1. Preoperative range of motion is measured and compared with the contralateral side.

padded, protecting all bony prominences and neurovascular structures. It is important to allow for plenty of access to both the front and the back of the shoulder for arthroscopic instrumentation. After this, anesthesia may be given. We prefer an interscalene or regional block to allow for an early, painless, aggressive range of motion postoperatively. Upon attaining satisfactory anesthesia, range of motion of both the affected and unaffected shoulders is measured in all directions, and the results are recorded (Figure 15.1). Next, a gentle manipulation under anesthesia may be attempted. If full motion (matching that of the opposite side) is obtained, we usually stop at this point unless the patient is diabetic. If the manipulation fails to restore normal range of motion, we proceed with an arthroscopic capsular release.

Instrumentation

The procedure can be undertaken with traditional arthroscopic instrumentation, including a 4 mm arthroscope, 5 mm cannulas, and standard tools. For the release itself, we prefer a 4.5 mm synovial resector blade as well as basket forceps of multiple angles and sizes. We prefer blunt-tapped capsular release basket forceps especially designed for this purpose (Figure 15.2). Incision of the capsuloligamentous complex can be accomplished in a number of ways, including a shaver blade, electrocautery, bipolar, or arthroscopic basket/scissors.

It is important to use a cannula system that allows for easy switching of the camera and the working instruments from front to back and vice versa. While

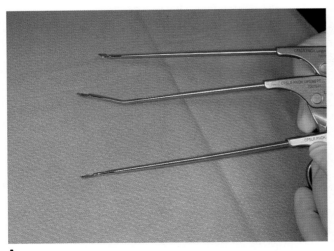

A

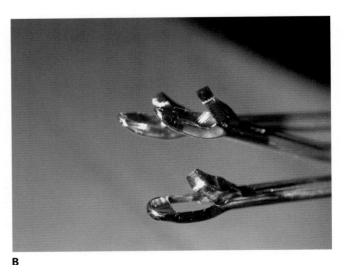

B

FIGURE 15.2. (A) Overview (Photograph courtesy of Smith & Nephew Dynonics.) and (B) close-up view of blunt-tipped capsular release forceps.

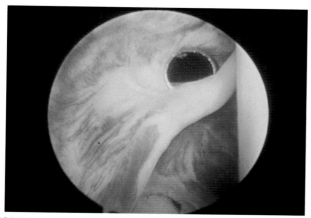

FIGURE 15.3. Intra-articular synovitis and adhesions are commonly seen initially (scope posterior, right shoulder, beach chair position).

the procedure can be done under gravity inflow, we prefer an arthroscopic pump for distension and hemostasis. However, as the capsule is progressively released, one needs to pay attention to fluid extravasation to limit overall shoulder swelling. Cautery is necessary in the uncommon cases in which excessive bleeding is encountered.

Surgical Technique

Landmarks are drawn out, including the clavicle, acromion, spine of the scapula, and coracoid process. This step is especially important given the potential for swelling, which may hinder the ability to palpate these landmarks and make appropriate portals later.

Initially, a posterosuperior portal is made in a standard fashion, approximately 1 cm below the spine of the scapula. Note that a thickened capsule can be dif-

ficult to penetrate and may require a conical obturator tip. Be careful not to violate the weakened osseous structures.

With the scope posterior, the shoulder is copiously irrigated with normal saline plus epinephrine. The joint is commonly quite inflamed, with extensive synovitis and/or adhesions (Figure 15.3). An antero-superior portal is made through the rotator interval at or above the level of the biceps tendon. This is done via an inside-out technique using a Wissinger rod, although an outside-in technique may be used as well. We have found that releasing the anterior structures first leads to a bit more swelling than is desirable. Therefore, we prefer to switch and view from the front, using the posterior portal as our initial working portal. We then release the entire posterior capsule, beginning with the posterosuperior capsule, continuing posteroinferiorly as far as possible, staying within 1 cm of the labrum, but being careful not to remove it (Figure 15.4). We incise the capsule, using the blunt-tipped broad basket forceps to first "channel" a space between the capsule and underlying extra-articular soft tissues, and then advance with the basket down the capsule, releasing it progressively. We prefer this broad basket instrument to remove a swath of tissue, although after the capsule and ligaments have been released, a shaver blade can accomplish the same task.

After the entire posterior capsule has been released, and/or if surgery becomes difficult, we will switch and release the anterior aspect of the shoulder while viewing from the back (Figure 15.5). We progressively incise the rotator interval, the superior glenohumeral ligament, the middle glenohumeral ligament, and the inferior glenohumeral ligament as far as is safely possible. The subscapularis is left intact, but all soft tissue, scar, and capsuloligamentous complex on the intra-articular aspect are excised, once again removing

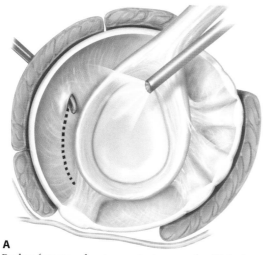

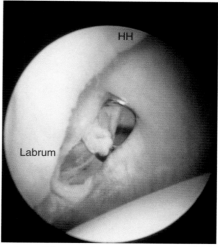

A   **B**

FIGURE 15.4. (A) Basket forceps releasing posterior capsule. (B) Arthroscopic view with scope in anterior portal, right shoulder, basket beginning posterior capsular release (beach chair position): HH, humeral head.

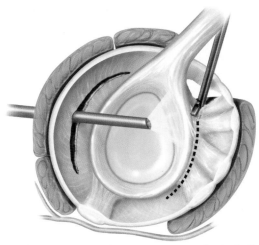

FIGURE 15.5. Structures to be released anteriorly, including rotator interval and superior, middle, and inferior glenohumeral ligaments.

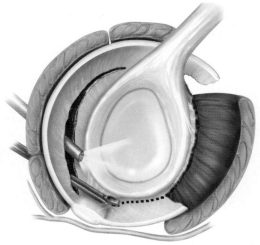

FIGURE 15.7. Inferior capsular release: note proximity of axillary nerve, approximately 1 cm inferior to glenoid.

a swath of tissue if possible. When adequately released, muscle fibers of the subscapularis should be easily visible along the glenoid rim's length (Figure 15.6). Inferiorly, one must remember that the axillary nerve is nearby, particularly in the posttraumatic or postsurgical situation, where scar tissue may make it somewhat adherent. The nerve may be encountered anteriorly at the inferior border of the subscapularis, as well as posteriorly just below the capsule, usually about 1 cm from the glenoid rim (Figure 15.7). Some advocate actually visualizing the nerve, though we do not do so routinely. Regardless, it is important to be careful in this area and to stay close to the glenoid rim, particularly when using heat or releasing blindly.

Upon completion of the anterior and posterior capsular release, we will then ensure that the inferior extents of the release are completed, using the already established portals, or making accessory portals about

1 to 2 cm inferiorly. The inferior extent of the capsular release is completed along the inferior axilla. Others advocate releasing anteriorly and posteriorly but manipulating the remaining inferior capsule owing to the risk of axillary nerve injury.

A complete arthroscopic capsular release can be done with two to four portals as needed. After releasing all or most of the capsular and ligamentous structures, we characteristically obtain a "drive-through" sign and inferior subluxation of the humeral head on the glenoid. After a complete release, we then use a shaver blade to trim back the cut edges, leaving a broad gap that is slow to heal (Figure 15.8). If adequate release of the entire capsule cannot be accomplished, the addition of a limited open approach, to incise any tissue that was difficult to visualize and/or safely release arthroscopically, must be considered.

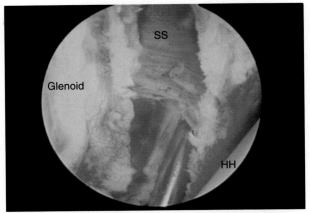

FIGURE 15.6. Arthroscopic view from posterior portal (beach chair position, right shoulder), demonstrating adequacy of anterior capsule release with visible muscle fibers of subscapularis muscle (SS): HH, humeral head.

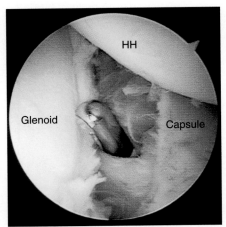

FIGURE 15.8. An arthroscopic shaver is used to trim the released capsule. (View from posterior portal, right shoulder, beach chair position): HH, humeral head.

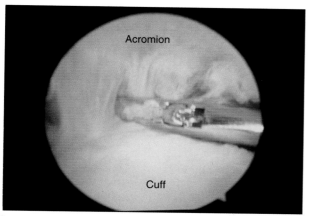

FIGURE 15.9. Subacromial adhesions must be released in posttraumatic and postsurgical stiff shoulders. (View from posterior portal, right shoulder beach chair, basket entering through lateral portal.)

Finally, in the postsurgical or posttraumatic situation, extracapsular scar tissue must be addressed as well. Thus, a complete release of the inside of the joint must be combined with adhesiolysis of subacromial–humeroscapular motion interface structures if necessary (Figure 15.9). This can be done arthroscopically or by open surgery. After as many impediments to motion as possible have been removed, a final, gentle manipulation is done to release any other soft tissue adhesions. Prior to removing the arthroscopic instruments, we generally place an intra-articular cortisone injection to slow the healing process and minimize early postoperative pain and inflammation. Arthroscopic portals are then closed with simple sutures and an absorbent dressing is applied.

POSTOPERATIVE MANAGEMENT

The procedure can be done on an inpatient or outpatient basis, but we prefer a short overnight stay. We place our patients in a simple, continuous passive motion machine in the recovery room, utilizing a limited arc of motion solely to keep things moving and to minimize spasms (Figure 15.10). Patients are given analgesics and anti-inflammatories postoperatively per protocol. We generally remanipulate the shoulder several hours postoperatively, after the swelling has dissipated, and record our postoperative range, comparing it with the preoperative motion. In addition, our therapist sees each patient later on the day of surgery as well as the next morning. Patients are instructed in a home stretching program, emphasizing aggressive range-of-motion exercises in all directions, to be done in the home five times per day, in addition to supplemental physical therapy as needed (Figure 15.11).

We encourage resumption of simple activities of daily living almost immediately, but avoid any strengthening or aggressive use. Basically, we recommend rest and stretching for 6 to 8 weeks while the shoulder heals, and then allow the slow, progressive resumption of activities as tolerated. Occasionally, during the initial 6- to 8-week postoperative period, patients begin to note a slight increase in pain and/or a downturn in flexibility. When this occurs, we generally take the patient back to the operating room for a gentle manipulation under anesthesia and repeat intra-articular cortisone injection in hope of boosting the situation and getting the patient back on track.

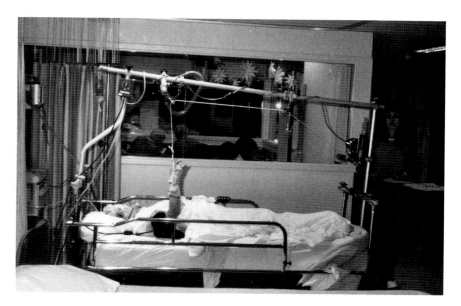

FIGURE 15.10. A continuous passive motion machine can be helpful initially to maintain motion.

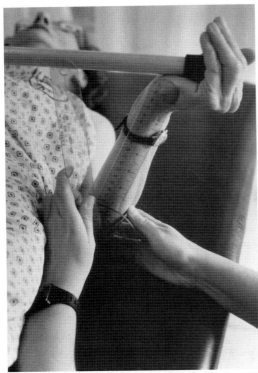

FIGURE 15.11. Regular patient-administered stretching is critical postoperatively.

RESULTS/OUTCOME

The results of arthroscopic release for stiff, recalcitrant shoulders have been quite good, though treating this condition remains a challenging problem. Success appears to depend largely on the diagnosis and the degree of stiffness. Diabetic frozen shoulders are perhaps the most difficult to manage. They are often the stiffest and are the most frequent to recur and/or cause continued pain. Indeed, some of the symptoms and difficulties of these patients may be related to neuropathy and other complicating factors associated with their disease. Early degenerative changes can diminish results as well.

COMPLICATIONS

Postoperative problems are relatively uncommon, although they can be severe. Routine complications as with any arthroscopic procedure include infection and other wound issues, blood loss, and nerve damage, particularly the axillary nerve because of its proximity to the inferior capsule. In addition, residual or recurrent stiffness is possible, and this occurs more frequently than other potential problems. Instability is a theoretical complication, though it has been noted only rarely in the literature. Finally, intraoperative fracture resulting from overzealous manipulation of osteopenic bone and late degenerative arthritis due to difficulties with arthroscopy may also occur.

Recommended Reading

Binder AI, Bulgen DY, Hazleman BL, Roberts S. Frozen shoulder: a long-term prospective study. *Ann Rheum Dis* 1984;43(3):361–364.

DePalma, AF. Loss of scapulohumeral motion (frozen shoulder). *Ann Surg* 1952;135:193.

Fisher L, Kurtz A, Shipley M. Association between cheiroarthropathy and frozen shoulder in patients with insulin dependent diabetes mellitus. *Br J Rheumatol* 1986;25:141–146.

Grey RG. The natural history of "idiopathic" frozen shoulder. *J Bone Joint Surg Am* 1978;60(4):564.

Harryman DT II. Arthroscopic management of the stiff shoulder: *Oper Tech Sports Med* 1997;5(4):264–274.

Harryman DT II, Matsen FA III, Sidles JA. Arthroscopic management of refractory shoulder stiffness. *Arthroscopy* 1997;13(2):133–147.

Harryman DT II, Lazarus MD, Rozencwaig R. The stiff shoulder. In: Rockwood CA, Matsen FA III, eds. *The Shoulder.* 2nd ed. Philadelphia; WB Saunders, 1998:1064–1112.

Helbig B, Wagner P, Dohler R. Mobilization of frozen shoulder under general anesthesia. *Acta Orthop Belg* 1983;49(1–2):267–274.

Kieras DM, Matsen FA III. Open release in the management of refractory frozen shoulder. *Orthop Trans* 1991;15(3):801–802.

Janda DH, Hawkins RJ. Shoulder manipulation in patients with adhesive capsulitis and diabetes mellitus: a clinical note. *J Shoulder Elbow Surg* 1993;2(1):36–38.

Lundberg BJ. The frozen shoulder. *Acta Orthop Scand* [suppl] 1969;119:1–59.

McLaughlin HL. On the frozen shoulder. *Bull Hosp Joint Dis* 1951;12:383–393.

Murnaghan GF, McIntosh D. Hydrocortisone in painful shoulder—a controlled trial. *Lancet* 1955;2:798.

Neviaser JS. Adhesive capsulitis of the shoulder. *J Bone Joint Surg* 1945;27:211–222.

Ogilvie HDJ, Biggs DJ, Fitsialos DP, MacKay M. The resistant frozen shoulder. Manipulation versus arthroscopic release. *Clin Orthop* 1995;319:238–248.

Ozaki J, Nakagawa Y, Sakurai G, Tamai S. Recalcitrant chronic adhesive capsulitis of the shoulder. *J Bone Joint Surg Am* 1990;71:1511–1515.

Pollock RG, Duralde XA, Flatow EL, Bigliani LU. The use of arthroscopy in the treatment of resistant frozen shoulder. *Clin Orthop* 1994;304:30–36.

Reeves B. The natural history of the frozen shoulder syndrome. *Scand J Rheum* 1976;4:193–196.

Shaffer B, Tibone JE, Kerlan RK. Frozen shoulder. A long-term follow-up. *J Bone Joint Surg Am* 1992;74(5):738–746.

Warner JJP, Allen A, Marks P, Wong P. Arthroscopic release of chronic, refractory capsular contracture of the shoulder. *J Shoulder Elbow Surg* 1995;5(2, pt 2):S7.

Wiley AM. Arthroscopic appearance of frozen shoulder. *Arthroscopy* 1991;7(2):138–143.

Subacromial Pathology and Rotator Cuff Tears

16

Arthroscopic Subacromial Decompression

James P. Tasto

Arthroscopic subacromial decompression (ASAD), modified from the open technique first described by Neer, is the procedure of choice for treating chronic shoulder impingement syndrome unresponsive to conservative care. Most of the current literature supports the value of arthroscopic over the conventional open technique and, in particular, for revision.

Advantages of the arthroscopic approach include complete evaluation of the glenohumeral joint and associated structures, ability to address other pathology, minimally invasive surgery without deltoid detachment and injury, and an earlier and more comfortable postoperative recovery.

INDICATIONS/CONTRAINDICATIONS

The indications for ASAD are basically the same that have classically been described for the open approach. A trial of nonoperative care is an absolute necessity before surgical intervention is considered. The majority of patients with impingement syndrome can be managed conservatively, and well over two-thirds of these patients should have a satisfactory result if there is no rotator cuff tear present. The nonoperative treatment program should consist of formal physical therapy or a home program, nonsteroidal anti-inflammatories, occasional judicious use of steroid injections in the subacromial space, and activity modification. Surgical intervention should not be entertained before a minimum of 6 months of conservative treatment. A prolonged history of symptoms, however, has been described as a predictor of a worse outcome. Other factors that may adversely influence outcome, and should therefore be considered in the evaluation of a patient for surgery, include diffuse calcific deposits, age under 20 and over 40, and an increased acromial angle.

One of the major contraindications to performing an ASAD is the presence of restricted motion. This problem is often unrecognized or overlooked, and when this happens, the outcome is almost universally a prolonged recovery or a poor result. The diagnosis of an impingement syndrome cannot be made in the presence of restricted motion because of the many complicating factors that are present, mimicking impingement. In fact, most patients with impingement (and even cuff tears) have little measurable restriction. The presence of such restriction warrants caution in presuming a diagnosis of impingement and may in fact reflect inflammatory and/or adhesive capsulitis. Suffice it to say that these patients invariably represent poor candidates for subacromial decompression.

Another contraindication to this procedure is secondary impingement due to underlying primary shoulder instability. This is a typical problem in the young overhead athlete and as such is seen in the throwing population or among swimmers (often bilateral "impingement"). The underlying instability issue obviously needs to be identified and addressed either conservatively or surgically. Not surprisingly, results of performing an ASAD in patients with underlying instability have been universally poor.

Some relative contraindications, or at least factors that should be considered as having a negative influence on outcome, include generalized hypermobility, a prolonged history of impingement or shoulder pain, diabetes, and a history of adhesive capsulitis. One must also differentiate between classic subacromial impingement and subcoracoid impingement. Patients with rotator cuff tears and os acromiale are also poor candidates for isolated subacromial decompression.

PREOPERATIVE PLANNING

In general, the preoperative evaluation (history and physical) continues to be the most accurate method of validating a diagnosis of subacromial impingement. The patient's history will usually consist of discomfort with overhead activity, lifting, reaching, or throwing a ball, and usually there will have been no associated traumatic event. The patient's age is most often in the range of 30 to 50. Pain usually occurs when the patient is reaching in the back of a car, serving a tennis ball, or doing some repetitive overhead work. The pain occurs over the anterolateral aspect of the shoulder. Patients often complain of pain radiating down to the deltoid insertion.

The physical exam should include evaluation for rotator cuff pathology, acromioclavicular (AC) joint involvement, instability, and cervical spine disorders. There are a number of specific tests for validating the impingement syndrome, most commonly the impingement signs described by Neer and Hawkins. Asking the patient to place the arm and shoulder into the provocative position that replicates the symptoms can be valuable.

Plain x-ray films are of great value and are necessary in gaining additional information. The traditional views that provide the most information are an anterior-posterior and internal rotation view of the shoulder, an outlet "Y" view, an axillary lateral, and a 15° cephalic of the AC joint. It is critical to evaluate acromial morphology and thickness, the presence of degenerative glenohumeral joint changes (best seen on the axillary film), the presence or absence of an os acromiale (also best seen with the axillary projection), and disease of the AC joint. Acromial morphology has been classified by Bigliani and is a useful exercise in preoperative planning (Figure 16.1).

Magnetic resonance image (MRI) scans have been very helpful in assessing rotator cuff pathology. However, I do not rely on MRI studies to validate the presence or absence of an impingement syndrome; this remains a clinical diagnosis. The MRI exam, when indicated, is helpful in ascertaining the extent of rotator cuff pathology for preoperative planning, and in describing to the patient the magnitude of the procedure that may be needed. It may also uncover other unexpected pathology. As a general rule, MRI data should *corroborate* the clinical picture rather than play an important role in *establishing* the diagnosis.

Differential injections may be of great help in ascertaining and validating the diagnosis of impingement syndrome. Injections can be either intra-articu-

lar (glenohumeral or AC joint), or subacromial. The most common indication for selective injection involves differentiating subacromial from AC joint pain. Injections may also be used in the biceps tendon sheath and at other soft tissue trigger point locations. These injections may or may not contain a steroid in conjunction with the local anesthetic. Any injection that includes a steroid should be given at a separate appointment, to facilitate evaluating both immediate and short-term effects.

SURGICAL TECHNIQUE

Positioning/SetUp

The ASAD procedure has been performed in the lateral decubitus position at our institution for the past 18 years. Advantages include avoiding the risks of a beach chair position, particularly in the elderly, and the absence of a requirement for assistance in a routine arthroscopic subacromial decompression. Arm position can be changed intermittently depending upon what portion of the shoulder is being approached. If necessary, conversion to an open procedure can be easily accomplished from the lateral decubitus position without prepping and draping again.

The patient is placed at a 60° angle to the floor (torso rolled "back" approximately 30° from true perpendicular) using an axillary roll, kidney rests, and a beanbag. If one starts at 90°, oftentimes the shoulder tends to fall away from the surgeon. Care is taken to appropriately pad the down leg and hip and to protect the peroneal nerve, as well as to place pillows between the hips and legs in an abducted position. Care is taken to protect the patient's head and to maintain a neutral head and cervical spine axis, to prevent undue traction or pressure on the brachial plexus when the arm is suspended. When traction is applied to the shoulder, the shoulder girdle and extremity generally assume the position that is perpendicular to the floor (Figure 16.2).

When the decubitus position is chosen, approximately 10 to 12 lb of traction is applied, and the patient's arm is placed in approximately 30° of abduction and 20° of forward flexion. Weight may be modified depending on the patient's size, but in general we do not refer to this as traction but "suspension" of the extremity. If the beach chair position is chosen by the surgeon, appropriate care needs to be taken to establish a stable head and neck support, and to protect against the extremes of head/neck rotation to avoid undue brachial plexus strain.

The anesthesiologist and his equipment is placed at either 60 or 90° perpendicular to the long axis of

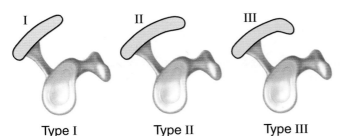

I   II   III

Type I   Type II   Type III

FIGURE 16.1. Classification of acromial morphology, as described by Bigliani.

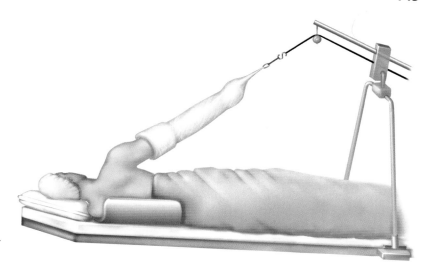

FIGURE 16.2. Patient positioning in the lateral decubitus position.

the patient to allow the surgeon appropriate working room to access all portals about the shoulder joint.

Instrumentation

Conventional arthroscopic equipment includes a 4.5 mm, 30° wide-angle arthroscope, appropriate cannulas, and an optical system for viewing. Our preference is to utilize the 30° arthroscope throughout the entire operation, and it is rare that a 70° arthroscope is necessary, but when visualization of the AC joint is difficult, as it sometimes is, one may chose to use the 70° lens. It is always helpful to have spare arthroscopes (30 and 70°) sterilized and ready to use if necessary.

A motorized shaver and burr are utilized, and these vary between 3.5 and 4.5 mm in diameter depending upon the area that is being treated. An Incisor (Smith & Nephew Dyonics, Andover, MA) or a full-radius blade may be used; my personal preference is to use the 3.5 mm rather than the 4.5 mm shaver because the fluid dynamics are more favorable with a smaller diameter device. It is necessary to have a high torque, high-speed bone-cutting instrument, and there are many to choose from in the marketplace. Our personal preference is a HeliCut blade (Smith & Nephew Dyonics), which allows a more precise bony resection and avoids some of the irregular skipping concavities one may encounter with a conventional round burr.

A pump is used in all of our arthroscopy work, and it is probably more important in subacromial decompression than in any other shoulder procedure. The pump permits control of both pressure and flow. With the use of some arthroscopic pumps, the surgeon can maintain flow and pressure independently, changing both readily and rapidly. Accurate sensor pressure

measurement is valuable in preventing swelling that can occur during this procedure.

Radiofrequency, which has been a great addition to our specialized surgical instruments, allows us to ablate and vaporize tissue very rapidly, as well as to identify bony landmarks and control bleeding with the same instrument. I prefer to use a bipolar radiofrequency device so that the procedure can be done in saline, with conductivity limited to the specific area that is being surgically addressed and with control over the depth of penetration. We have used the ArthroWand (Arthrocare Corp., Sunnyvale, CA) for the past five years. The procedure is done with normal saline, but with 1 ampule of 1:100,000 units of epinephrine in each 3 liter bag.

Surgical Procedure

The patient is given either a general anesthetic or an interscalene block, depending upon the surgeon's preference. We have done the majority of these procedures under general anesthesia. To avoid complications with regional anesthesia, it is critical that the anesthesiologist have extensive experience. We generally ask the anesthesiologist to keep the systolic blood pressure at approximately 95 mmHg pressure unless there is a medical contraindication.

An examination under anesthesia is carried out with the patient in the lateral decubitus position, which is particularly useful in detecting any signs of occult instability or palpable/audible signs of labral disruption. The shoulder is prepped and draped, and the traction/suspension apparatus is connected.

The osseous landmarks about the shoulder are clearly delineated with a marking pencil. This aids in establishing portals later on in the procedure when swelling can otherwise interfere with one's ability to palpate osseous landmarks. The acromion, clavicle, and AC joint are clearly delineated.

The portal sites are not injected. A posterior portal is chosen at the soft spot approximately 1.5 cm inferior and 1.5 cm medial to the posterolateral corner of the acromion. The arthroscope is placed directly into the glenohumeral joint, and a complete diagnostic arthroscopy is carried out. Initially, unless one has a triple-stopcock sheath, an anterior portal is established with a 14-gauge angiocatheter to allow for inflow and outflow. This avoids making a large rent in the rotator interval if no glenohumeral pathology is encountered. If an anterior portal is necessary, it is then established with an inside-out technique through the rotator interval. Any glenohumeral surgery that is felt to be necessary is carried out at this time. Following this, one withdraws the cannula and arthroscope and, through the same posterior incision, redirects the arthroscope sheath with blunt obturator into the subacromial space.

The cannula and blunt obturator are then passed directly through to the anterior portal (if previously established), and a cannula of appropriate size is placed over the obturator and brought back into the subacromial space. Flow is started immediately, with the cannula and the arthroscope in close proximity to each other, to establish appropriate flow and visualization.

At this stage, one can place a full-radius blade or an incisor blade through the anterior cannula and debride some of the bursa if necessary, to achieve better visualization. We establish our lateral portal immediately, keeping the outflow cannula patent. Our lateral portal is established almost directly in line with the anterior border of the acromion. If one were to err, one would like to err 1 or 2 mm posteriorly. The portal is located approximately 1 to 1.5 cm inferior to the lateral border of the acromion (Figure 16.3). We have chosen a portal laterally that places us parallel with the acromial undersurface and directly in line with the anterior portion of the acromion to be resected. If one deviates too far anterior or posterior, there is great risk for cutting the anterior acromial prominence on a bias cut and thereby not replicating what is done in the open procedure. The lateral portal is a critical portal, and if it does seem to be so misplaced that a precise cut is not being obtained, one should not hesitate to make an alternative portal. After the portal has been made, a bright orange trocar is inserted to facilitate optical identification. Clear visualization is quite necessary at this stage of the procedure to prevent excessive extravasation (Figure 16.4). Once the orange cannula can be visualized, one can proceed with shaver placement and perform a bursectomy. The scope is oriented such that the acromion is superior and the cuff inferior throughout.

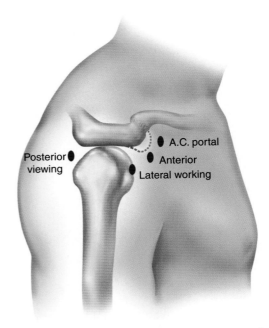

FIGURE 16.3. Scope portal locations used in subacromial decompressions.

Adequate flow and pressure must be maintained throughout the procedure. Delays in instrumentation or interruption of flow can lead to a swollen shoulder that will make the rest of the procedure much more difficult. A partial bursectomy is carried out with a conventional shaver until one can visualize the rotator cuff inferiorly and the coracoacromial (CA) ligament superiorly (Figure 16.5). To avoid bleeding, we complete the bursectomy *after* the ASAD. We then place a Covac (Arthrocare Corp., Sunnyvale, CA) bipolar radiofrequency device through the lateral portal. This bipolar unit allows us to ablate the periosteum, fascia, and CA ligament, while simultaneously suctioning out bubbles and debris. The soft tissue is re-

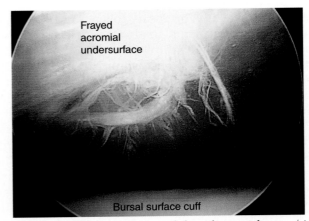

FIGURE 16.4. Arthroscopic view of the subacromial space (right shoulder, beach chair perspective).

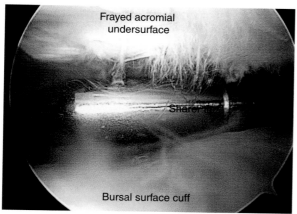

FIGURE 16.5. A shaver removing the subacromial bursa from the lateral scope portal (right shoulder, beach chair perspective).

moved from the anterior third of the acromion (Figure 16.6). This unit also allows us to simultaneously coagulate bleeders as they are encountered.

If a conventional ASAD is going to be carried out, we choose to subperiosteally dissect the CA ligament off the acromion and do not attempt to ablate it completely. If this subperiosteal dissection is carried out appropriately, the acromial branch of the thoracromial artery usually can be avoided. If this artery is encountered, however, one should immediately switch to coagulation, dampen the portals, stop the outflow to reduce turbulence, and coagulate. This technique can be used throughout the surgery if bleeding is encountered. Excessive inflow, outflow, and turbulence will make visualization much more difficult.

If one is not going to be doing an arthroscopic Mumford, we suggest trying not to violate the adventitia, fatty tissue, and synovium in juxtaposition to and immediately inferior to the AC joint. Cutting in this highly vascularized area usually causes unneces-

sary and sometimes troublesome bleeding. If we are not doing an AC resection, we attempt to keep as much integrity of the AC joint's inferior capsule as possible when planing the acromion and resecting the anterior edge. We do not coplane the AC joint, for fear of creating patholaxity and destabilization, or creating a symptomatic AC joint. Once the fascia and periosteum have been removed and the bony landmarks have been clearly delineated, particularly on the anterior and the anterolateral third of the acromion, we place the shaver blade in to remove debris and to get full visualization of the rotator cuff. A thorough examination of the rotator cuff's bursal surface is critical to determine the presence of cuff pathology such as partial or complete tears.

The entire procedure is performed while visualizing through the posterior portal. If we are only doing an ASAD, the anterior portal is used for outflow and the lateral portal is our working portal throughout. We do not employ a cutting block technique, which has the potential of inadequate or excessive bone resection and is somewhat dependent on posterior acromial morphology (Figure 16.7).

The most critical portion of this operation is adequate resection of the anterior and anterolateral components of the acromion. The amount resected depends upon preoperative imaging (acromial morphology and structures based on the "outlet" views obtained preoperatively) and intraoperative visualization. The anterolateral corner must be exposed to prevent inadequate resections. This is the site at which most contact pressure is applied to the rotator cuff

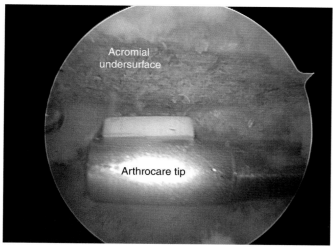

FIGURE 16.6. A bipolar device ablating the periosteum and fascia from the acromion (View from right shoulder, beach chair perspective).

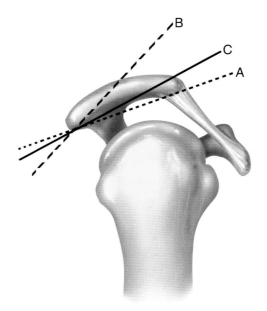

FIGURE 16.7. Cutting block technique may be inadequate (plane A) or may result in excessive bone resection (plane B). Plane C shows optimal resection.

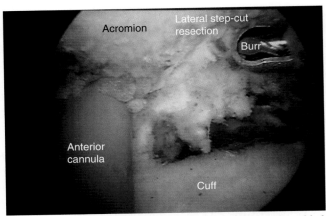

FIGURE 16.8. Creating the anterolateral notch with a Helicut blade rotator cuff. (View from right shoulder, beach chair perspective.)

during forward elevation, abduction, and most functional positions of the shoulder.

In general, after direct visualization of the osseous morphology, we place the Helicut blade in the lateral portal and perform the amount of bony resection decided on, making a lateral step cut in the acromion at this site (Figure 16.8). An accurate estimate of this can be obtained because the diameter of the arthroscopic cannula is known. Generally, we will take a minimum of one diameter of the 6 mm diameter cannula, perhaps taking as much as two diameters (12 mm). Once the step cut has been created, we proceed with the resection from lateral to medial, usually coming level with the sagittal plane of the AC joint. Care is taken to smooth the anterior acromial surface and preserve soft tissue attachments. Final resection yields a smooth, even surface (Figure 16.9). One will usually see continuity of fibers where the periosteum and deltoid fascia begin to coalesce together. It is not unusual

to see some fibers of the deltoid. Great care is taken not to excessively dissect off soft tissue attachments to the acromion from the deltoid musculature. With this technique, we have not encountered any partial disruption of deltoid fibers even in the performance of a rather aggressive anterior resection. Spinal needles can be placed for appropriate orientation, although we have not found this necessary.

If distal clavicle resection is going to be performed arthroscopically, a bipolar radiofrequency device is used to delineate the anatomical landmarks underneath the AC joint, coagulate all bleeders in the adventitia, and carry out a distal clavicular resection. This procedure is covered in detail in Chapters 22 and 23.

There is some controversy regarding AC joint coplaning. It is our opinion that if no AC surgery is contemplated, the AC joint should not be violated to any significant degree, in an effort to reduce the possibility of residual instability. Rarely will there be more than a small rent or buttonhole in the inferior capsule following satisfactory decompression.

Following completion of the decompression, the surgeon may choose to place the arthroscope in the lateral portal to get an "outlet" perspective (Figure 16.10). If this subacromial decompression is a new procedure and one is not entirely sure that an adequate resection has been done, merely extend the length of lateral portal incision and introduce the index finger to confirm the decompression adequacy by palpations. Thorough irrigation must follow this procedure because of the amount of bony debris that is generated and might otherwise remain within the adventitia and bursal tissue.

The portals are closed with Steri-Strips. We feel that the ability of the shoulder to drain spontaneously through some of these portals is advantageous. A Pain Care 2000 pain pump (Breg, Inc., Carlsbad, CA) is

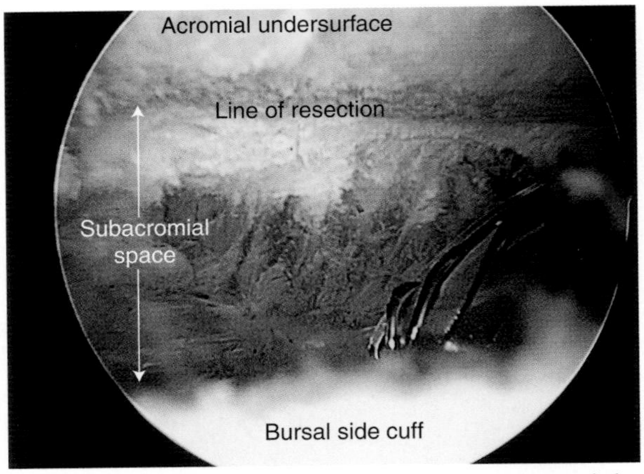

FIGURE 16.9. Postacromioplasty view of the resection of the anterior and anterolateral portion of the acromion.

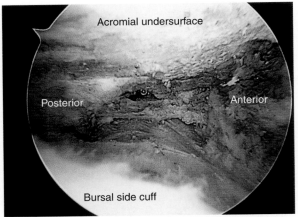

FIGURE 16.10. This final "outlet" perspective is achieved with the scope placed in the lateral portal (right shoulder, lateral decubitus perspective). Note the even line of resection.

sometimes placed into the subacromial space, particularly if concomitant AC resection or rotator cuff repair is performed. A bulky dry sterile dressing is applied along with the application of a Polar Care unit (Breg, Inc.) or an ice pack.

The patient is placed in a sling with a bolster, sent to the recovery room, and discharged home within 2 hours. It is critical to assess the patient's neurovascular status before discharge from the recovery room.

POSTOPERATIVE MANAGEMENT

The patient is discharged from the outpatient recovery room and sent home with appropriate instructions. If a pain pump has been inserted for additional pain relief, the patient is given instructions in how to deliver up to 10 mL of medication every 4 hours, in divided doses as necessary. Generally, conventional pain control can be obtained through the use of oral medication. The patient is then seen in the office within 24 to 48 hours. At this stage, the dressing is removed, the wounds are inspected, and the pain pump can be removed. Conversely, the patient may remove this at home with appropriate instructions within the following 24 to 48 hours.

Pendulum exercises are started within 2 to 3 days after surgery, with the patient instructed to bend over, both with the sling and without the sling, and perform passive range-of-motion pendulum program to the point of pain and slightly beyond four or five times a day. If a rotator cuff repair was performed in conjunction with the decompression, pendulum exercises may be started a little later, but almost always within the first 5 days, to avoid stiffness. Formal physical therapy is usually employed on about the seventh to tenth day, with very careful instructions for the therapist to begin with passive range-of-motion exercises for the first 7 to 10 days, active assistance at about 14 days, and active at about 3 to 4 weeks (for decompression without cuff repair). Muscle-strengthening programs are not employed early in the regime, but isometrics can begin at about week 2 to 3. Active range-of-motion work can begin at about week 4, and light weights at about 6 weeks. Although we do not particularly fear disruption of the operative procedure or detachment of the deltoid, it does appear that early strengthening or aggressive rehabilitation with this operation merely leads to more pain, restricted motion, and a slower rehabilitative process.

In general, the earliest an overhead athlete should return to overhead activities is 3 months. The average time for complete recovery is probably closer to 6 months.

RESULTS/OUTCOME

Outcomes following ASAD have been quite good, with most series ranging from 80 to 90% good to excellent results. This compares quite favorably with the open procedure, although there are more data in the arthroscopic literature today than in the earlier open literature. There certainly appear to be fewer complications.

Outcomes are somewhat influenced by the status of the rotator cuff and other factors that can negatively affect the results. These include patients who have had workplace injuries, such that workers' compensation is involved, and patients with prolonged prodromal histories, patients under the age of 20 and over the age of 60, patients with restricted motion, and patients with multifocal calcification.

The success rate of subacromial decompression in the presence of partial articular and bursal-sided tears is still somewhat unclear. Although the published data are sparse, recent reports seem to indicate that a partial cuff tear that approaches 50% on the articular side and perhaps even less on the bursal side may, when repaired, favorably influence the long-term outcome of a subacromial decompression (Chapter 17).

COMPLICATIONS

Complications associated with arthroscopic subacromial decompression are quite similar to those experienced with the open procedure. The most prevalent of these appears to be inaccurate diagnosis and incorrect technique: excessive or inadequate bone resection, either anteriorly, anterolaterally, or at the AC joint (Figure 16.11). Excessive scarring, frequently

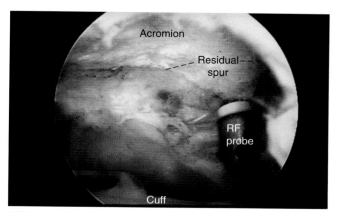

FIGURE 16.11. Flawed acromioplasty secondary to a residual anterolateral spur. Bipolar radiofrequency probe is introduced via the lateral portal. (View from right shoulder, beach chair perspective.)

noted, responds very well to debridement and cannot be diagnosed in any other fashion. Postoperative stiffness is a relatively common residual effect of all shoulder surgery and sometimes not a direct consequence of the operative procedure per se. It certainly is directly related to unrecognized adhesive capsulitis.

Iatrogenic fractures of the acromion and clavicle have been reported with both aggressive acromioplasties and surgical disorientation. Failure to recognize substantial partial tears in the rotator cuff is less a failure of the decompression than a failure to recognize concomitant pathology. Infections are very uncommon and appear to represent less than 1% of all complications. Reflex sympathetic dystrophy is rare but may occur in patients with a predisposing tendency who have reported prodromal radicular symptoms or feelings of paresthesia extending beyond the elbow. Some series have reported AC joint symptomatology after successful ASAD when aggressive coplaning had taken place at the time of surgery.

Recommended Reading

Anderson NH, Sojbjerg JO, Johannsen HV, et al. Self-training versus physiotherapist-supervised rehabilitation of the shoulder in patients treated with arthroscopic subacromial decompression: a clinical randomized study. *J Shoulder Elbow Surg* 1999;8(2):99–109.

Buford D Jr, Mologne T, McGrath S, et al. Midterm results of arthroscopic co-planing of the acromioclavicular joint. *J Shoulder Elbow Surg* 2000;9(6):498–501.

Ellman H. Arthroscopic subacromial decompression: analysis of one- to three-year results. *Arthroscopy* 1987;3(3):173–181.

Fisher BW, Gross RM, McCarthy JA, et al. Incidence of acromioclavicular joint complications after arthroscopic subacromial decompression. *Arthroscopy* 1999;15(3):241–248.

Morrison DS, Frogameni AD, Woodworth P. Non-operative treatment of subacromial impingement syndrome. *J Bone Joint Surgery Am* 1997;79(5):732–737.

Neer CS. Impingement lesions. *Clin Orth* 1983;173:70–77.

Patel VR, Singh D, Calvert PT, et al. Arthroscopic subacromial decompression: results and factors affecting outcome. *J Shoulder Elbow Surg* 1999;8(3):231–237.

Paulos LE, Franklin JL. Arthroscopic shoulder decompression development and application. A five year experience. *Am J Sports Med* 1990;18(3):235–244.

Roberts RM, Tasto J. The effects of acromioclavicular joint stability after arthroscopy co-planing. *Arthroscopy* 1998;14(2)suppl.1:12.

Roye RP, Grana WA, Yates CK. Arthroscopic subacromial decompression: two- to seven-year follow-up. *Arthroscopy* 1995;11(3):301–306.

17

Arthroscopic Treatment of Partial-Thickness Rotator Cuff Tears

Wesley M. Nottage and Charles J. Ruotolo

Arthroscopy has improved our diagnostic assessment of rotator cuff disease, especially in the understanding of the different patterns of articular surface partial-thickness tears. Articular or bursal partial-thickness rotator cuff tears may be a primary cause of shoulder pain and dysfunction or may occur in secondary to a primary pathological condition of the shoulder. Partial-thickness rotator cuff tears may be categorized into those arising on the bursal surface, those arising on the articular surface, and those that are purely intratendinous. Controversy surrounds the management of partial-thickness rotator cuff tears, especially articular-sided lesions.

The rotator cuff represents the confluence of the tendon fibers from the subscapularis, supraspinatus, infraspinatus, and teres minor muscles. This tendinous cuff is reinforced superficially and deeply at its insertion on the humerus by 1 mm thick fibers from the coracohumeral ligament, particularly on the supraspinatus and infraspinatus tendons. On the articular side, the deepest layer of the rotator cuff is reinforced at its attachment by the joint capsule, which is 1.5 to 2.0 mm thick. The normal rotator cuff varies in thickness, being greatest at the muscle tendon junction (8.5–11 mm wide) and least at the rotator interval.[1]

The rotator cuff changes with age, with a localized thin area adjacent to the supraspinatus attachment, known as the "rotator crescent"; the thickened area of cuff surrounding this is termed the "rotator cable" (Figure 17.1).

Intratendinous tearing of the rotator cuff may be related to age and repetitive trauma. Intratendinous tears refer to local disruptions within the tendon itself between the superficial and deep layers of a degenerative rotator cuff, presumably due to shear within the tendon. Concomitant subacromial bursitis commonly occurs.

The natural history of articular-sided, partial-thickness rotator cuff tears is believed to reflect a lack of healing response and commonly may progress to a larger tear. An arthrography study on 40 articular partial-thickness rotator cuff tears followed for a mean of 412 days with repeat arthrogram, demonstrated disappearance of the torn portion in only four instances (10%), reduction of the tear size in 10%, enlargement of the tear size in 52%, and progression to full-thickness cuff tear in 28%. This group was believed to represent primarily degenerative tendon disease, with the prognosis for progression of the joint side tear with age and larger original tear size.[3]

ETIOLOGY

It is important to determine whether the rotator cuff lesion represents either a primary or a secondary disease condition. The anatomical location of the partial-thickness tear can be the key guide to confirming the suspected etiology.

The etiology of partial-thickness rotator cuff tears includes extrinsic impingement on the undersurface of the acromion or coracoacromial ligament, as well as internal abrasion along the glenoid rim anteriorly or posteriorly, tensile failure, or traumatic avulsion. Differentiating the cause for a partial-thickness rotator cuff tear should be guided by patient age, history, physical examination, and arthroscopic findings.

Partial-thickness rotator cuff tears occurring due to *extrinsic* impingement are found on the bursal side of the rotator cuff. To make the diagnosis of extrinsic impingement, there must be ulceration or fraying of the coracoacromial arch (Figure 17.2). An articular-sided lesion may lead to cuff weakness, inability to depress the humeral head, and secondary extrinsic impingement.

Although the majority of partial-thickness cuff tears occur in the supraspinatus tendon, partial-thickness tears may occur on the articular surface between the subscapularis and the supraspinatus or posteriorly be-

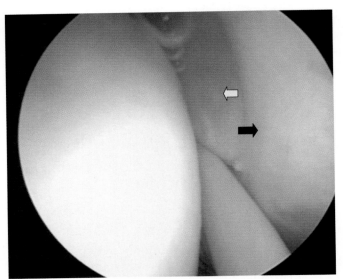

FIGURE 17.1. The rotator cable–crescent complex (left shoulder, viewing from posterior scope portal, lateral decubitus position): white arrow points to the thin crescent; black arrow points to the thickened cable.

tween the supraspinatus and infraspinatus. Identifying the normal anatomy of the rotator cuff, including rotator cable and crescent configuration, rotator interval, and the specific location of the cuff lesion, aids both in defining the etiology and in the specific management.

Partial-thickness rotator cuff tears in younger individuals, and specifically overhead athletes, may occur for a variety of reasons. Younger patients generally have tensile failure or abrasion as the cause of their partial-thickness lesion. Tensile failure results from a combination of shearing and tearing of the cuff tendons during the deceleration phase of activity. Tensile failure of the cuff can also occur as a result of underlying instability from capsular laxity, labral deficiency, or from abnormal obligate translation in patients with posterior–inferior capsular contracture (loss of internal rotation).[4,5] The rotator cuff itself may also abrade on either the anterior or posterior portion of the glenoid rim as a result of glenohumeral instability or internal impingement.[6] In overhand athletes with a posterior–superior labral tear, the partial-thickness tear is usually found on the posterior aspect of the supraspinatus or may include a portion of the infraspinatus. Associated arthroscopic findings should include a posterior SLAP (superior labrum anterior/posterior) tear or fraying of the posterior labrum, which is demonstrated by abduction and external rotation of the arm, arthroscopically confirming this etiology.[4] Partial-thickness cuff tears can occur in the anterior aspect of the supraspinatus associated with an underlying microinstability pattern, typically as a SLAC lesion (i.e., an anterior SLAP tear and an anterior partial-thickness rotator cuff tear).[7]

Anterior capsular laxity has been associated with tensile failure of the cuff as well, although plastic deformity of the anterior capsule can be difficult to assess arthroscopically. Morgan uses the criterion of greater than 130° of external rotation with the arm abducted 90° as evidence of anterior capsular laxity.[8]

Acute trauma, including weight lifting or forceful rotator cuff contraction, can account for partial-thickness rotator cuff tears, specifically a tear with an avulsion of a portion of the supraspinatus directly from the proximal humerus. This lesion has been described as the PASTA lesion, a partial articular supraspinatus tendon avulsion.[9] Rarely are there bursal-sided changes in the rotator cuff or coracoacromial arch in this group.

In patients over 60 years of age, articular fraying of the rotator cuff may occur as a degenerative phenomenon. Simply fraying of the rotator cuff itself is not necessarily the primary pathology and may reflect an ongoing degenerative process.

INDICATIONS/CONTRAINDICATIONS

The indication for operative treatment of partial-thickness rotator cuff tears is persistent pain affecting activities of daily living, sport, or work. Patients should have been initially treated nonoperatively, which may include modification of activities, subacromial corticosteroid injections, or an exercise program emphasizing range of motion, painless shoulder strengthening exercises, and scapular stabilizing exer-

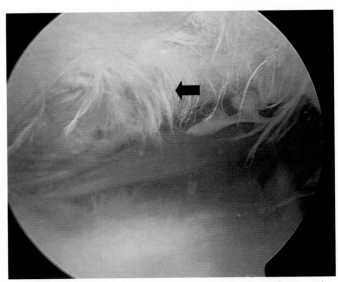

FIGURE 17.2. Black arrow points to the impingement lesion. This fraying or ulceration along the undersurface of the acromion and coracoacromial ligament must be seen before the diagnosis of impingement can be made. (View from posterior scope portal, right shoulder, beach chair position.)

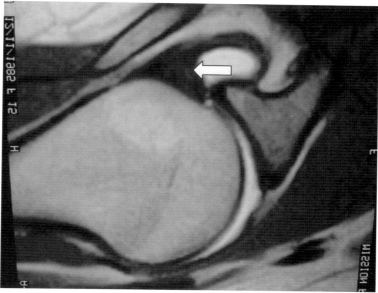

FIGURE 17.3. Magnetic resonance arthrogram with the shoulder in the ABER position: white arrow points to the normal supraspinatus footprint. Note the clear visualization of the undersurface of the supraspinatus tendon.

cises. Relative contraindications to operative treatment of partial-thickness rotator cuffs include advanced age, stiffness, and osteoarthritis.

PREOPERATIVE PLANNING

A complete history and physical examination, including radiographs, is necessary. Scapulothoracic motion should be assessed as well as the total arc of motion of the shoulder, with the shoulder abducted 90°. Radiographic examination should include anterior-poste-

rior, axillary, and supraspinatus outlet views. Magnetic resonance (MR) arthrography may add sensitivity and specificity to partial-thickness rotator cuffs better than unenhanced MR imaging and is probably the test of choice for patients suspected of having partial-thickness articular or bursal cuff tears.[10] Articular surface rotator cuff tears are best visualized when the extremity is positioned in the ABER (**ab**duction **e**xternal **r**otation) or "behind the head" position, which clearly shows the insertion of the supraspinatus on the greater tuberosity and also brings the articular surface of the cuff away from the humeral head (Figures 17.3, 17.4).

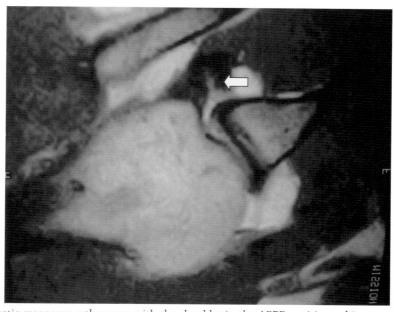

FIGURE 17.4. Another magnetic resonance arthrogram with the shoulder in the ABER position: white arrow points to an articular-sided, partial-thickness rotator cuff tear.

Although a positive finding is helpful, the sensitivity for diagnosis of partial tears in several studies is reportedly poor, making the partial-thickness cuff tear frequently best (or only) diagnosed at arthroscopy.

SURGICAL TECHNIQUE

Positioning/Setup

The patient is placed in the lateral decubitus position, using a beanbag positioner, with the head aligned with the torso. Five to seven pounds of balanced suspension is utilized on the involved arm. The patient's systolic blood pressure is maintained between 85 and 95 mmHg to improve visualization (unless contraindicated), and a fluid pump is used with lactated Ringer's without epinephrine and inflow pressure set at 60 mmHg.

Instrumentation

Standard arthroscopic instrumentation is utilized, including a 4 mm, 30° offset arthroscope, motorized shaver and burr, 90 mm long by 8.25 mm diameter clear-threaded cannulas (Arthrex, Naples, FL), switching sticks, Wissinger rod, an arthroscopic probe, arthroscopic baskets, suture and loop grabbers, and arthroscopic graspers. Specialized instruments for rotator cuff repair include the Linvatec Spectrum Suture Hook System (Linvatec, Largo, FL) and Shut-

tle Relay (Smith/Nephew Dyonics, Andover, MA), as well as 30 and 45° suture transport devices. For tying arthroscopic knots, single- and double-hole knot pushers are used, as well as an arthroscopic suture cutter.

Surgical Technique

Prior to performing the arthroscopic procedure, the shoulder should have a full examination under anesthesia for both range of motion and laxity. The most important part of the EUA is a comparison of the total arc of motion with the contralateral extremity, measuring external and internal rotation with the shoulder abducted 90°. Stiffness, or capsular contracture as a primary pathological process associated with partial-thickness cuff tears, needs to be identified, since it could significantly alter a patient's postoperative course and management. Similarly, the load and shift test should be performed to identify asymmetric laxity indicative of instability.

The arthroscopic examination starts in the glenohumeral joint from a utility posterior portal. A complete examination of the glenohumeral joint and subacromial space should be performed before treatment is decided upon. Once an articular partial-thickness tear has been identified, its location and thickness should be assessed. Debridement is recommended prior to assessing actual thickness, since the thickness of the cuff tear is difficult to determine beforehand only the clearly pathologic tissue is removed. Similarly, the amount of exposed bone between the articular carti-

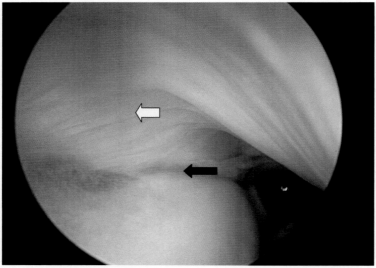

FIGURE 17.5. Intra-articular view of the normal supraspinatus insertion (left shoulder, posterior viewing portal, lateral decubitus position): white arrow points to the normal rotator cuff tendon; black arrow points to the margin between the articular cartilage and the supraspinatus footprint. Note that only 1 to 2 mm of bone is seen between the cartilage and the tendon insertion.

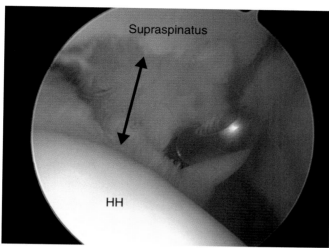

FIGURE 17.6. Intra-articular view of a supraspinatus articular-sided, partial-thickness tear after debridement (Left shoulder, posterior viewing portal, lateral decubitus position). The amount of exposed bone, as indicated by the arrow, helps in determining the amount of tendon loss: HH, humeral head.

lage and supraspinatus footprint can be a helpful guide for the magnitude of a cuff avulsion (Figures 17.5, 17.6). Normal cuff thickness at the supraspinatus attachment averages 12.1 mm. Normal exposed bone averages 1.7 mm. A 50% tear is estimated at approximately 7 mm of exposed bone. The system of Ellman and Gartsman is used to grade the partial-thickness tear as grade 1 (fraying), grade 2 (<50% of the tendon substance), or grade 3 (>50% of the tendon substance). A spinal needle is used to pass a monofilament suture percutaneously as a "marking stitch" through the central portion of the tear (Figure 17.7).

The arthroscope is then directed into the subacromial space through the same posterior skin incision portal. An anterolateral portal is established, through which a motorized shaver is introduced to remove bursal tissue and evaluate the rotator cuff. The marking suture is identified and the corresponding area inspected for cuff pathology. Abnormal cuff tissue is debrided, noting that diseased tissue is removed far more easily than normal tissue. The presence of considerable bursitis or bursal tissue suggests intratendinous or bursal-side disease, which sometimes requires a thorough subacromial bursectomy. Other bursal findings may include ulceration along the coracoacromial ligaments' (or acromial) undersurface, which further suggests a diagnosis of extrinsic impingement. If such findings are not present, a "routine" acromioplasty, as an adjunct to treating the partial-thickness rotator cuff tear, is not recommended. Intratendinous involvement, which can be considerable, may be underappreciated from articular-side viewing. Preoperative MR imagery may provide the best opportunity to appreciate intratendinous pathology.

At this time, having definitively evaluated the cuff from below and above, and debrided as necessary, a decision may be made on how to proceed with treatment. This is based on the surgeon's assessment of the location and extent of involvement. The most difficult decision in treating partial-thickness rotator cuff tears is estimating the true thickness of the tear. One must be aware that the cuff varies in thickness, being thinner anteriorly in the interval, and laterally in the crescent, and increasing in thickness at its humeral

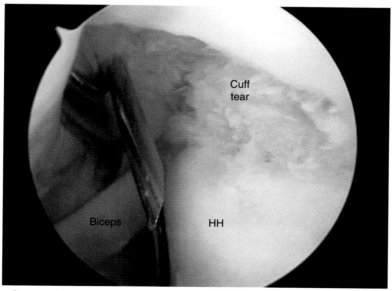

FIGURE 17.7. Suture marker placement (via spinal needle) through the center of an articular-sided rotator cuff tear: HH, humeral head.

insertion. The tear may be an avulsion from the tuberosity, or it may just be a loss of intratendinous tissue.

LESIONS LESS THAN 50% THICKNESS

For lesions less than 50% of the thickness of the supraspinatus tendon (grade 2) but with significant intratendinous tissue loss, it is recommended that the tear defect be debrided and closed by using a side-to-side suture approximation technique. For bursal-sided tears, this can be performed under direct vision in the subacromial space. For articular-sided tears that are between 30 and 50%, I will sometimes reapproximate the healthy remnant cuff tendon against the tuberosity in a technique described by Savoie. In this approach, the adjacent bare footprint area of the tuberosity is abraded to stimulate a healing response. While the cuff is visualized from within the glenohumeral joint, a monofilament suture is passed percutaneously via a spinal needle through the cuff medial/posterior to the defective tissue (Figure 17.8). A suture retriever passed anteriorly through the rotator interval, then grasps the percutaneously placed suture and is withdrawn from the anterior portal, thereby creating a simple "side-to-side" cuff repair suture near its terminal insertion (Figure 17.9). The sutures from the subacromial space and rotator interval area are then tied "blindly" down the anterior portal, while the surgeon views the supraspinatus pull up against the abraded tuberosity. This may be repeated as many times as necessary to actually close the defect and to approximate the cuff tear to the humeral head (Figure 17.10). Care is taken to avoid overtightening the rotator interval; the aim is to approximate tendon apposition, without overconstraint.

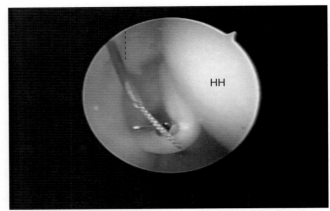

FIGURE 17.9. Arthroscopic view showing suture retriever entering anteriorly to grasp superior suture. This constitutes the first (or at times only) repair suture to reapproximate a partial-thickness tear: HH, humeral head.

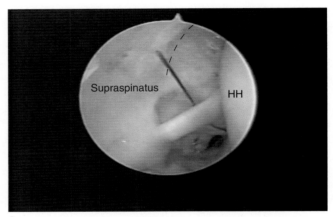

A

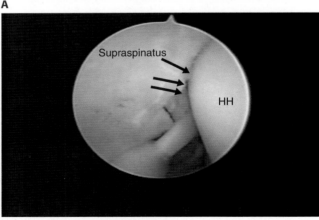

B

FIGURE 17.10 (A) Arthroscopic view (right shoulder, posterior scope portal) of suture that has been placed through the supraspinatus just medial to the partial undersurface cuff defect, grasped, and pulled through the rotator interval. (B) The suture has been tied down an anterior arthroscopic cannula with pulling of the tendon to the abraded tuberosity. Note the opposition of tendon against the abraded tuberosity (arrows): HH, humeral head.

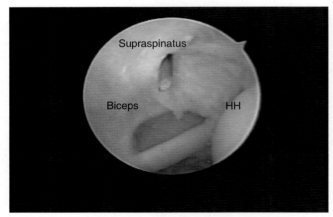

FIGURE 17.8. Arthroscopic view of a glenohumeral joint: spinal needle with suture is passed posterior to partial-thickness tear into the joint. The tuberosity at the area of detachment has been abraded to stimulate a healing response: HH, humeral head.

LESIONS MORE THAN 50% THICKNESS

It is recommended that any rotator cuff tear that involves close to 50% or more of the thickness of the cuff (grade 3) be taken down and repaired, either arthroscopically or by open surgery. Arthroscopic repairs can be performed via either a transtendon technique or by simply completing the tear and then performing the equivalent procedure for a full-thickness tear of the rotator cuff (see Chapter 18 on full-thickness cuff repairs). The transtendon repair technique has been described by Snyder.[8] In this approach, one or more suture anchors are placed into the tuberosity through the superior surface of the rotator cuff tear, and the sutures are tied on the bursal surface in the subacromial space.[9] We have found this transtendinous approach, however, technically challenging, since it is necessary to switch back and forth between the glenohumeral joint and the subacromial space to visualize anchor placement through the tendon and into the tuberosity. Our preference is to complete the tear from the subacromial (bursal) side and then proceed with an arthroscopic repair. Usually this can be easily accomplished with a motorized shaver, using a suture marker as a guide to the tear location. If necessary, the cuff tear can be mobilized with a knife, incising parallel to the tendon fibers and then debriding the area with a shaver to remove all degenerative tissue.

If repair is entertained, the arthroscope is moved to the lateral portal viewing from the subacromial space, and anterior and posterior working portals are created, using 8.25 mm by 90 mm clear cannulas. One is placed in the posterior portal, and a Wissinger rod is used to make an anterior portal superior and lateral to the coracoid process in line with the rotator cuff tear and greater tuberosity. The cuff tear is then manipulated with a clamp device from both anterior and posterior directions, to visualize the correct placement of the suture anchors as well as the proper way the cuff tear should lie down. A tear may initially require side-to-side sutures, or it may require a direct reapproximation to bone. The majority of partial-thickness cuff tears that are taken down and repaired will require both side-to-side suture repair and suture anchor reattachment to the greater tuberosity footprint adjacent to the articular margin.[10]

Next, viewing from the lateral portal, one uses a spinal needle to mark the location of anchor placement into the tuberosity. The needle should enter just lateral to the acromion and should have the correct angle of approach into the humeral head. A small nick is made in the adjacent skin, and a small straight hemostat is used to spread a pathway through the deltoid. The needle is then removed, and under direct vision, a screw-in, double-loaded anchor is placed percutaneously into bone, which is loaded with no. 2 nonabsorbable suture. After anchor placement, the suture is routed through the rotator cuff, commonly by means of suture shuttles passing either anteriorly or posteriorly and tied with sliding arthroscopic knots to reattach the cuff near the articular margin. Once the suture anchor tying has been completed at this level, and to support this repair, several side-to-side sutures are recommended *lateral* to the anchor, reapproximating any defect and unloading the tension on the rotator cuff repair at the articular margin (Figure 17.11).

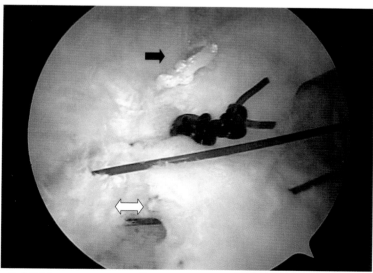

FIGURE 17.11. Significant partial-thickness rotator cuff tear arthroscopically repaired to bone: black arrow points to the suture anchor reapproximating the tendon to bone; white arrow demonstrates how two sutures placed side to side lateral to the anchor placement can easily restore the entire supraspinatus footprint. (View from the lateral portal, right shoulder, beach chair position.)

TABLE 17.1. Summary of Results.

Study	Number of patients	Follow-up	Debrided	Repaired	SAD[a]	Results	Miscellaneous
Snyder et al[11]	31	Average 23 months	31	0	18	84% satisfied	Size of tear did not affect outcome
Esch et al[12]	34	Average 19 months	34	0	34	76%	All tears >50%, 88% articular
Weber[22]	65	2–7 years	32	33	65	Debrided, 14/32; Repaired, 31/32	
Budoff, Nirschl et al[17]	76	Average 53 months	76	0	0, but 40% had acromion debrided	87%	65 athletes with 80% return to same level
Fukuda et al[13]	66	Average 31.7 months	0	All, open	All, open acromioplasty	94%	
Ellman[18]	20	Short	All	0	All	75%	
Gartsman[19]	40	28.9 months	All	0	All	33/40	32/40 articular 93% satisfied not workers comp 58% who were workers' comp
Wright/Cofield[14]	39	55 months	0	All	All	59% excellent 26% satisfactory	Open technique
Gartsman[5]	106	32.3 months	I: 85 II: 14 III: 0	III: 12	I: 85 II: 0 III: 0	88%	I: impingement II: athlete with cap recon or rehabilitation III: trauma
Payne et al[20]	43	Average 48 months	40 A: 12/14 B: 28	2 A: 2/14 B: 0	26	72% A: 86% B: 66%	All athletes <40 years old 91% articular A: trauma, 64% return to sports B: insidious; 45% return to sport same level
Morgan et al[4]	20	1 year	All	0	Not stated	Negative impact on results	All patients with SLAP repairs, all articular
Andrews et al[21]	51	2 years	All	0	Not stated	A: 61% at same or higher level of comp. B: 86%	All baseball pitchers A: debride, −TACS B: debride, +TACS

This can easily be accomplished by passing sutures from posterior to anterior using the Rotator Crescent Spectrum needle (Linvatec) and no. 1 polydioxanone sutures. The crescent needle is passed through both the anterior and posterior cuff margins, using the cannula to help stabilize the tissue as it is passed, and then the tissue edges are reapproximated by means of a sliding knot.

POSTOPERATIVE MANAGEMENT

In patients who have had simple debridement of the rotator cuff lesion, immediate active assisted range-of-motion therapy is begun on the first postoperative day, with scapular-stabilizing exercises. Resistive exercises are not initiated until the shoulder is pain free.

Following rotator cuff repair, the shoulder is immobilized in a 15° abduction sling for approximately 3 weeks, associated with passive range of motion of the shoulder and active range of motion of the wrist and elbow. Active range-of-motion work is allowed at 6 weeks, withholding resistive exercises until pain free.

RESULTS

Results of 12 studies are summarized in Table 17.1.

DEBRIDEMENT

Multiple authors have respectively reviewed the results of debridement alone for partial-thickness rotator cuff tears. Snyder reviewed his results in 31 patients, noting 84% to have a satisfactory outcome, with tear size not related to outcome at 23 months.[11] Esch published the results in 34 patients at average follow-up of 19 months, with a satisfaction rate of only 76%.[12]

REPAIR

The literature contains descriptions of the repair of partial-thickness rotator cuff tears, including excision of the diseased tissue and repair of the defect with side-to-side sutures or directly to bone by either open or mini-open arthroscopic techniques. Open and mini-open repairs have success rates ranging between 82.5 and 96.8%.[5,13–16] Noojin et al. presented results comparing debridement, abrasion of the humerus with side-to-side repair, and arthroscopic or mini-open repair in 107 patients with an articular-sided tear with

a follow-up of 24 to 52 months.[16] The average UCLA score for all groups was 33, but the results of the debrided group had a tendency to deteriorate over time.[16] Weber describes a comparative study of debridement versus repair for partial-thickness rotator cuff tears.[15] Thirty-two patients underwent debridement and 32 underwent repair of the partial-thickness rotator cuff tear; all tears involved over 50% of the tendon thickness. All patients had a concomitant subacromial decompression, and follow-up ranged from 2 to 7 years. A satisfactory result was had by 96.8% of the repair group, compared with only 43.7% of those with just a debridement and decompression. Based upon this study, it is recommended that all partial-thickness cuff tears involving 50% or greater of the thickness of the cuff be repaired.

SUBACROMIAL DECOMPRESSION

Most authors believe that bursal-sided lesions are best served by a concomitant arthroscopic decompression, expecting good results. Controversy surrounds the role of subacromial decompression in management of articular-sided rotator cuff lesions. No study published to date directly compares the results of partial thickness cuff tear treatment with and without acromioplasty. Budoff et al. published results of 76 patients who underwent debridement of their partial-thickness cuff tears with an 87% success rate (average of 53 months of follow-up).[17] Difficulties in interpreting the data include the great number of patients (40%) who had some form of "acromion debridement" and the absence of a description of the thickness of the partial tears for this series. Other authors believe that extrinsic impingement can cause an articular-sided tear without bursal findings of abrasion and recommend arthroscopic subacromial decompression for all articular-sided partial-thickness rotator cuff tears to reduce the compressive and shearing forces on the rotator cuff. The role of subacromial decompression in the treatment of articular partial-thickness rotator cuff tears remains controversial. In general, patients who have been treated with isolated arthroscopic decompression for significant partial-thickness, articular-sided lesions without repair do not fare well, and a significant risk of tear progression has been noted.[15]

COMPLICATIONS

Partial-thickness rotator cuff tears may be associated with underlying instability, adhesive capsulitis, osteoarthritis, or suprascapular neuropathy. Failure to recognize the primary reason for shoulder dysfunction associated with the partial-thickness cuff tear may lead to failure of the procedure and a less than satisfactory result. Failure to debride and repair a significant partial-thickness cuff tear can also lead to failure with extension to a full-thickness tear. Technical errors may include failure to appropriately seat anchors in bone and failure to tie appropriate knots.

SUMMARY

Bursal-sided lesions that are minor (<10–20% of the rotator cuff) can be treated by debridement and a subacromial decompression. Larger bursal-sided, partial-thickness lesions, including flaps and splits, should be treated by suture repair and decompression.

We recommend that articular partial-thickness rotator cuff tears, if minor in a relatively young individual, be treated by debridement and rehabilitation. Debride all frayed degenerative tissue in the partial-thickness tear before assessing the size of the tear. An extensive partial-thickness tear, defined as approaching 50% or greater after debridement, should be treated by repair, examining the younger patient for ligamentous deficiencies. When one is uncertain, it is better to take down and repair a significant partial-thickness cuff tear rather than simply debride it.

References

1. Clark JM, Harryman DT. Tendons, ligaments, and capsule of the rotator cuff. *J Bone Joint Surg Am* 1992;74(5): 713–725.
2. Burkhart SS, Esch JC, Jolson RS. The rotator crescent and rotator cable: an anatomic description of the shoulder's "suspension bridge". *Arthroscopy* 1993;9(6):611–616.
3. Yamanaka K, Matsumoto T. The joint side tear of the rotator cuff. *Clin Orthop* 1994;304:68–73.
4. Morgan CD, Burkhart SS, Palmeri M, Gillespie M. Type II SLAP lesions: three subtypes and their relationships to superior instability and rotator cuff tears. *Arthroscopy* 1998;14(6):553–565.
5. Gartsman GM, Milne JC: Articular surface partial-thickness rotator cuff tears. *J Shoulder Elbow Surg* 1995;4(6):409–415.
6. Walch G, Boileau P, Noel E, Donell ST. Impingement of the deep surface of the supraspinatus tendon on the posterior glenoid rim: an arthroscopic study. *J Shoulder Elbow Surg.* 1992;1:238–245.
7. Savoie FH, Field LD, Atchinson S. Anterior superior instability with rotator cuff tearing: SLAC lesion. *Oper Tech Sports Med* 2000;8(3):221–224.
8. Morgan CD. The thrower's shoulder: spectrum of pathology. Paper presented at: *American Academy of Orthopaedic Surgeons/American Orthopedic Society for Sports Medicine Comprehensive Sports Medicine: The Athletic Perspective to Treatment, Controversies and Problem Solving*, February 2, 2001; Lake Tahoe, NV.
9. Snyder SJ. Arthroscopic treatment of partial articular surface tendon avulsions. Paper presented at: *American Academy of Orthopaedic Surgeons/American Orthopedic Society for Sports Medicine Comprehensive Sports Medicine: The Athletic Perspective to Treatment, Controversies and Problem Solving*; February 2, 2001; Lake Tahoe, NV.
10. Hodler J, Kursunoglu-Brahme S, Snyder SJ, et al. Rotator cuff disease: assessment with MR arthrography versus standard MR imaging in 36 patients with arthroscopic confirmation. *Radiology* 1992;182:431–436.
11. Snyder SJ, Pachelli AF, Del Pizzo W, et al. Partial thickness rotator cuff tears: results of arthroscopic treatment. *Arthroscopy* 1991;7:1–7.
12. Esch JC, Ozerkis LR, Helager JA, et al. Arthroscopic subacromial decompression: results according to the degree of rotator cuff tear. Arthroscopy 1988;4:241–249.
13. Fukuda H, Hamada K, Nakajima T, et al. Partial-thickness tears of the rotator cuff. *Int Orthop* 1996;20:257–265.
14. Wright SA, Cofield RH. Management of partial-thickness rotator cuff tears. *J Shoulder Elbow Surg* 1996;5(6):458–466.
15. Weber SC. Arthroscopic debridement and acromioplasty versus miniopen repair in the management of significant partial thickness tears of the rotator cuff. *Orthop Clin North Am* 1997;28:79–82.
16. Noojin FK, Savoie FH, Field LD. Arthroscopic treatment of partial thickness articular-sided rotator cuff tears. Paper presented at: *Arthroscopy Association of North America 20th Annual Meeting*; April 19, 2001; Seattle, WA.
17. Budoff JE, Nirschl RP, Guidi EJ: Debridement of Partial-Thickness Tears of the Rotator Cuff without Acromioplasty. *J Bone Joint Surg* 1998;80A(5):733–748.
18. Ellman H. Diagnosis and treatment of incomplete rotator cuff tears. *Clin Orthop* 1990;(254):64–74.
19. Gartsman G. Arthroscopic acromioplasty for lesions of the rotator cuff. *J Bone Jont Surg Am* 1990;72(2):169–180.
20. Payne LZ, Altchek DW, Craig EV, Warren RF. Arthroscopic treatment of partial rotator cuff tears in young athletes. A preliminary report. *Am J Sports Med* 1997;25(3):299–305.
21. Andrews JR, Dugas JR. Diagnosis and treatment of shoulder injuries in the throwing athlete: the role of thermal-assisted capsular shrinkage. *Instr Course Lect* 2001;50:17–21.
22. Weber SC. Arthroscopic debridement and acromioplasty versus mini-open repair in the treatment of significant partial-thickness rotator cuff tears. *Arthroscopy* 1999;15:126–131.

18

Arthroscopic Repair of Full-Thickness Tears of the Rotator Cuff

Peter M. Parten and Stephen S. Burkhart

The last decade has seen a dramatic progression in the arthroscopic management of rotator cuff tears. Arthroscopic cuff debridement, favored in the 1990s, has yielded to the sophisticated arthroscopic cuff repairs (including large and massive tears) performed today. The refinement of suture anchor techniques and the continued development of arthroscopic skills have ushered in the current era of arthroscopic repair for virtually all rotator cuff tears.

Rotator cuff tears that have done well with arthroscopic debridement are tears with balanced force couples in the transverse and coronal planes (Figure 18.1). Shoulders with balanced force couples, despite large rotator cuff tears, generally demonstrate good function despite pain, hence their description as "functional rotator cuff tears."[1] Conversely, cuff tears that are not balanced do not respond well to arthroscopic debridement alone, with a number of authors demonstrating unsatisfactory results, especially in younger, more active patients. In these patients, the results of rotator cuff debridement deteriorate over time.[2-9]

One of the advantages of arthroscopic surgery is that the surgeon can approach a pathological area from any direction (anterior, posterior, medial, or lateral) with equal facility. Conversely, open cuff repair through an anterolateral incision obligates bringing the torn edge of the cuff into one's field of view within the incision to see and repair it. This medial-to-lateral mind-set has dominated (and compromised) open rotator cuff surgery. Traditional teaching has emphasized cuff mobilization to permit lateral translation toward the greater tuberosity for repair.[10-17] Unfortunately this often incorrect medial-to-lateral perspective has delayed the progress of rotator cuff repair by limiting the recognition of one of the most useful concepts in the repair of massive rotator cuff tears: *margin convergence.*[18] Margin convergence, used for side-to-side closure of U-shaped tears, greatly reduces the

strain at the "converged" margin, thereby helping to protect the cuff repair (Figure 18.2).

Arthroscopy allows visualization of the rotator cuff defect as well as assessment of the tear pattern and mobility. Recognition of the unique pattern of each tear allows the surgeon to choose the appropriate combination of techniques to accomplish a tension-free repair for all tears, small to massive.

INDICATIONS/CONTRAINDICATIONS

Arthroscopic rotator cuff repair is indicated for most patients with rotator cuff tears. Diagnosis in the majority of cases can by achieved by appropriate history, plus physical and radiographic examinations. Operative treatment is preferred for patients with documented rotator cuff tears to provide pain relief, to improve strength and function, and to decrease the risk of progression of the rotator cuff tear.

Patients with prior failed rotator cuff repair, either open or arthroscopic, can also be successfully treated with arthroscopic rotator cuff repair. The cause of the initial failed repair often is failure to have recognized the true tear configuration, with predictable subsequent retear due to excessive tension on the repair. Arthroscopic repair allows the surgeon optimal visualization of the rotator cuff defect, and recognition of the appropriate repair technique.

Arthroscopic rotator cuff repair is contraindicated for elderly patients without significant pain and for patients with associated medical problems that present unacceptable risks for surgical anesthesia.

PREOPERATIVE PLANNING

Routine preoperative radiographs are obtained for all patients, including true anteroposterior (AP) views of

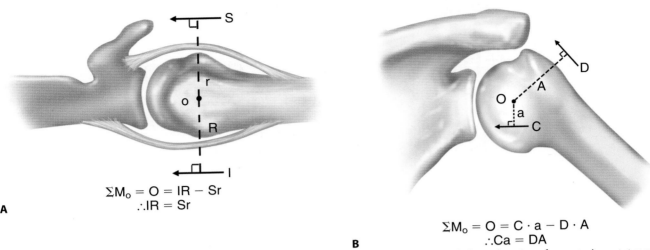

FIGURE 18.1. (A) Transverse (axial) plane force pair in which the anterior rotator cuff (S) is balanced against the posterior rotator cuff (I). (B) Coronal plane force pair between the deltoid (D) and the rotator cuff (C).

the glenohumeral joint (30° posterior oblique view) in internal and external rotation, axillary view, outlet view and 30° caudal tilt view. We prefer that every patient have a magnetic resonance imaging (MRI) exam prior to surgery. The MRI views can provide information on tear size, configuration, and tendon involvement, as well as suggest whether a large or massive rotator cuff tear is potentially repairable by margin convergence techniques. In a large U-shaped tear that can be repaired by margin convergence, MRI will show the apex of the tear to be located just above the glenoid with evidence of an intact subscapularis and an intact posterior-inferior cuff margin (teres minor alone or teres minor in addition to a partially intact infraspinatus).

MRI is also essential in diagnosis of a spinoglenoid ganglion cyst, which can mimic rotator cuff tear symptoms.

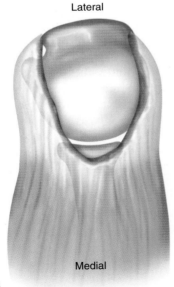

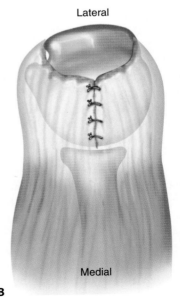

FIGURE 18.2. (A) U-shaped rotator cuff tear, "aerial" view. (B) Margin convergence is accomplished by using side-to-side sutures to "converge" the cuff margin toward the greater tuberosity. This maneuver greatly reduces strain at the "converged" margin and helps to protect the repair.

TECHNIQUE

Positioning/Setup

Rotator cuff repair is performed under general endotracheal anesthesia. A warming blanket prevents hypothermia. The patient is placed in the lateral decubitus position and secured with a suction beanbag. Balanced suspension of 5 to 10 lb is used to maintain the arm in 30° abduction and 20° forward flexion with the Star Sleeve traction system (Arthrex, Naples, FL). The amount of abduction can be varied intraoperatively by an assistant to maximize exposure and visualization. An arthroscopic pump is used to maintain the subacromial pressure at 60 mmHg. The pump pressure can be incrementally adjusted up to 95 mmHg temporarily if bleeding compromises visualization. However, elevated pressures (> 90 mmHg) for more than 15 min is to be avoided because increased swelling can result. A more effective method of controlling bleeding and improving visualization is to maintain turbulence control.[19] This is simply accomplished by blocking all escaping fluid flow from the noncannulated portals with digital pressure from an assistant, thus regulating turbulence within the closed system and facilitating a clear view (Figure 18.3).

The two key elements to any arthroscopic shoulder procedure are maintaining adequate visualization (achieved by electrocautery and turbulence control) and obtaining the appropriate angle of approach through proper portal placement and instrumentation.

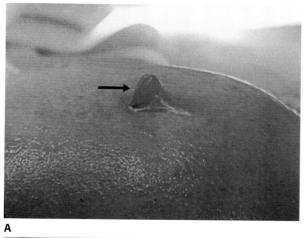

A

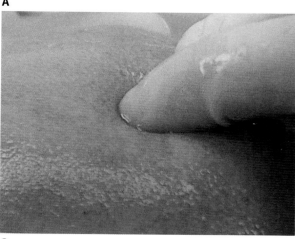

C

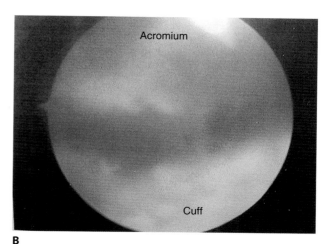

B

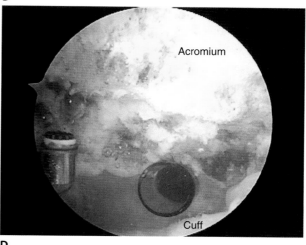

D

FIGURE 18.3. Turbulence control is accomplished by blocking escaping fluid flow from the portals. Fluid escaping from lateral portal (arrow) (A) causes turbulence and a bloody subacromial field (B). Digital pressure over the portal (C) eliminates turbulent flow and provides a clear field of view (D). Posterior scope view, left shoulder, beach chair perspective. (B and D represent the same arthroscopic view, with and without turbulence.)

Instrumentation

In addition to standard arthroscopic instrumentation, (4.0 mm scope with 5.5 mm sheath, motorized shaver, and burr system), specialized arthroscopic instruments are necessary to facilitate suture passing through tendon, suture retrieval and management, and suture tying. Arthroscopic suture passers can be used for antegrade and retrograde passage of suture through the rotator cuff tendon, both as free suture for margin convergence and to retrieve sutures of inserted anchors. Preferred instruments include the Penetrator and BirdBeak suture passers (Arthrex), each of which can be used for both methods. An atraumatic arthroscopic tendon grasper is useful for grasping the free tendon edge to assess tendon mobility. A cannula system with clear cannulas allows improved visualization of the cuff around the cannula and is especially helpful for viewing sutures for arthroscopic knot tying in tight spaces. A spinal needle (18 gauge) is useful to localize accessory portals prior to skin incision.

Surgical Technique

After standard arthroscopic inspection of the glenohumeral joint and appropriate treatment of any intraarticular pathology, the rotator cuff is inspected from the intra-articular aspect. The normal footprints of the supraspinatus and infraspinatus insertions are inspected, as well as that of the subscapularis tendon. To optimize visualization of the subscapularis footprint, the shoulder can be internally rotated to relax the anterior capsule and enlarge the potential space anteriorly. When the intra-articular inspection (and any necessary debridement) is complete, the arthroscope is placed in the subacromial space through the posterior portal. A lateral working and viewing portal is then established parallel to the undersurface of the acromion. An anterior portal is also established to function as an inflow portal as well as an accessory working portal.

The first step is to clear all bursal and fibrofatty tissues from the subacromial space and cuff margins to permit proper identification and classification of the tear pattern. This is accomplished initially with the scope posterior and the shaver in the lateral working portal. To fully clear the posterior gutter and visualize the posterior aspect of the cuff, the scope is changed to the lateral portal and the shaver positioned in the posterior portal. Adequate visualization for repair also requires a clear view into the lateral gutter and involves removal of the lateral shelf of the subacromial bursa.

For repairable tears less than 5 cm, standard subacromial decompression including coracoacromial (CA) ligament release is performed, using a cutting block technique.[20] If the tear is greater than 5 cm, a subacromial smoothing as recommended by Matsen et al. is used rather than true subacromial decompression, preserving the CA ligament.[21]

Next, the bone bed on the humeral tuberosity is prepared through the lateral portal, using a shaver. The bone is lightly debrided up to the articular margin to remove any soft tissues and provide a bleeding surface, without decorticating the bone bed. Decortication should be avoided to maximize bone resistance to suture anchor pullout. Animal studies have demonstrated that tendon healing to a bleeding surface of cortical bone is equivalent to tendon healing to cancellous bone.[22]

The first critical step in carrying out an arthroscopic repair involves tear pattern recognition. Most rotator cuff tears can be broadly classified into two patterns: crescent-shaped tears and U-shaped tears. Crescent-shaped tears, even large and massive ones, typically pull away from bone but do not retract far (Figure 18.4A). Therefore, they can be repaired directly to bone with minimal tension (Figure 18.4B). U-shaped tears generally extend much farther medially than crescent-shaped tears, with the apex of the tear located above the glenoid or even medial to the glenoid (Figure 18.5A). It is important to realize that this medial extension of the tear does not represent retraction, but rather represents the shape assumed by an L-shaped tear under physiological load from its muscle–tendon components. Closing such a tear is much like closing a tent flap; one must reconstitute the two limbs of the L (Figure 18.5B–E). One must not make the mistake of trying to mobilize the medial margin of the tear from the glenoid and scapular neck enough to pull it over to the humeral bone bed. Even if such a tear could be mobilized and pulled laterally to the tuberosity, the large tensile stresses in the middle of such a repaired cuff margin would doom it to failure.

The Crescent-Shaped Tear

The tear pattern is assessed by testing the mobility of the tear margin with an atraumatic tendon grasper. If the tear can be easily brought over the bone bed with minimal tension, it can be repaired directly to bone with suture anchors without margin convergence techniques.

The next step is to place suture anchors to secure the cuff to the prepared bone bed. Through a posterior viewing portal, suture anchors of the screw-in type are placed approximately 1 cm apart on the bone bed. The anchors are emplaced in the bone bed through percutaneous incisions lateral to the acromion at a 45° "deadman angle" approximately 5 mm from the ar-

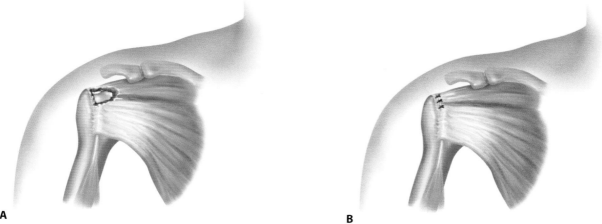

FIGURE 18.4. (A) Crescent-shaped tear without significant retraction can be repaired directly to bone with minimal tension. (B) Repair of crescent-shaped tears directly to bone should respect the crescent-shaped margin of the tear to avoid tension overload.

ticular margin[23] (Figure 18.6). The crescent-shaped margin of the tear must be respected in the repair, and therefore the suture anchors should be placed in a crescent array just 5 mm off the articular surface to avoid tension overload at any of the fixation points. Tension overload has been shown experimentally to cause failure of cuff repairs subjected to physiological cyclic loads.[24,25]

The authors' preference is to use a biodegradable DL-polylactic acid screw-in type of anchor (Bio-

Corkscrew from Arthrex). The BioCorkscrew suture eyelet consists of no. 4 Ethibond suture insert molded into the body of the anchor, allowing the suture to glide easily through the eyelet no matter what the anchor's direction of orientation (Figure 18.7). This flexible eyelet minimizes friction within the eyelet and prevents entanglement of sutures within the eyelet, even with two sutures loaded per anchor.

After anchor placement, a suture passer, such as a Penetrator or BirdBeak, is passed through the superior

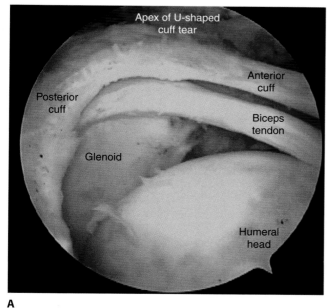

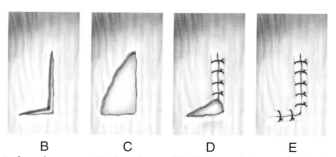

FIGURE 18.5. (A) U-shaped rotator cuff tear whose apex extends toward the glenoid, the "Grand Canyon view" when viewed through the lateral portal (right shoulder). (B) L-shaped tear. (C) Elasticity of the musculotendinous units causes deformation of the L-shaped tear to a U-shaped tear. (D) Closure of the vertical limb of the tear by side-to-side sutures. (E) Closure of the horizontal limb of the tear by tendon-to-bone sutures.

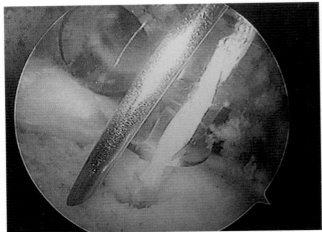

FIGURE 18.6. The anchors are placed into the bone bed at a 45° "deadman angle" approximately 5 to 10 mm from the articular margin. A spinal needle is used to locate/ensure the optimal position of the anchors prior to placement.

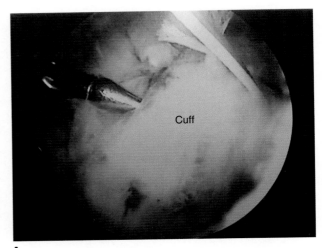

A

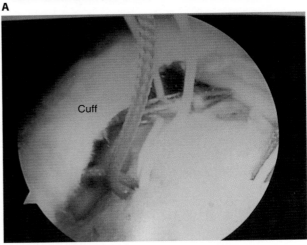

B

FIGURE 18.8. Suture passage is performed by "lining up the putt" (A) so that the suture passer penetrates the cuff to (B) emerge close enough to the anchor to easily capture the suture. (Viewing from lateral portal, right shoulder, beach chair perspective.)

aspect of the cuff in line with the anchor, grasping the suture beneath the cuff and easily pulling the suture back out through the cuff.

The posterior aspect of the cuff is best visualized while one is viewing through the lateral portal to obtain a panoramic view of the suture anchor, posterior cuff, and suture passer. Suture passage is performed by "lining up the putt" so that the suture passer penetrates the cuff to emerge close enough to the anchor to easily capture the suture (Figure 18.8).

A modified Neviaser portal as described by Nord is the best approach to the anterior and central portion of the cuff in crescent shaped tears (Figure 18.9).[26]

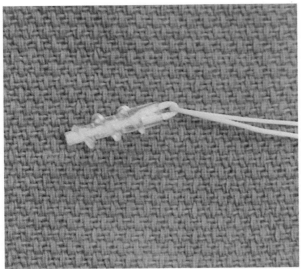

FIGURE 18.7. BioCorkscrew anchor with flexible braided suture eyelet minimizes friction and prevents entanglement of sutures within the eyelet.

This portal requires a small 3 mm puncture incision located approximately 1 cm posteromedial to the acromioclavicular (AC) joint in the "soft spot" bordered by the posterior clavicle, medial acromion, and the scapular spine. A spinal needle is used to determine the proper location of the portal, and then the suture passer is placed adjacent to the needle as the surgeon observes its entry into the subacromial space. Suture passage is performed as described earlier, and one limb of each suture pair (simple rather than mattress configuration sutures) is passed individually through the cuff to obtain separate soft tissue fixation points for each suture.

Occasionally the most anterior aspect of the crescent requires an additional angle of approach through the anterior cannula. This approach is most easily accomplished with an angled suture passer such as the

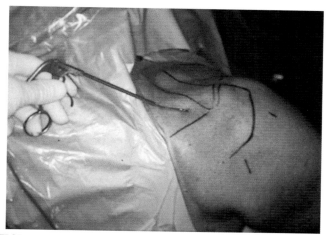

FIGURE 18.9. The modified Neviaser portal is located approximately 1 cm posteromedial to the AC joint in the "soft spot" bordered by the posterior clavicle, medial acromion, and the scapular spine. This portal provides a good angle of approach to the anterior and central portion of the cuff in crescent-shaped tears.

BirdBeak, with the shoulder held in maximal external rotation.

One limb of each of the suture anchors placed should be passed before any knots are tied. By passing all sutures prior to tying, it is easier to manipulate the suture retriever under the cuff margin, since the cuff is not bound down by previously tied sutures. The sutures are tied beginning with those nearest to the intact cuff insertions and proceeding toward the central part of the tear, usually posterior to anterior. This progression sequentially decreases the amount of tension the central sutures will have to withstand.

A potential drawback to passing all the sutures before tying is that a tangled web of sutures may result. However this situation can be easily resolved as the suture pairs are retrieved for knot tying. Grasping the suture pairs proximal to the entanglement, at the level of the anchor or directly on the cuff surface, one can pull each suture pair through a dedicated cannula (usually lateral) for knot tying. Each pair is then tied sequentially, and entanglement is never an issue. It is important that only the two suture limbs being tied are within the working cannula to avoid "fouling" the sutures as the knot is tied.

The rotator cuff can be secured to the bone bed by using complex sliding knots or a nonsliding knot to tie the sutures. Because we wish to avoid damaging the tendon as the suture slides through the tendon, and to avoid the abrasion of the suture against the eyelet of the anchor (which could weaken the suture), we do not routinely use a sliding knot.[27] We prefer a static nonsliding knot, to use a double-diameter knot pusher (Surgeon's Sixth Finger, from Arthrex) (Figure

18.10).[28,29] The static locked knot is composed of a base knot consisting of three stacked half-hitches that is locked by three additional half-hitches in which the post is reversed for each throw.

The minimal configuration that will lock a base knot is three reversed-post half-hitches: that is, three half-hitches applied on top of the base knot so that the post is switched on three consecutive throws. The three reversed-post half-hitches will always lock the base knot and convert its mode of failure from slippage to breakage, thereby reliably maximizing knot security.[30] Therefore this is the recommended locking configuration, regardless of which base knot is used.

The suture limb that passes through the cuff is threaded through the lumen of the knot pusher (the initial post) so that the knot will be positioned on top of the cuff rather than over the bone. For better loop security, continuous tension is maintained on the post limb as the knot is tied, to prevent loosening of the soft tissue loop. Post switching is accomplished without rethreading the knot pusher simply by tensioning the wrapping suture limb (the initial loop suture) at the same time tension is released on the post suture limb.[31] By flipping the post three consecutive times in this manner, maximal knot security is achieved.[30] The completed repair should generate a crescent shape to the repaired cuff margin to avoid tension overload centrally, with a separate soft tissue fixation point for each suture.

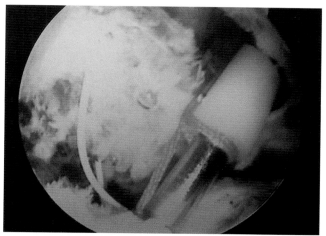

FIGURE 18.10. Arthroscopic view demonstrating our technique for knot tying using the Surgeon's Sixth Finger knot pusher (Arthrex). A nonsliding knot is preferred, and we use a double-diameter knot pusher with knot composed of a base knot of three stacked half-hitches locked by three additional half-hitches in which the post is reversed for each throw. For better loop security, continuous tension is maintained on the post limb, since the knot is tied to prevent loosening of the soft tissue loop.

The U-Shaped Tear

After glenohumeral arthroscopy and initial subacromial bursectomy have been completed, inspection of the rotator cuff margins is performed with the scope in the lateral portal. With large U-shaped tears, the abundant bursal tissue in the posterior gutter of the subacromial space often obscures the posterior margin of the rotator cuff. This bursal tissue is removed with a shaver brought in through the posterior portal. Often the bursal tissue is very thick and may be mistaken for rotator cuff tendon. To properly identify the tissue, the surgeon must follow the edge of the tissue laterally to determine whether the tissue inserts onto the humerus (Figure 18.11). If the tissue inserts onto the humerus, it is rotator cuff tendon. Tissue that continues *past* the humerus to blend into deltoid fascia is bursa and must be removed.

Once the anterior and posterior cuff margins have been fully exposed, one must determine whether the tear is a mobile U-shaped tear that can be repaired by means of the margin convergence technique.[18] If the apex is located at or medial to the glenoid articular surface, the tear is usually a U-shaped tear. Placing the scope in the lateral viewing portal allows the apex of the tear to be identified medially. The tear pattern is assessed by grasping the cuff margin with an atraumatic tendon grasper, testing the mobility of the anterior leaf through the posterior portal, and testing the posterior leaf through the anterior portal. If the tear is mobile, the anterior and posterior leaves can be approximated by side-to-side sutures to achieve margin convergence.

If one remains uncertain of the configuration, a single side-to-side suture can be placed a centimeter from the apex of the tear and tensioned to see if partial closure of the tear is accomplished. The margin convergence effect of a single suture can be dramatic, causing the two leaves of the cuff to "converge" the cuff to a tension-free state above the bone bed (Figure 18.12).

Mobilization of the rotator cuff from the glenoid margin is rarely necessary, although in previously operated shoulders, adhesions between the cuff and deltoid or between the cuff and acromion may need to be excised. If the cuff is scarred to the deltoid, the proper plane of dissection can be identified by finding the fatty layer above the cuff at the apex of the tear. If this fatty stripe is followed posteriorly with a shaver,

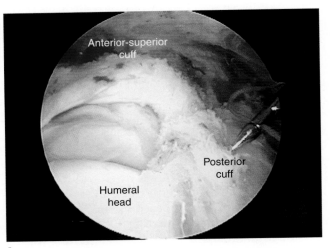

A

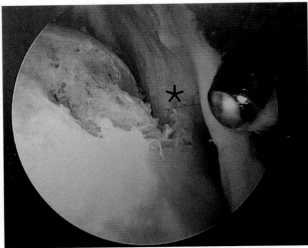

FIGURE 18.11. The superior edge of the posterior cuff is identified and cleared of bursal tissue prior to repair with shaver through the posterior portal (scope in lateral portal, left shoulder, beach chair perspective). Tissue inserting into humerus is rotator cuff tendon (*), but tissue that continues past the humerus to blend into the deltoid fascia is bursa and must be removed.

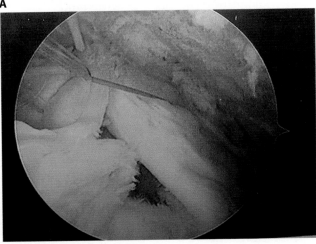

B

FIGURE 18.12. (A) The first limb of a single margin convergence stitch is being placed to evaluate whether the tear pattern is appropriate for the margin convergence technique (lateral viewing portal, left shoulder, beach chair perspective). (B) Tensioning a single side-to-side stitch can provide dramatic partial closure of a massive U-shaped tear, confirming that margin convergence is the proper technique for closing the tear.

the cuff can be dissected free from the deltoid to the periphery of the cuff margin. The adhesions between the peripheral cuff and the deltoid are then released by the shaver or with electrocautery.

For large or massive U-shaped tears, a standard arthroscopic acromioplasty is not performed. Instead of a true subacromial decompression, a subacromial smoothing, as recommended by Matsen et al., is performed.[21] This smoothing entails a debridement of the soft tissues on the undersurface of the acromion and removal of small bony irregularities, but the CA ligament is preserved. The CA arch is preserved to maintain the restraint against proximal humeral migration if the repair should fail.

The bone bed on the humerus is prepared through the lateral portal with a shaver. The bone is lightly debrided up to the articular margin to remove any soft tissues and to provide a bleeding surface without decorticating the bone bed.

Margin convergence is the next step. The scope is placed in the lateral portal for the "Grand Canyon" view to optimize viewing of side-to-side suture placement (Figure 18.5A). Two suture passers (Penetrator or BirdBeak) one for each leaf of the cuff, are utilized to "hand off" the suture from one leaf to the other (Figure 18.13). A no. 2 Ethibond free suture is loaded into one of the suture passers, and the loaded suture passer is brought through the posterior portal to penetrate the posterior leaf of the cuff near the apex of the tear. The second (empty) suture passer is then brought through the anterior leaf via the anterior portal, and a "hand off" of the suture from posterior to anterior is performed. The anterior suture passer is withdrawn, pulling the free suture through the anterior leaf and out the anterior portal. This "handoff" step is repeated as many times as necessary, placing

sutures at 5 to 10 mm intervals and alternating white with green sutures to facilitate suture management. Typically an average of four side-to-side sutures is used if the apex of the tear overlies the glenoid (Figure 18.14A).

The sutures are then tied sequentially from medial to lateral to accomplish margin convergence (Figure 18.14B). The apex suture is tied first, bringing its two limbs out the posterior portal. All other suture limbs are transferred out an alternate cannula (usually anterior). To avoid "fouling" the sutures as the knot is tied, it is important that only the two suture limbs being tied occupy the working cannula.

A clear, 7 mm "fishbowl" cannula is preferred for knot tying to improve visualization. The knots are tied over the posterior leaf of the cuff to avoid the theoretical problem of knot impingement on the undersurface of the acromion. In performing margin convergence, it is important to achieve both loop security

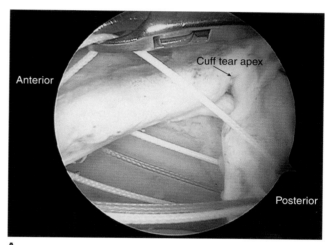

A

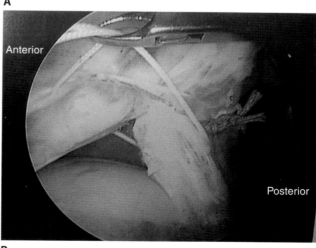

B

FIGURE 18.14. Lateral viewing portal, left shoulder. (A) Side-to-side sutures placed for U-shaped tear. (B) Anterior and posterior cuff margins "converge" as side-to-side sutures are tied.

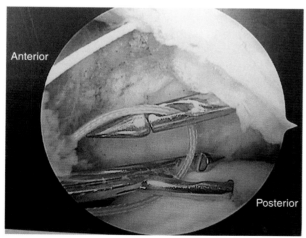

FIGURE 18.13. Side-to-side sutures passed through anterior and posterior leaves of the rotator cuff tear; two suture passers are used to "hand off" the suture from one leaf to the other.

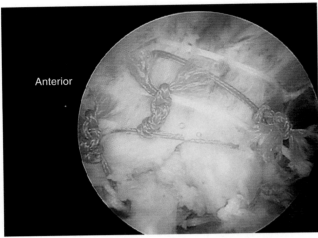

Anterior

Posterior

Lateral

FIGURE 18.15. Arthroscopic view of completed repair, viewed through the lateral viewing portal (left shoulder, beach chair perspective).

(maintenance of a tight suture loop around the enclosed soft tissue) and knot security (resistance of the knot to failure by slippage or breakage).[28–30]

After margin convergence has been accomplished with the side-to-side repair of the anterior and posterior leaves, the rotator cuff must be secured to the bone bed with suture anchors. The use of a posterior viewing portal allows the placement of screw-in suture anchors approximately 1 cm apart on the bone bed. The anchors are placed into the bone bed at a 45° "deadman angle" approximately 5 to 10 mm from the articular margin. The suture anchors are placed 1 cm from the anterior and posterior leaves of the cuff, to shift the cuff to the anchors as the knots are tied. Typically two biodegradable DL-PLA screw-in type anchors are used, one for each leaf of the cuff. A spinal needle is used to locate the optimal position of the anchors to create the "deadman angle," and each anchor is placed through a 3 mm puncture incision adjacent to the lateral acromion.

After anchor placement, suture passage is accomplished by passing a suture passer such as a Penetrator or a BirdBeak through the superior aspect of the cuff in line with the anchor, grasping the suture beneath the cuff, and easily pulling the suture back out through the cuff.

For the posterior aspect of the cuff, this is best visualized through the lateral portal to obtain a panoramic view of the suture anchor, posterior cuff, and suture passer, and to "line up the putt" so that the suture passer penetrates the cuff close to the anchor and easily captures the suture (Figure 18.8).

This sequence is repeated for the anterior leaf through the anterior cannula. This approach is most easily accomplished with an angled suture passer (e.g., BirdBeak) with the shoulder held in maximal external rotation.

Again, all the anchor sutures should be passed before any knots are tied. The sutures are tied through a clear cannula through the lateral portal while the surgeon is viewing through the posterior portal. As the knots are tied, the cuff is shifted to the anchors, maximizing contact of the cuff with the bone bed.

After the knots have been secured, the arm is rotated to view the entire repair and assess the strength and security of the completed repair (Figure 18.15).

POSTOPERATIVE MANAGEMENT

The arm is placed at the side in a sling with a small pillow attached (Ultrasling, D-J Ortho; Vista, CA) for 6 weeks. All procedures are performed on an outpatient basis.

Passive external rotation is started immediately, as well as elbow flexion and extension. To minimize excessive stress on the repair, however, no overhead stretching is initiated until 6 weeks after surgery. This 6-week period maximizes tendon-to-bone healing, with reestablishment of as much of the rotator cuff footprint as possible. The postoperative stiffness associated with immobilization in open and mini-open shoulder surgery does not seem to occur in arthroscopic patients as long as early passive external rotation is maintained, possibly because deltoid damage is minimized.

At the end of 6 weeks, the sling is discontinued and passive overhead stretching is started, using supine flexion stretches as well as a rope and pulley in the sitting position. Internal rotation stretching is also initiated.

At 12 weeks after surgery, muscle strengthening is started for the rotator cuff, deltoid, biceps, and scapular stabilizers. Sonnabend et al. observed in a primate study of rotator cuff repair that strong, Sharpey-type fibers did not form until 12 weeks after surgery. Therefore to minimize the risk of early retear, resistive exercises are not started until after 12 weeks.[32]

Activities are progressed as strength allows. However particular activities that require angular acceleration of the shoulder, such as overhead sports (tennis, baseball, golf), are not allowed until at least 6 months after surgery.

RESULTS/OUTCOME

Published outcomes of arthroscopic rotator cuff repair for small and medium-sized tears have reported good or excellent results in approximately 90% of patients.[33,34]

Tauro presented the results of 53 patients who underwent arthroscopic rotator cuff repair with minimum 2-year follow-up.[33] All patients were evaluated by means of a modified UCLA rating system, with a maximum score of 45, adapted to include additional points for abduction range of motion and strength. The author reported 92% good or excellent results (49 of 53) and overall improvement from an average preoperative rating of 17 to a postoperative rating of 41.

Gartsman presented the results of arthroscopic repair of the rotator cuff in 73 patients with minimum 2-year follow-up evaluated by means of the standard UCLA rating scale and with the American Shoulder and Elbow Surgeons (ASES) shoulder index.[34] The study included 11 small, 45 medium, 11 large, and 6 massive tears. The average UCLA score improved from 12.4 to 31.1 points and the average ASES index score from 30.7 to 87.6. None of the shoulders were rated as good or excellent preoperatively, whereas 84% (61 of 73) were rated as good or excellent at final follow-up evaluation.

Despite these promising results, the conventional thinking has been that arthroscopic rotator cuff repair may produce excellent results in smaller tears but open repair is necessary to repair large to massive tears. However, contrary to this line of thought, we have found that arthroscopic cuff repair for large to massive tears yields an even greater improvement compared to open techniques.

A recent series compiled by the senior author (SSB) reviewed the results of 59 rotator cuff repairs performed between 1993 and 1997, with average follow up of 3.5 years.[35] The tears were subdivided into groups according to tear diameter using the classification system of DeOrio and Cofield and included 13 tears classified as massive (>5 cm).[36] Average UCLA scores improved from 14.0 to 29.9, and average forward flexion improved from 90° to 132°. Improve-

ments in forward flexion and UCLA scores were both significant ($p < 0.0001$), and good or excellent results were achieved in 92% of the entire patient group. Between-group comparisons for the four groups of tear sizes showed no differences in the results, such that the massive tears did as well as the small, medium, and large tears. This finding is strikingly different from the reported results of open rotator cuff repair, where larger size tears have been shown to have poorer results than smaller size tears.

COMPLICATIONS

Complications of arthroscopic rotator cuff repair are relatively uncommon. Postoperative complications associated with open rotator cuff repair, such as infection, stiffness, and deltoid detachment are rarely observed in arthroscopic surgery. Elevated arthroscopic pump pressures (> 90 mmHg) for extended periods of time are avoided to prevent excessive swelling. The postoperative stiffness associated with immobilization in open and mini-open shoulder surgery is uncommon.

References

1. Burkhart SS. Reconciling the paradox of rotator cuff repair vs. debridement: a unified biomechanical rationale for the treatment of rotator cuff repairs. *Arthroscopy* 1994;10:1–16.
2. Burkhart SS. Arthroscopic treatment of massive rotator cuff tears. Clinical results and biomechanical rationale. *Clin Orthop* 1991;(267):45–56.
3. Burkhart SS. Arthroscopic debridement and decompression for selected rotator cuff tears. Clinical results, pathomechanics, and patient selection based on biomechanical parameters. *Orthop Clin North Am* 1993; 24:111–123.
4. Ellman H. Arthroscopic subacromial decompression: analysis of one- to three-year results. *Arthroscopy* 1987; 3:173–181.
5. Ellman H, Kay SP, Wirth M. Arthroscopic treatment of full-thickness rotator cuff tears: 2- to 7-year follow-up study. *Arthroscopy* 1993;9:195–200.
6. Esch JC, Ozerkis LR, Helgager JA, Kane N, Lilliott N. Arthroscopic subacromial decompression: results according to the degree of rotator cuff tear. *Arthroscopy* 1988;4:241–249.
7. Gartsman GM. Arthroscopic acromioplasty for lesions of the rotator cuff. *J Bone Joint Surg Am* 1990;72(2):169–180.
8. Zvijac JE, Levy HJ, Lemak LJ. Arthroscopic subacromial decompression in the treatment of full thickness rotator cuff tears: a 3- to 6-year follow-up. *Arthroscopy* 1994;10:518–523.
9. Melillo AS, Savoie FH 3rd, Field LD. Massive rotator cuff tears: debridement versus repair. *Orthop Clin North Am* 1997;28(1):117–124.

10. Bigliani LU, Cordasco FA, McIlveen SJ, et al. Operative treatment of massive rotator cuff tears: long term results. *J Shoulder Elbow Surg* 1992;1:120–130.

11. Codman EA. Complete rupture of the supraspinatus tendon: operative treatment with report of two successful cases. *Boston Med Surg J* 1911;164:708–710.

12. Cofield RH. Rotator cuff disease of the shoulder. *J Bone Joint Surg Am* 1985;67:974–979.

13. Ellman H, Hanker G, Bayer M. Repair of the rotator cuff: end result study of factors influencing reconstruction. *J Bone Joint Surg Am* 1986;68:1136–1144.

14. Harryman DT, Mack LA, Wang KY, et al. Repairs of the rotator cuff: correlation of functional results with integrity of the cuff. *J Bone Joint Surg Am* 1991;73:982–989.

15. Iannotti JP, Bernot MP, Kuhlman JR, et al. Postoperative assessment of shoulder function: a prospective study of full-thickness rotator cuff tears. *J Shoulder Elbow Surg* 1996;5:449–457.

16. Neer CS, Flatow EL, Lech O. Tears of the rotator cuff: long term results of anterior acromioplasty and repair. *Orthop Trans* 1988;12:735.

17. Neviaser JS. Ruptures of the rotator cuff of the shoulder: new concepts in the diagnosis and operative treatment of chronic ruptures. *Arch Surg* 1971;102:483–485.

18. Burkhart SS, Athanasiou KA, Wirth MA. Margin convergence: a method of reducing strain in massive rotator cuff tears. *Arthroscopy* 1996;12:335–338.

19. Burkhart SS, Danaceau SM, Athanasiou KA. Technical note: turbulence control as a factor in improving visualization during subacromial shoulder arthroscopy. *Arthroscopy* 2001;17:209–212.

20. Sampson TG, Nisbet JK, Glick JM. Precision acromioplasty in arthroscopic subacromial decompression. *Arthroscopy* 1991;7:301–307.

21. Matsen FA III, Lippitt SB, Sidles JA, et al. Surgical approach to roughness at the non-articular humeroscapular motion interface. In: Matsen FA III, Lippitt SB, eds. *Practical Evaluation and Management of the Shoulder.* Philadelphia: WB Saunders; 1994:176–178.

22. St Pierre P, Olson FJ, Elliott JJ, et al. Tendon healing to cortical bone compared with healing to a cancellous trough: a biomechanical and histological model evaluation in goats. *J Bone Joint Surg Am* 1995;77:1858–1866.

23. Burkhart SS. The deadman theory of suture anchors: observations along a South Texas fence line. *Arthroscopy* 1995;11:119–123.

24. Burkhart SS, Diaz-Pagan JL, Wirth MA, et al. Cyclic loading of anchor based rotator cuff repairs: confirmation of the tension overload phenomenon and comparison of suture anchor fixation with transosseous fixation. *Arthroscopy* 1997;13:720–724.

25. Burkhart SS, Johnson TC, Wirth MA, et al. Cyclic loading of transosseous rotator cuff repairs: Tension overload as a possible cause of failure. *Arthroscopy* 1997;13:172–176.

26. Nord K. Modified Neviaser portal and subclavian portal in shoulder arthroscopy. Paper presented at: 19th Annual Meeting of the Arthoscopy Association of North America; Miami FL; April 14, 2000.

27. Bardana DD, Burks RT, West JR. The effect of suture anchor design and orientation on suture abrasion: an in-vitro study. Submitted to *Arthroscopy.*

28. Burkhart SS, Wirth MA, Simonich M, et al. Knot security in simple sliding knots and its relationship to rotator cuff repair: how secure must a knot be? *Arthroscopy* 2000;16:202–207.

29. Burkhart SS, Wirth MA, Simonich M, et al. Loop security as a determinant of tissue fixation security. *Arthroscopy* 1998;14:773–776.

30. Chan KC, Burkhart SS, Thiagarajan P, Goh JC. Optimization of stacked half-hitch knots for arthroscopic surgery. *Arthroscopy* 2001;17:752–759.

31. Chan KC, Burkhart SS. Technical note. How to switch posts without rethreading when tying half-hitches. *Arthroscopy* 1999;15:444–450.

32. Sonnabend DH, Jones D, Walsh WR. Rotator cuff repair in a primate model: observations and implications. *Proceedings of the 14th Annual Closed Meeting, American Shoulder and Elbow Surgeons; Manchester, VT, September* 1997:27.

33. Tauro JC. Arthroscopic rotator cuff repair: analysis of technique and results at 2 and 3 year follow up. *Arthroscopy* 1998;14:45–51.

34. Gartsman GM. Arthroscopic acromioplasty for lesions of the rotator cuff. *J Bone Joint Surg Am* 1990;72(2):169–180.

35. Burkhart SS, Danaceau SM, Pearce CE. Arthroscopic rotator cuff repair: analysis of results by tear size and by repair technique, margin convergence versus direct tendon to bone technique. *Arthroscopy.* In press.

36. DeOrio JK, Cofield RH. Results of a second attempt at surgical repair of a failed initial rotator-cuff repair. *J Bone Joint Surg Am* 1984;66:563–567.

19

Arthroscopic Management of Massive Rotator Cuff Tears

Stefan J. Tolan, Felix H. Savoie III,
and Christopher K. Jones

Arthroscopic rotator cuff repair has emerged as a successful alternative to open repair and can be considered an option for most patients being evaluated for surgical intervention. The main advantage of arthroscopic rotator cuff repair is the avoidance of deltoid detachment. Since the deltoid does not need to be protected postoperatively, physical therapy can be accelerated, potentially decreasing postoperative stiffness. Arthroscopy is also associated with decreased postoperative pain, allowing the procedure to be performed on an outpatient basis.[1]

Arthroscopic repair of the rotator cuff has been generally indicated in small to medium tears (<3 cm diameter) with adequate bone and tendon quality. These tears are usually repairable to their original position on the tuberosity without significant tension. As the tear size increases, treatment becomes much more difficult. With advanced techniques, however, the principles of open repair of massive rotator cuff tears can be applied to arthroscopic repairs.

Cofield's classification is most often used, but the definition of a massive rotator cuff tear is not universally agreed upon.[2] Cofield separated tears by size into four categories: small (≤1 cm), medium (1–3 cm), large (3–5 cm), and massive (>5 cm). Gerber et al. proposed that rotator cuff tears be defined as massive only if they involved detachment of two or more entire tendons.[3] The arthroscopic appearance is a large inverted U-shaped tear with an exposed humeral head and greater tuberosity (Figure 19.1). These tears are complex, consisting of a progressive transverse component with significant medial extension. Physiological load from the muscle–tendon components converts an L-shaped tear into this characteristic U-shaped configuration.[4] Most massive tears involve the supraspinatus and infraspinatus, but anterosuperior tears involving the supraspinatus and subscapularis may also occur. With time, these tears may extend medial to the glenoid and form significant adhesions on the cuff's bursal and articular surfaces.

The arthroscopic management of massive tears is still evolving. Current arthroscopic procedures include limited debridement and decompression, partial repair, mini-open repair, and arthroscopic repair.[5–13] Successful arthroscopic debridement and decompression has been reported in select patients if the deltoid vector can be balanced by the force couple of the anterior and posterior cuff. Arthroscopic partial repair has also been recommended when the tear is felt to be too large for a complete repair, and the anterior cuff is intact. With this technique the infraspinatus is mobilized and repaired to the greater tuberosity, but the superior defect is not closed. The goal of this partial repair is to restore the balance between the posterior cuff and the anterior cuff, creating a stable fulcrum for glenohumeral motion. The arthroscope can also be used as an adjunct to open repair of a massive tear. In this technique, the arthroscope is used to evaluate the glenohumeral joint, to perform the subacromial decompression and, when necessary, distal clavicle excision, and to prepare the greater tuberosity. A deltoid splitting incision is used for cuff mobilization and fixation to bone. This chapter details a technique for an all-arthroscopic repair of massive rotator cuff tears.

INDICATIONS/CONTRAINDICATIONS

Initially, a trial of conservative treatment should be instituted. This usually consists of oral anti-inflammatory medication, rotator cuff and scapular stabilizer strengthening exercises, and subacromial cortisone injections. Massive tears are usually chronic and may have been exacerbated by a recent event. If acute symptoms can be helped, and the patient is satisfied

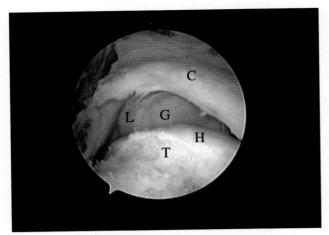

A

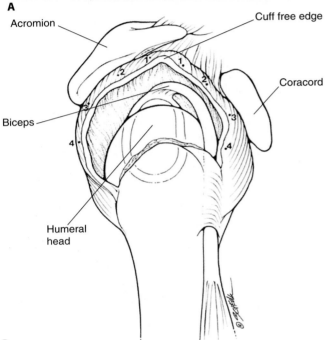

B

FIGURE 19.1. View of massive rotator cuff tear from lateral portal. (A) There is complete detachment of the supraspinatus and infraspinatus tendons, and the maximum diameter of the tear is greater than 5 cm: C, cuff; H, humeral head; G, glenoid; L, labrum; T, trough. (B) Drawing corresponding to photograph in (A). (Note numbers that will correspond to side-to-side repair sutures.)

with the function of the injured shoulder, nonoperative measures may suffice.

The primary indications for arthroscopic repair of massive rotator cuff tears are refractory pain, decreased shoulder strength, and loss of active motion. No definitive contraindications to arthroscopic repair of massive tears exist. Operative repair is indicated in both acute and chronic tears, and in patients of all age groups. Advanced age is not a contraindication to sur-

gical repair, and successful results have been demonstrated with open procedures in patients older than 70 years of age with massive rotator cuff tears.[14,15]

PREOPERATIVE PLANNING

History and physical examination remain important diagnostic tools and aid in preoperative planning of the rotator cuff repair. A long duration of symptoms suggests likely retraction and scarring, and weakness signifies loss of the cuff's mechanical advantage. With massive tears, it is important to identify and document the strength of the infraspinatus and the subscapularis muscles. Good active external rotation strength with the arm abducted 30° suggests an intact infraspinatus muscle, and the "liftoff test" is used to assess the subscapularis muscle. The integrity of these two muscles is an important element of the planned repair of the rotator cuff.

Radiographs of the affected shoulder are routinely obtained, and include an anteroposterior, axillary, and outlet view. The radiographs are screened for the presence of osteoarthritis and acromioclavicular arthritis, and for the shape and thickness of the acromion. A high-riding humeral head suggests a massive tear of chronic duration. In this situation the surgeon must be prepared to release the inferior capsule of the glenohumeral joint, allowing reduction of the humeral head after the cuff has been repaired.

Magnetic resonance imaging (MRI) has replaced shoulder arthrography because of the ability to preoperatively characterize the tear according to size and to assess the quality of the remaining cuff tissue. Fatty infiltration of the rotator cuff musculature, visible on MRI, suggests poor tissue quality and bodes poorly for operative success.

SURGICAL TECHNIQUE

Positioning/Setup

General anesthesia is induced, and controlled hypotension, with systolic blood pressure around 90 mmHg, is maintained throughout the procedure. Hypotension is extremely important to maintain hemostasis, allowing clear visualization. The patient is placed in the lateral decubitus position and supported with a beanbag. The pelvis is held perpendicular to the table and the affected shoulder is allowed to roll posteriorly 30°. A sterile traction stockinet is applied to the forearm with 10 lb of traction. The shoulder is abducted 30° and forward flexed 15°.

Instrumentation

An arthroscope (Smith & Nephew Dyonics, Andover, MA) with attachable 4.5 and 5.5 mm metal cannulas is used. A motorized full-radius resector (Dyonics) is used for soft tissue debridement and cuff mobilization. The Helicut Bur (Dyonics) is very versatile and is used for the acromioplasty, distal clavicle excision (when necessary), and preparation of the tuberosity. A 60° retrograde suture retriever (Innovasive, Johnson & Johnson, New Brunswick, NJ) is used for the margin convergence sutures and to retrieve the anchor sutures through the rotator cuff. Gravity inflow is used, and epinephrine (1:250,000) is added to each 5 L bag of lactated Ringer's solution to aid in hemostasis.

Surgical Technique

A posterior portal is created at the equator of the glenohumeral joint, and diagnostic arthroscopy of the glenohumeral joint is performed. The rotator cuff tear is easily visualized from the glenohumeral joint. If additional intra-articular pathology is identified, it is addressed prior to rotator cuff repair.

A 5.5 mm metal cannula and trochar is inserted into the subacromial space through the posterior portal. The trochar is pushed anteriorly along the inferior aspect of the acromion until it encounters the coracoacromial (CA) ligament. The trochar is then directed laterally, around the CA ligament, and advanced into the anterior soft tissues until the anterior skin is tented. An incision is made over the tip of the trochar and a second 5.5 mm metal cannula, with attached inflow tubing, is placed over the tip of the trochar and guided into the subacromial space. Both cannulas are

directed laterally to the area of the subdeltoid bursa, and the arthroscope remains positioned posteriorly.

A lateral portal is created approximately three fingerbreadths distal to and in line with the anterolateral corner of the acromion. A spinal needle is used to confirm adequate position prior to creation of this portal. A 4.5 mm metal cannula is directed into the subacromial space and the motorized resector is used to perform a bursectomy (Figure 19.2). The mobility of the cuff is assessed by applying traction to the cuff and examining the cuff tear pattern from different portals. When the presence and degree of restriction have been determined, a release is performed if necessary. The release is carried out stepwise by first introducing the motorized resector between the inferior aspect of the cuff and the glenoid, releasing the undersurface of the cuff circumferentially around the glenoid (Figure 19.3). Adhesions are next removed between the superior cuff surface and the scapular spine. Mobi-

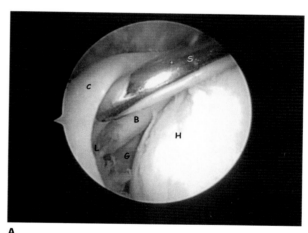

A

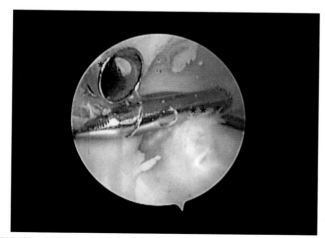

FIGURE 19.2. Looking from posterior portal (right shoulder, beach chair perspective), the 5.5 mm metal cannula (*) and conical trochar (**) are inserted through the lateral working portal into the subacromial space.

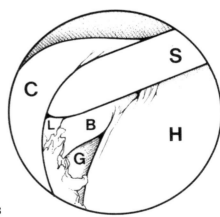

B

FIGURE 19.3. Release of the rotator cuff, viewing from posterior portal (right shoulder, beach chair perspective). (A) The motorized shaver is introduced between the bursal surface of the rotator cuff and the glenoid labrum. The teeth of the shaver are directed away from the cuff and are used to release adhesions circumferentially around the glenoid. C, cuff; S, motorized shaver; B, biceps tendon; L, labrum; G, glenoid; H, humeral head. (B) Drawing corresponding to photograph in (A).

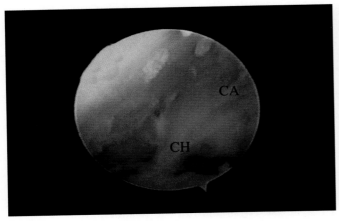

A

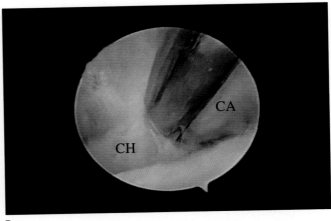

B

FIGURE 19.4. Coracohumeral ligament release. (A) View with arthroscope in posterior portal (right shoulder, beach chair perspective) showing coracoacromial ligament (CA) and coracohumeral ligament (CH). (B) Motorized shaver entering from lateral portal releasing coracohumeral ligament (right shoulder, beach chair perspective).

lization is continued anteriorly as necessary, following the coracoacromial ligament down to the base of the coracoid. The coracohumeral ligament is identified and released (Figure 19.4).

The arthroscope is next moved to the lateral portal, and the Helicut Burr is placed posteriorly. The greater tuberosity is decorticated, and a trough is created in the greater tuberosity near the articular margin (Figure 19.5). The coracoacromial ligament is elevated from the anterior acromion, allowing visualization of the anterolateral corner of the acromion. The acromioplasty is performed with the arthroscope in the lateral portal and the Helicut blade placed posteriorly, using the posterior slope of the acromion as a cutting block. Acromial bone is resected in layers until the anterior acromial edge lies posterior to the anterior margin of the clavicle. An arthroscopic Mumford procedure is next performed if indicated. For this procedure, the camera remains in the lateral portal but is rotated so that an "end-on" view of the acromioclavicular (AC) joint is obtained. The Helicut blade is then used to remove the clavicular facet of the acromion, followed by removal of the distal clavicle until a 10 mm AC resection has been achieved (approximately two shaver blade widths).

Rotator cuff repair begins by replacing the small arthroscopic cannula currently in the lateral portal with a larger diameter (5.5 mm) cannula, allowing greater fluid flow. The posterior portal is used for passage of the 60° retrograde retriever. A 5.5 mm plastic cannula (Accufex, Andover, MA) is placed in the anterior portal for suture passage and management. Additional bursal tissue is removed from the area around

the anterior and posterior portal to facilitate suture passage. Initial repair of massive tears consists of side-to-side cuff reapproximation using multiple no. 5 Ethibond convergence sutures[16] (Figure 19.6). The 60° retrograde retriever (Innovasive) is passed from the posterior portal and directed through the cuff from posteromedial to anterolateral. Usually, three to four margin convergence sutures are passed, converting the U-shaped tear into a crescent-shaped tear that can be sutured to the tuberosity without significant tension (Figure 19.7).

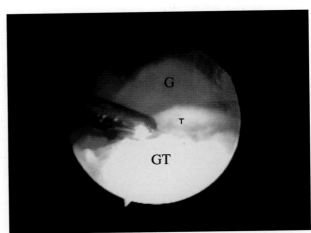

FIGURE 19.5. The scope has been repositioned in the lateral portal, with the shaver entering posteriorly for abrasion of the greater tuberosity and creation of a vascular trough (right shoulder, beach chair perspective). The motorized full-radius resector is used to debride the soft tissue and lightly abrade the greater tuberosity, creating a trough at the articular margin to stimulate bleeding: G, glenoid; T, trough; GT, greater tuberosity.

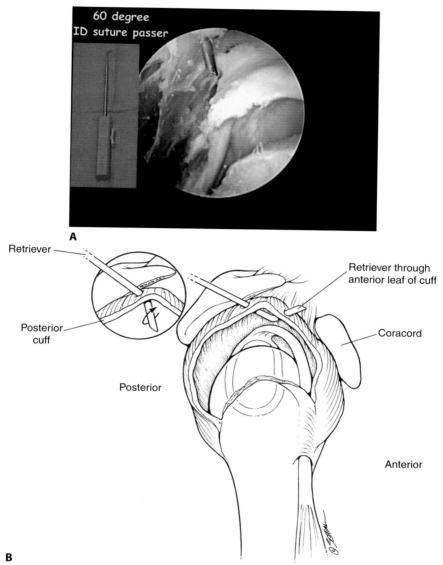

FIGURE 19.6. Placement of convergence suture (scope in lateral portal, right shoulder, beach chair perspective). (A) A 60° retrograde retriever is passed through posterior portal and then rotated and passed through the posterior leaf of the rotator cuff. (B) The retriever is next passed over the biceps tendon and out through the anterior cuff.

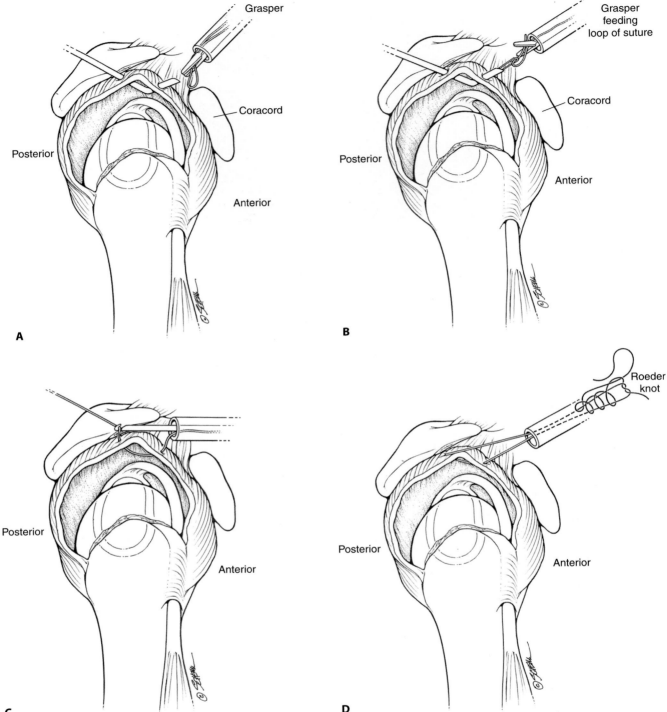

A

B

C

D

FIGURE 19.7. Placement of convergence suture continued (lateral viewing, right shoulder, beach chair perspective). (A) A grasper is used to deliver a no. 5 Ethibond suture with a small loop to the retrograde retriever. (B) The retriever is deployed, grasping the loop and shuttling the suture back through both leaves of the rotator cuff. (C) Crochet hook subsequently used to retrieve the posterior limb through the anterior cannula. (D) An arthroscopic knot (modified Roeder knot) is tied, using the posterior limb as a post. (E) Arthroscopic view through lateral portal (right shoulder, beach chair perspective) of first convergence side-to-side suture. (F) First convergence suture with placement of suture retriever subsequently passed a second time to place next more lateral margin convergence stitch. (G) Arthroscopic view through lateral portal of multiple convergence sutures approximating the anterior and posterior leaves of the rotator cuff.

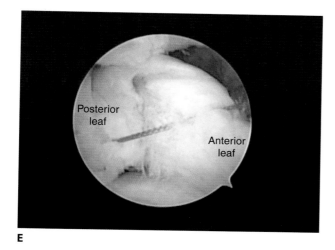

E

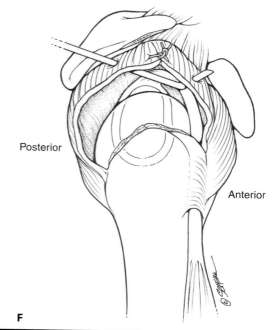

F

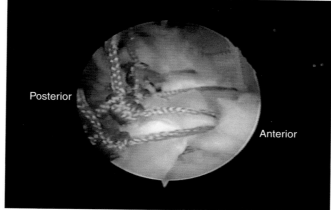

G

FIGURE 19.7. *Continued*

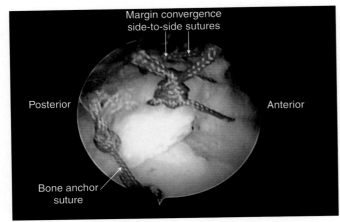

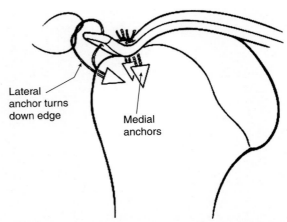

FIGURE 19.9. Alternate anchor placement. Anchors may be placed in the trough adjacent to the articular margin. With this technique a mattress stitch pulls the cuff tissue down to the trough, and a lateral anchor with a simple stitch is used to turn down the edge of the cuff tendon.

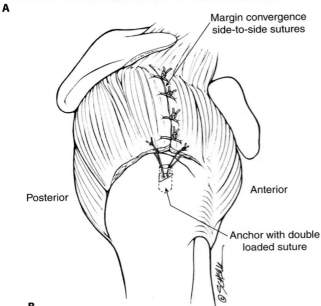

FIGURE 19.8. (A) Suture anchors are placed as needed through an accessory lateral portal, and the sutures are passed through the lateral margin of the cuff to secure the cuffs' edge to the tuberosity. (B) The final arthroscopic appearance, as seen through the lateral viewing portal (right shoulder, beach chair perspective) with a single anchor suture placed through posterior and anterior leaves of cuff tear.

Viewing from the posterior (or anterior) portal, double-loaded suture anchors (Panalock RC, Mitek, New Brunswick, NJ) are then passed through an accessory lateral portal and are used to secure the lateral margin of the cuff down to the prepared area of the tuberosity (Figure 19.8). Usually simple sutures are used because they effectively turn down the edge of the cuff onto the tuberosity.

Alternatively, medial anchors can be placed in the trough created at the articular margin, and a mattress stitch (or stitches) can be used to pull the cuff tissue down into the trough (or onto the abraded tuberosity). This maneuver, however, tends to evert the most lateral cuff margin, and we therefore will place an anchor laterally to turn the margin down to bone with a simple suture (Figure 19.9).

POSTOPERATIVE MANAGEMENT

The majority of rotator cuff repairs are performed on an outpatient basis. Postoperative pain is managed with a combination of an interscalene nerve block and oral analgesics. Additionally, a pain pump may be placed in the subacromial space, and it can deliver a local anesthetic for 48 to 72 h postoperatively.[17] The repair is protected by a large abduction pillow, which is worn continuously except to bathe or dress. After one week, the patient is started on passive forward flexion exercises and the abduction pillow is worn at night. During the day, an abduction sling is worn for comfort.

Over the next several weeks, the patient is advanced to active-assisted forward flexion and external rotation. It is stressed to the patient and the physical therapist that performance of the exercises must be pain free. Full passive range of motion is initiated during the fourth postoperative week, along with active rotator cuff exercises. The patient is allowed full active range of motion after 8 weeks, with return to functional activities after 12 weeks.

RESULTS/OUTCOME

Long-term results of open repair of massive tears have demonstrated a significant decrease in pain, along with significant improvement in function and range of motion.[3,18–22] Strength has also been shown to improve postoperatively in the majority of patients, although more than a year may be required for complete restoration.[18,19]

The number of reports that deal with arthroscopic repair of massive tears is limited; however, current studies indicate that outcomes following arthroscopic repair of massive tears are equal to or better than those reported for open techniques.[1,22] We recently reviewed the arthroscopic treatment of 37 large and 13 massive tears.[23] We were able to perform an anatomic repair in all patients following extensive mobilization. Good or excellent results were attained in 88% of these patients. There was no difference in outcomes between the large tears and the massive tears. Bittar reported on a group of 74 patients with massive, retracted rotator cuff tears.[22] He obtained an anatomic repair in all patients, and 83% of his patients had a good or excellent outcome. Up to 18 months of supervised rehabilitation was required for patients to restore normal strength and function of their shoulder. Tauro performed arthroscopic repair or partial repair in 37 patients with chronic retracted rotator cuff tears.[1] All these patients required a rotator interval slide to facilitate a repair. Good or excellent outcomes were obtained in 89.5% of Tauro's patients at average follow-up of 31 months.

COMPLICATIONS

Complications related to arthroscopic treatment are rare. Structural failure of the repair is the most likely complication. Rates of rerupture range from 13 to 68%.[24–28] However, not all structural failures are clinical failures, and it has been shown that a watertight repair is not necessary for a successful rotator cuff repair.[29] In our arthroscopic series, clinical failure occurred in one out of 13 massive rotator cuff repairs.

No wound infections or areas of persistent drainage occurred, and there were no neurological injuries. No deltoid detachment occurred with arthroscopic repair, although there have been reports of this complication with open repairs.[30–34]

References

1. Tauro JC. Arthrscopic rotator cuff repair: analysis of technique and results at 2 and 3 years follow-up. *Arthroscopy* 1998;14(1):45–51.
2. Cofield RH. Current concepts review. Rotator cuff disease of the shoulder. *J Bone Joint Surg Am* 1985;67:974–979.
3. Gerber C, Fuchs B, Holder J. The results of repair of massive tears of the rotator cuff. *J Bone Joint Surg Am* 2000;82:505–515.
4. McLaughlin H. Lesions of the musculotendinous cuff of the shoulder. The exposure and treatment of tears with retraction. *J Bone Joint Surg Am* 1944;24:31.
5. Burkhart SS. Arthroscopic treatment of massive rotator cuff tears: clinical results and biomechanical rationale. *Clin Orthop* 1991;267:45–56.
6. Esch JC, Ozerkis LR, Helgager JA, et al. Arthroscopic subacromial decompression: results according to the degree of rotator cuff tear. *Arthroscopy* 1988;4:241–249.
7. Burkhart SS. Arthroscopic treatment of massive rotator cuff tears: clinical results and biomechanical rationale. *Clin Orthop* 1991;267:45–56.
8. Burkhart SS. Partial repair of massive rotator cuff tears: the evolution of a concept. *Clin Orthop* 1997;28:125–132.
9. Burkhart SS, Nottage WM, Ogilvie-Harris D, et al. Partial repair of irreparable rotator cuff tears. *Arthroscopy* 1994;10:363–370.
10. Pollock RG, Flatow EL. Full-thickness tears: mini-open repair. *Orthop Clin North Am* 1997;28(2):169–177.
11. Norberg FB, Field LD, Savoie FH. Repair of the rotator cuff: mini-open and arthroscopic repairs. *Clin Sports Med* 2000;19(1):77–99.
12. Levy H, Fordner R, Lemak L. Arthroscopic subacromial decompression in the treatment of full thickness rotator cuff tears. *Arthroscopy* 1991;7:8–13.
13. Snyder, SJ. Evaluation and treatment of the rotator cuff. *Orthop Clin North Am* 1993;24:173–192.
14. Worland RL, Aredondo JA, Angles F, et al. Repair of massive rotator cuff tears in patients older than 70 years. *J Shoulder Elbow Surg* 1999;8(1):26–30.
15. Grondel JR, Savoie FH, Field LD. Rotator cuff repairs in patients 62 years of age or older. *J Shoulder Elbow Surg* 2001;10(2):97–99.
16. Burkhart SS, Athanasiou KA, Wirth MA. Margin convergence: a method of reducing strain in massive rotator cuff tears. *Arthroscopy* 1996;12(3):335–338.
17. Savoie FH, Field LD, Jenkins RN, et al. The pain control infusion pump for postoperative pain control in shoulder surgery. *Arthroscopy* 2000;16(4):339–342.
18. Rokito AS, Cuomo F, Zuckerman JD, et al. Strength after surgical repair of the rotator cuff. *J Shoulder Elbow Surg* 1996;5:12–17.
19. Bigliani LU, Cordaso FA, McIlven SJ, et al. Operative repair of massive rotator cuff tears: long-term results. *J Shoulder Elbow Surg* 1992;1:120–130.
20. Hawkins RJ, Misamore GW, Hobeika PE. Surgery for full thickness rotator cuff tears. *J Bone Joint Surg Am* 1985;1349–1355.
21. Essman JA, Bell RH, Askew M. Full thickness rotator cuff tear. An analysis of results. *Clin Orthop* 1991;265:170–187.
22. Bittar E. Arthroscopic repair of massive rotator cuff tears. Paper presented at: 20th Annual Meeting of the Arthroscopy Association of North American; April 19–20, 2001; Seattle, WA.
23. Jones CK, Savoie FH, Tolan SJ. Arthroscopic repair of large and massive rotator cuff tears. Paper presented at: 20th Annual Meeting of the Arthroscopy Association of North America; April 19–20, 2001; Seattle, WA.

24. Gazielly P, Gleyze P, Mongtagnon C. Functional and anatomical results after rotator cuff repair. *Clin Orthop* 1994;304:43–53.

25. Goutallier D, Postel J, et al. Fatty muscle degeneration in cuff ruptures. Pre and postoperative evaluation by CT scan. *Clin Orthop* 1994;304:78–83.

26. Harryman DT II, Mack LA, Wang KY, et al. Repairs of the rotator cuff. Correlation of functional results with integrity of the cuff. *J Bone Joint Surg Am* 1991;73:982–989.

27. Mansat P, Cofield RH, et al. Complications of rotator cuff repair. *Orthop Clin North Am* 1997;28:205–213.

28. Thomazeau H, Boukobza E, et al. Prediction of rotator cuff repair results by magnetic resonance imaging. *Clin Orthop* 1997;344:275–283.

29. Jost B, Pfirrmann CW, Gerber C. Clinical outcome after structural failure of rotator cuff repairs. *J Bone Joint Surg Am* 2000;82(3):304–314.

30. Bigliani LU, Corsdaso FA, McIlveen SJ, et al. Operative treatment of failed repairs of the rotator cuff. *J Bone Joint Surg Am* 1992;74:1505–1515.

31. DeOrio JK, Cofield RH. Results of a second attempt at surgical repair of a failed initial rotator cuff repair. *J Bone Joint Surg Am* 1984;66:563–567.

32. Ianotti JP. Full-thickness rotator cuff tears: factors affecting surgical outcome. *J Am Acad Orthop Surg* 1994;2:87–95.

33. Neer CS II, Marberry T. On the disadvantages of radical acromionectomy. *J Bone Joint Surg Am* 1981;63:416–419.

34. Neviaser RJ, Neviaser TJ. Reoperation for failed rotator cuff repair: analysis of fifty cases. *J Shoulder Elbow Surg* 1992;1:283–286.

20

Arthroscopic Repair of the Subscapularis Tendon

Stephen S. Burkhart, Peter M. Parten,
and Armin M. Tehrany

Tears of the subscapularis tendon are the least common of all rotator cuff tears, and they are the most technically demanding to repair arthroscopically. The combination of "least common . . . most demanding" makes it difficult for an individual arthroscopic surgeon to gain enough experience to feel comfortable with this operation. Yet subscapularis repair can be done quite effectively if one approaches it systematically. The goal of this chapter is to convey an approach that has worked well for us.

INDICATIONS/CONTRAINDICATIONS

Indications for subscapularis repair are similar to those of other rotator cuff tears: pain, weakness, and dysfunction associated with the tear. In the case of the subscapularis, the dysfunction can be profound if more than the upper two thirds of the tendon is torn.

We have found the Napoleon test, described by Imhoff[1] as a variation of the Gerber belly-press test,[2,3] to be the best indicator of subscapularis function. In addition, this test provides a quantitative estimate of the percentage of the subscapularis tendon that is torn. The Napoleon test is named after the position in which Napoleon held his hand (against the stomach) for portraits. The patient is asked to place the hand on the side being tested against the stomach and move the elbow anteriorly. The test is considered to be negative when the patient is able to keep the wrist straight and move the elbow in front of the plane of the body. The negative belly-press test (Figure 20.1A) indicates integrity of the subscapularis. With a completely subscapularis-deficient shoulder, the only way to perform a belly press is to flex the wrist 90°, to orient the arm so that the posterior deltoid can extend the shoulder, thereby allowing the hand to press against the belly (Figure 20.1B). Patients with partial subscapularis tears may exhibit an intermediate

Napoleon sign, in which the wrist flexes 30 to 60° when a belly press is performed (Figure 20.1C).

The Napoleon test is quite useful in predicting the extent of the subscapularis tear. Tears of less than 50% of the tendon have a negative Napoleon sign; those with tears between 50 and 100% of the tendon have an intermediate Napoleon sign; and those with complete tears exhibit a positive Napoleon sign.[4]

In our experience, magnetic resonance imaging (MRI) for subscapularis tears, particularly partial tears, has been less reliable than for tears of the supraspinatus and infraspinatus. In our series,[4] we were able to correctly identify 79% of subscapularis tears preoperatively on MRI, but the radiologist's report identified these tears in only 38% of the cases. Since MRI often does not show the tear, the defect may be unexpectedly discovered at the time of diagnostic arthroscopy, in which case repair may be appropriate. It is noteworthy that partial-thickness tears can be seen only from an intra-articular view, so that proper diagnosis demands arthroscopic evaluation.

Some authors have stated that contraindications to repair of a torn subscapularis are as follows:

1. Proximal migration of the humerus[2]
2. Fatty infiltration of greater than 50% of the subscapularis muscle belly as demonstrated by MRI or CT scan.[5]

We disagree with these contraindications based on our clinical results in 25 consecutive arthroscopic subscapularis repairs.[4] Of those 25 patients, 10 had proximal migration of the humerus and 8 had greater than 50% fatty infiltration of the muscle by MRI. Even so, 8 of the 10 had reversal of proximal migration. These 8 patients all improved their forward flexion from a preoperative "shoulder shrug" of 50.8° to a postoperative average of 135.2°.

Gerber et al.[2,3] have suggested that a delay in repair of a torn subscapularis tendon may produce less

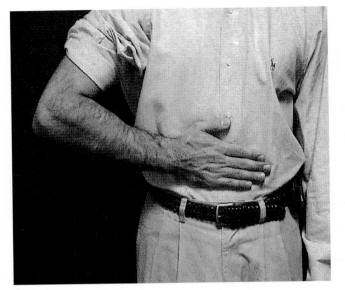

A

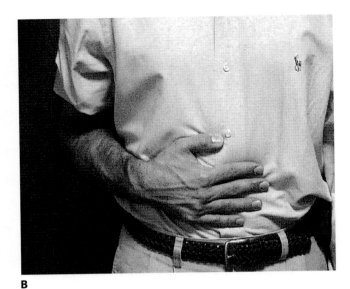

B

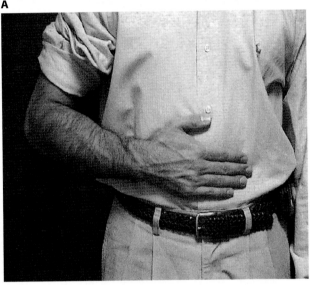

C

FIGURE 20.1. Napoleon test. (A) A negative Napoleon sign indicates normal subscapularis function. The patient is able to maintain wrist extended while pressing on belly. (B) A positive Napoleon sign indicates a nonfunctional subscapularis. The patient can press on the belly only by flexing the wrist 90°, using the posterior deltoid muscle rather than the subscapularis for this function. (C) An intermediate Napoleon sign indicates partial integrity of the subscapularis. As the patient presses on the belly, the wrist flexes 45 to 60° because of partial tearing of the subscapularis.

satisfactory results owing to fatty degeneration of the muscle. Although we agree that repairs should be done as soon as possible, we do not believe that long-standing tears with associated fatty degeneration are a contraindication to surgical repair. The delay from injury to surgical repair in one series averaged 1.5 years and was as long as 6 years in one patient. Even if the muscle is not fully functional, there is strong clinical and electromyographical evidence that much of the subscapularis function is due to a tenodesis effect,[6,7] so

that repairing the tendon to bone may be beneficial even if motor function of the torn subscapularis is poor.

PREOPERATIVE PLANNING

The Napoleon test, belly-press test, and lift off[2,8] tests are performed on preoperative clinical exam when possible. However, we have found that many patients have so much pain with full internal rotation that they are unable to position the hand behind the back to perform the liftoff test.

Our standard x-ray series includes two anteroposterior (AP) views (one taken in internal rotation and the other in external rotation), axillary view, outlet view, and 30° caudal tilt view. Proximal humeral migration is best judged on the AP views and should meet the following criteria:

1. Acromiohumeral interval of less than 5 mm
2. Greater than 5 mm proximal migration of the inferior articular margin of the humerus relative to the inferior articular margin of the glenoid

We obtain MRI scans on all patients preoperatively; subscapularis tears can be identified 79% of the time.

SURGICAL TECHNIQUE

Positioning/Setup

We perform arthroscopic subscapularis repair with the patient in the lateral decubitus position, supported by a vacuum beanbag. The head is supported so that the neck is in line with the body and not laterally flexed. We place the arm in balanced suspension of 5 to 10 lbs, depending on the size of the arm, oriented at 20° abduction and 20° forward flexion. General anesthesia with endotracheal intubation is always used. The anesthesiologist attempts to maintain the systolic blood pressure in the 90 to 100 mmHg range to minimize bleeding, thereby enhancing arthroscopic visualization.

Instrumentation

Standard instrumentation for all shoulder surgery includes 30° and 70° arthroscopes, power shaver and burr, bipolar electrocautery for ablation, and monopolar pencil-tip electrocautery for dissection (particularly if the torn subscapularis is scarred down to the deltoid). We utilize an arthroscopic pump and generally keep it set at 60 mmHg, although if necessary pump pressure is raised as high as 90 mmHg for short periods (no more than 15 min at a time) until visualization improves.

Surgical Technique

Some subscapularis tears are partial-thickness tears involving the articular surface, analogous to the PASTA lesions (i.e., **pa**rtial-thickness **s**ubscapularis

tears) involving the supraspinatus. These tears are likely to be missed unless the arthroscopic surgeon views the subscapularis tendon all the way to its insertion on the lesser tuberosity. When one is viewing through a posterior portal, this area is best seen with the arm in approximately 45° of abduction and 30° internal rotation.

When the surgeon encounters a subscapularis tear, it is important to repair that tear before any other work is done in the shoulder, since the space available for instrumentation is very tight, and swelling of the deltoid can compromise the space even more.

PASTA-type tears should be converted to full-thickness tears by means of electrocautery or a mechanical shaver and then repaired as full-thickness tears.

The full-thickness tears may involve a variable amount of the subscapularis tendon (e.g., from proximal third to entire tendon); they may be isolated or combined tears (e.g., associated with tears of supraspinatus and infraspinatus). Large combined chronic tears generally require mobilization of the subscapularis tendon, whereas isolated tears involving less than 50% of the net length of the tendon insertion do not.

In arthroscopically repairing the subscapularis tendon, we use four portals (Figure 20.2). We prefer the posterior portal for viewing, bringing the bone bed into view with internal rotation of the arm. If visualization of the insertion of the subscapularis at the lesser tuberosity is difficult, one can either change to a 70° scope and remain in the posterior portal or switch to

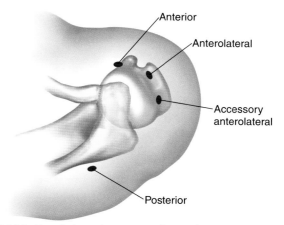

FIGURE 20.2. Portals for arthroscopic subscapularis repair. The anterior portal is used for anchor placement and suture passage. The anterolateral portal is used for subscapularis mobilization and preparation of the bone bed. The accessory anterolateral portal is used for the traction sutures. The posterior portal is used as the arthroscopic viewing portal.

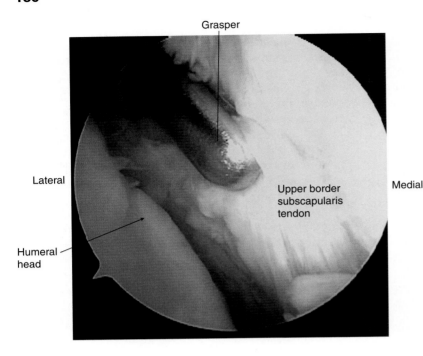

Grasper

Lateral

Humeral head

Upper border subscapularis tendon

Medial

FIGURE 20.3. Lateral traction on the subscapularis tendon with an arthroscopic grasper can assist in the identification of the superior border of the subscapularis tendon (left shoulder, posterior viewing portal, beach chair perspective).

an anterolateral viewing portal. There are two anterolateral portals, one that enters the joint anterior to the biceps tendon (anterolateral portal) and another that enters the joint posterior to the biceps tendon (accessory anterolateral portal). The accessory anterolateral portal is used for traction sutures, and the anterolateral portal is used for passage of arthroscopic elevators, shavers, and knot pushers, needed to mobilize and repair the tendon.

The first step is to identify the subscapularis tendon (Figure 20.3). This is easy in the case of a partial tear but a chronic complete tear may be retracted to the glenoid rim and may even be scarred to the anterior deltoid (Figure 20.4). In chronic complete subscapularis tears, the tendon usually displays a "comma sign," in which the superior glenohumeral ligament avulses from its humeral attachment adjacent to the subscapularis footprint and remains attached to the lateral upper margin of the subscapularis tendon, forming a comma-shaped extension above the superolateral subscapularis (Figure 20.5). Traction sutures (usually two monofilament no. 1 Ethilon) are passed through the tendon by means of a spinal needle (placed percutaneously from anteriorly into the free edge of the tendon) and retrieved through the accessory anterolateral portal (Figure 20.6). In the case of a chronic retracted tear, the tendon is pulled as far lateral as possible while the traction sutures are

passed by means of a tendon grasper through the accessory anterolateral portal.

Next, while one is pulling laterally on the traction sutures, the retracted tendon is mobilized by means

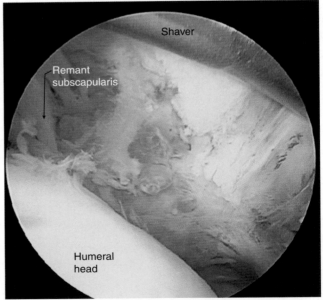

Shaver

Remant subscapularis

Humeral head

FIGURE 20.4. The retracted subscapularis tendon can be difficult to identify (left shoulder as viewed through the posterior portal, beach chair perspective).

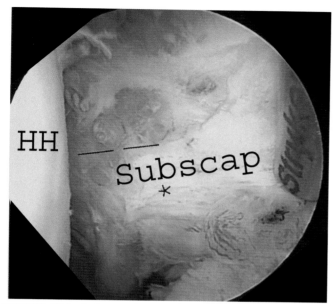

FIGURE 20.5. Arthroscopic view from the posterior portal (left shoulder) demonstrating the difficulty in orientation when a chronic complete tear of the subscapularis tendon is present. A "comma sign" is seen in chronic retracted subscapularis tears. The arc of the comma (*) is formed by the detached superior glenohumeral ligament, which extends proximal to the superolateral border of the subscapularis tendon (lines): HH, humeral head.

of a 15° arthroscopic elevator (Arthrex, Inc., Naples, FL) freeing the tendon anteriorly, posteriorly, and superiorly until it can be pulled laterally to its bone bed on the lesser tuberosity (Figure 20.7). We do not use the elevator inferiorly, and we generally do not dissect medial to the coracoid, which can be easily pal-

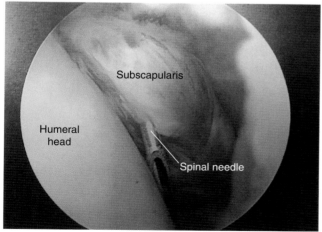

FIGURE 20.6. View from posterior scope portal (left shoulder, beach chair perspective) in which a spinal needle is being passed from anteriorly and monofilament suture is being shuttled through to be used as a traction suture through the subscapularis tendon.

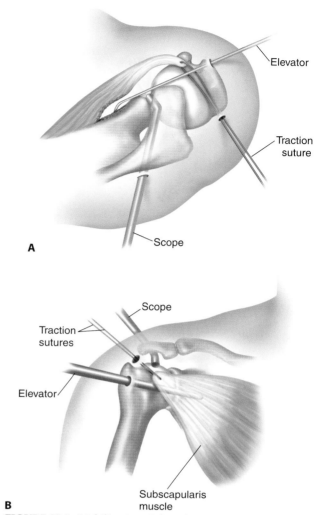

FIGURE 20.7. Mobilization of the subscapularis tendon is achieved by using an arthroscopic elevator. (A) superior view and (B) anterior view.

pated. Dissection is quite safe posterior to the tendon, in the interface between subscapularis and glenoid neck, but dissection anterior to the tendon becomes dangerous if carried medial to the coracoid. One must avoid any uncontrolled dissecting or plunges medially, anteromedially, or inferomedially with the elevator.

Once the tendon has been freed up enough to reach the lesser tuberosity, the bone bed is prepared with a burr through the anterolateral portal (Figure 20.8). We usually medialize the bone bed approximately 5 mm, by removing the adjacent 5 mm of articular cartilage to provide a broad "footprint" for subscapularis healing to bone.

At this point, we determine whether a coracoplasty will be required. We have found that in many sub-

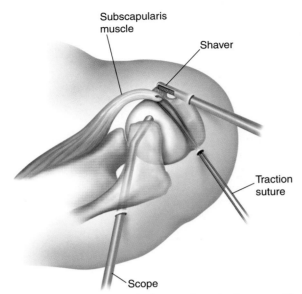

FIGURE 20.8. The bone bed on the lesser tuberosity is prepared by using a high-speed shaver (superior view).

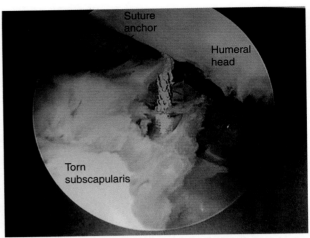

FIGURE 20.9. Anchor insertion into lesser tuberosity (left shoulder, posterior viewing portal, beach chair perspective).

scapularis tears, the coracoid encroaches tightly onto the bone bed to which the tendon will be repaired. To avoid coracoid impingement, the guideline that we use is that there must be at least 7 mm of space between the subscapularis tendon (when it is held reduced over its bone bed) and the coracoid. If there is less than 7 mm of space, we do an arthroscopic coracoplasty. The palpable soft tissues on the posterolateral tip of the coracoid are made up entirely of the coracoacromial ligament. These soft tissues are removed with a combination of electrocautery and power shaver, and then bone is removed in the plane of the subscapularis tendon by means of a high-speed burr until there is a 7 mm space between the coracoid and the subscapularis.

An anatomic study of 18 cadaver shoulders has shown that the average subscapularis tendon footprint is 2.5 cm long, from superior to inferior. This information is useful in judging how much of the subscapularis is torn. If there is an exposed footprint of 1.25 cm, for example, then 50% of the tendon has been torn. To repair the tendon to bone, we use one or two suture anchors, depending on the percentage of tendon that has been torn. If the tear involves 50% or less of the tendon, we use one anchor; and if it involves more than 50%, we use two anchors.

In placing the biodegradable screw-in anchors (Bio-Corkscrew, Arthrex), we use a spinal needle to determine the angle of approach to the bone bed. We try to place the anchors at a 30 to 45° "deadman angle," approximately 5 mm from the articular margin (Figure 20.9).

Sutures can be passed in one of two ways. If the tendon is quite mobile and the space is not compromised excessively by swelling, a Penetrator or Bird-Beak (Arthrex) suture passer can be brought through the tendon from an anterior portal, retrieving the suture directly. Simple sutures are used for the repair, passing one limb through the tendon edge and one limb "around" the free edge" (Figure 20.10).

If the space is very tight and visualization on both sides of the tendon is poor due to swelling, we prefer to use the "traction shuttle" technique, in which the sutures are shuttled from the anchor through the tendon by means of traction sutures. For the lower anchor, the posterior limb of the lowermost traction stitch is retrieved through the accessory anterolateral portal along with one limb of each suture pair from the anchor. The anterior limb of the traction stitch is

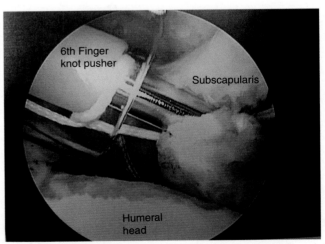

FIGURE 20.10. Arthroscopic view showing suture tying of second knot using "sixth finger" knot pusher (left shoulder, posterior scope viewing, beach chair perspective).

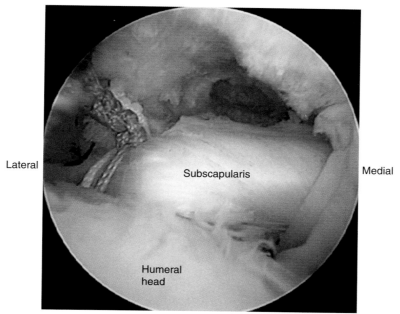

FIGURE 20.11. Arthroscopic view of a completed subscapularis repair of a left shoulder as viewed through a posterior portal (beach chair perspective).

retrieved out the anterolateral portal. A loop is tied in the posterior limb of the traction stitch, and the no. 2 Ethibond suture limbs are threaded through the loop. Then the anterior limb of the traction stitch is pulled by the surgeon to "shuttle" the anchor sutures through the cuff. At this point, the sutures are tied. If the surgeon places the upper anchor before the sutures in the lower anchor have been tied, it will be very difficult to visualize the lower sutures for tying.

If necessary, the second (upper) BioCorkscrew anchor is next implanted, and the sutures are passed and tied in the same manner as for the lower anchor (Figure 20.11).

After subscapularis repair, associated rotator cuff tears are repaired.

POSTOPERATIVE MANAGEMENT

Postoperative management of subscapularis repairs differs from that of other full-thickness rotator cuff tears in one important respect: early external rotation must be limited for 6 weeks, since it will stress the repair. For partial tears (in which there was no retraction), we will allow 20 to 30° of external rotation during the first 6 weeks, since the tendon is supple and the repair is protected to some extent by the intact lower portion of the tendon. However, for complete tears, particularly those that have been chronically retracted, we do not allow external rotation beyond 0° for 6 weeks. After that, the patient may

progress with active and active-assisted external rotation as tolerated, in addition to overhead stretching. Strengthening exercises are delayed until the twelfth postoperative week, as with other varieties of full-thickness tear.

RESULTS/OUTCOME SUMMARY

The only report of arthroscopic subscapularis repair has been that of Burkhart and Tehrany. The senior author (SSB) performed arthroscopic subscapularis repair in 32 shoulders between August 1996 and May 2000.[4] We have evaluated 25 shoulders at least 3 months after surgery, with an average follow-up of 10.7 months (range: 3–48 months). The average time from onset of symptoms to surgery was 18.9 months (range: 1–72 months), indicating a significant delay before surgical repair.

For the entire group of patients, UCLA scores increased from a preoperative average of 10.7 to a postoperative average of 30.5 ($p < 0.0001$). Forward flexion increased from an average 96.3° preoperatively to an average 146.1° postoperatively ($p = 0.0016$). By UCLA criteria, good or excellent results were obtained in 92% of patients, with one fair and one poor result.

Seventeen of the 25 shoulders had massive rotator cuff tears that involved the subscapularis, supraspinatus, and infraspinatus, with an average tear size of 5 cm × 8 cm. Ten of these 17 shoulders had proximal humeral migration as demonstrated by an acromiohumeral interval of less than 5 mm and superior translation of the inferior articular margin of the humerus relative to the inferior articular margin of the glenoid of > 5 mm on AP x-rays. Eight of these 10 shoulders have had radiographically proven reversal of their proximal humeral migration. In addition, these eight shoulders improved their overhead function from a preoperative "shoulder shrug" with attempted elevation of the arm to functional overhead use of the arm postoperatively. Specifically, forward flexion improved significantly from $50.8°$ to $135.2°$ ($p < 0.0001$). The UCLA scores improved significantly from 8.4 to 27.7 ($p < 0.0001$). In one of the two patients whose proximal migration recurred, active forward elevation was unchanged at only $45°$ postoperatively, and in the other patient active forward elevation improved from $90°$ to $110°$. By the UCLA criteria, these two patients with recurrence of proximal migration had poor and fair results, respectively, with little or no change in range of motion, in contrast to the significant improvement in UCLA scores and range of motion demonstrated by patients with durable reversal of proximal migration. In this series, recurrence of proximal humeral migration led to a poor outcome.

COMPLICATIONS

One patient in our series failed to improve and had only $45°$ of forward flexion and a humeral head palpable just beneath the anterior deltoid. This patient presented with a preoperative proximal humeral migration and loss of the coracoacromial arch from a prior acromioplasty. For long-standing contracted subscapularis tears that require mobilization, there is the potential for neurovascular injury, although there were no such complications in our series. In dissecting scarred, contracted tendons, we dissect with a blunt elevator anteriorly, superiorly, and posteriorly. We do not dissect the inferior aspect of subscapularis, and we do not dissect medial to the coracoid. Uncontrolled plunges medial, anteromedial, or inferomedial to the coracoid, even with a blunt elevator, must be avoided.

References

1. Schwamborn T, Imhoff AB. Diagnostik und Klassifikation der rotatorenmanschettenlasionen. In: Imhoff AB, Konig U, eds. Schulterinstabilitat-Rotatorenmanschette. Darmstadt: Steinkopff Verlag, 1999;193–195.
2. Gerber C. Massive rotator cuff tears. In: Iannotti JP, Williams GR Jr., eds. Disorders of the shoulder: diagnosis and management. Philadelphia. Lippincott, 1999: 57–92.
3. Gerber C, Hersche O, Farron A. Isolated rupture of the subscapularis tendon. *J Bone Joint Surg (Am)* 1996;78: 1015–1023.
4. Burkhart SS, Tehrany AM. Arthroscopic subscapularis repair: Technique and preliminary results. Accepted for publication by *Arthroscopy*.
5. Goutallier D, Postel JM, Lavau L, Bernageau J. Fatty muscle degenerations in cuff ruptures. *Clin Orthop* 1994;78–83.
6. Speer, KP. Personal communication, 1999.
7. Jobe FW, Tibone JE, Perry J, et al. An EMG analysis of the shoulder in throwing and pitching: A preliminary report. *Am J Sports Med* 1983;11:3–5.
8. Gerber C, Krushell RJ. Isolated rupture of the tendon of the subscapularis muscle. Clinical features in 16 cases. *J Bone Joint Surg (Br)* 1991;73:389–394.

21

Arthroscopic Management of Calcific Tendonitis

Mark I. Loebenberg and Andrew S. Rokito

Calcific tendonitis of the rotator cuff is a distinct pathological entity that occurs when calcium deposits accumulate within the substance of the rotator cuff tendons. This condition should be distinguished from the degenerative calcifications seen in association with the edges of a torn rotator cuff. Calcific tendonitis can present with varying degrees of severity. In some patients, deposits will be noted as an incidental finding on radiographic examination. In other patients, these deposits appear to be responsible for significant functional disability. The surgeon's task is to determine when intratendinous calcium deposits are the source of the patient's symptoms, and to diminish or shorten the duration of those symptoms with appropriate intervention.

INDICATIONS/CONTRAINDICATIONS

The vast majority of patients with calcific tendonitis are successfully treated with nonoperative management. The clinical presentation of calcific tendonitis and the surgical indications for this entity must be understood within the pathophysiology of the process. Most authors refer to two major phases of calcific tendonitis, formative (chronic) and resorptive (acute). The clinical presentation varies with the stage of the disease. The formation of calcium deposits in the tendons of the rotator cuff is understood by most authors to inflict minimal if any symptoms, and when discovered in the formative phase, it is usually an incidental finding. An area of the tendon, usually 1.5 to 2 cm from the insertion, undergoes a cell-mediated fibrocartilaginous dysplasia. Tenocytes undergo a metaplasia into chondrocytes, with an associated increase in proteoglycan production. The inciting factors of this process remain unclear, and a variety of factors have been suggested, including hypoxia, microtrauma, and disuse.

In the formative, or chronic, phase, calcium crystals are deposited in matrix vesicles and eventually coalesce into larger deposits. If these deposits are large enough, they may cause impingement-type symptoms. Usually, however, there are very few symptoms associated with formation. When the condition enters a more chronic stage, the incidence of symptoms may increase. Typically, pain is the cardinal symptom. The patient is usually able to localize a point of maximal tenderness with pain referred to the deltoid insertion. Sometimes patients are unable to sleep on their affected side and have a painful arc of motion between 70 and 110° of forward elevation. Occasionally, there can be associated atrophy of the spinati.

The resorptive or acute phase is characterized by the sudden onset of worsening pain, which is often quite severe. The pain may be characterized as having a "hot" or "burning" quality. Patients may refuse to move the shoulder, and the symptoms may mimic infection. Treatment of the resorptive phase is nonoperative, and should be supportive, with pain and anti-inflammatory medication given as necessary. Since the time course of the acute phase is relatively short (days or weeks), symptoms usually resolve regardless of the initiatives undertaken. Some authors, however, have reported the efficacy of needling the deposit, along with lavage of the subacromial space. Corticosteroid injections may also provide dramatic relief.

Treatment of the formative phase is initially nonoperative, including daily exercises to maintain mobility and moist heat as needed. Several studies have concluded that over 90% of patients with calcific tendonitis can be treated without surgery. Some authors caution against the use of corticosteroids in treating this phase. Uthoff has recommended that a single injection be considered, but only in the face of prolonged, refractory symptoms.[1] Other authors, however, have noted marked improvement in symptoms with one or two injections, especially in patients who have been symptomatic for less than 6 months.

Radiation, needling, and lavage of the subacromial space, and extracorporeal shock wave therapy have also been used with varying degrees of success. When nonoperative treatment fails, surgical management of calcific tendonitis should be considered if criteria including the following are met: progressive symptoms, pain that interferes with activities of daily living, and failure of nonoperative treatment.

The efficacy of surgical excision of the calcium was established with standard open surgical techniques through a deltoid splitting approach. These techniques were subsequently adapted to arthroscopic surgery such that this is now the predominant operative approach to calcific tendonitis.

PREOPERATIVE PLANNING

Plain radiographs are the single most valuable tool in establishing the diagnosis of calcific tendonitis and must be obtained prior to any surgical procedure. Anteroposterior views in both external and internal rotation, as well as supraspinatus outlet and axillary views, should be obtained to allow for proper assessment of the glenohumeral joint, acromioclavicular joints, and the subacromial space. Two anteroposterior views are obtained, since the humeral head may obscure a calcific deposit with varying degrees of rotation (Figure 21.1). Advanced imaging studies such as arthrography, ultrasonography, and magnetic resonance imaging may allow for further characterization of the size and location of the deposit (Figure 21.2). These studies can also provide valuable preoperative assessment of the integrity and quality of the rotator

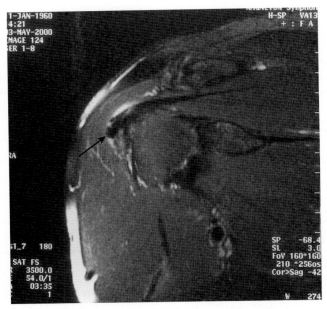

A

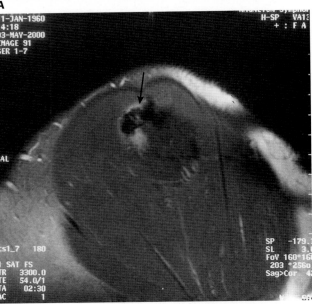

B

FIGURE 21.2. MRI images in the coronal (A) and sagittal (B) views demonstrate the presence of a large calcium deposit in the distal anterior supraspinatus tendon. The decreased signal intensity in the T1 images is typical of calcium deposition.

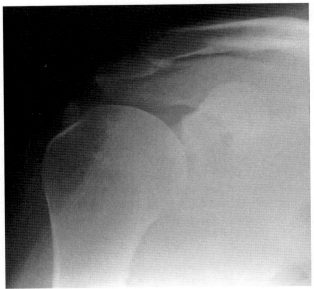

FIGURE 21.1. Anteroposterior view of the glenohumeral joint demonstrates the presence of a large calcific deposit in the region of the supraspinatus tendon. It is important to obtain both internal and external rotation views because calcium deposits can be obscured by the humeral head in some projections.

cuff. Complete preoperative assessment of the extent of the pathology not only allows for adequate surgical planning, but also enhances patients' level of understanding of their disease. This information helps prepare for reasonable outcome expectations.

The issue of whether excision of the calcific deposit should be accompanied by an acromioplasty remains controversial. Many of the symptoms of calcific tendonitis resemble those of impingement, and it can often be difficult to determine the primary etiology of the patient's symptoms. In our practice an acromioplasty is performed only if there is significant radiographic evidence of subacromial impingement in addition to the calcium deposits.

SURGICAL TECHNIQUE

Positioning/Setup

Excision of calcific depostis can be accomplished under general, regional, or a combination of anesthetics. Once adequate anesthesia has been obtained, the patient can be appropriately positioned, either beach chair or lateral decubitus. If the beach chair or semi-sitting position is chosen, it is helpful to utilize a commercially available table attachment that allows the patient to be placed in a seated or upright position with full access to the posterior scapula. A Philadelphia collar can be utilized to stabilize the neck during the procedure, and the head is placed in a stable headrest and gently secured in place with an elastic bandage. The bed should be flexed slightly and the legs elevated on several pillows to prevent the patient from sliding into a more supine position during the procedure. The entire extremity, including the shoulder girdle, is prepped and draped freely.

The lateral decubitus position may also be utilized for this procedure. The patient is positioned with the uninvolved side down and the involved extremity is suspended in a standard shoulder arthroscopy traction device. An exhausted beanbag and kidney rest attachments help secure the patient in a stable position. An axillary roll should be placed to protect the dependent extremity, and all bony prominences must be carefully padded.

Instrumentation

The procedure requires basic arthroscopic instrumentation including a standard 30° arthroscope and a complete set of hand instruments. An 18-gauge spinal needle is needed for localization of the lesion. Arthroscopic knives and curettes may be used for excision of the deposits, along with a motorized shaver system. More recently, radiofrequency ablation devices have been used for this purpose.

Surgical Technique

Following the administration of anesthesia, a systematic examination of both shoulders should be performed. Any restriction in range of motion should be noted and a gentle manipulation performed as needed.

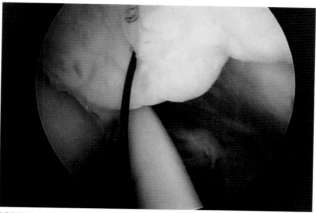

FIGURE 21.3. Arthroscopic photograph of the glenohumeral joint viewed from a posterior portal (right shoulder, lateral decubitus position). The undersurface of the rotator cuff is carefully examined, and any areas that appear to be thickened or erythematous can be marked with an absorbable monofilament suture passed through a spinal needle. This will facilitate localization of the deposit in the subacromial space.

The major bony anatomical landmarks are outlined with a surgical marker. These include the acromion, clavicle, acromioclavicular joint, scapular spine, and the coracoid process. A standard posterior viewing portal is then created, and a complete arthroscopic inspection of the glenohumeral joint is performed. Any intra-articular pathology (articular surface rotator cuff tears and labral tears or degeneration) can be addressed at this time. A careful evaluation of the rotator cuff is carried out, and any thickened or erythematous areas can be marked with an absorbable monofilament suture passed through a spinal needle (Figure 22.3). The end of the suture is brought out through a standard anterior portal in the rotator interval region. The suture is useful in identifying the corresponding area of cuff on the bursal surface, which will be carefully inspected for calcific deposits.

Following the glenohumeral portion of the procedure, the arthroscopic sheath and blunt trochar are redirected into the subacromial space. A gentle sweeping motion can assist in releasing any bursal-side adhesions. A lateral portal is established approximately 2 to 3 cm from the lateral margin of the acromion. Placement of this portal can be adjusted to correspond to the suspected location of the calcific deposits. Other accessory portals can be created as needed.

A partial bursectomy allows complete visual access of the rotator cuff. This can be best accomplished with the use of an arthroscopic shaver or radiofrequency ablation device. The previously placed suture marker can then be located and attention directed to the area of the calcific deposit. A spinal needle can be utilized to "needle" the deposit, often creating a

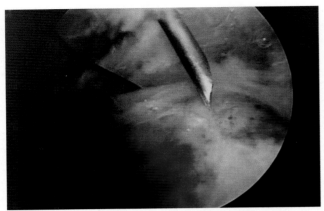

FIGURE 21.4. Arthroscopic photograph of the subacromial space viewed from a posterior portal (right shoulder, beach chair orientation). Once the suture marker has been localized, a spinal needle can be used to "needle" the deposit, often creating a "snowstorm" effect from released calcium, which should be irrigated out of the joint.

"snowstorm" effect in the subacromial space (Figure 22.4). An arthroscopic shaver is introduced to debride the appropriate areas of residual deposits. In many cases it is necessary to incise the rotator cuff to gain access to the deposit. The rotator cuff should be incised in a longitudinal direction along the line of the tendon fibers. A curette or arthroscopic shaver can then be placed into the incision and the residual calcium removed (Figure 22.5). Once the calcium has been completely removed, the subacromial space is copiously irrigated to remove any remaining debris. An acromioplasty is performed if the preoperative assessment indicated clinical or radiographic signs of impingement.

Several studies have demonstrated that the best clinical results are associated with complete removal of the calcium deposits from the rotator cuff tendons. Once this has been accomplished, the surgeon must survey the area of debridement and assess the integrity of the rotator cuff. Any significant partial- or full-thickness defect should be repaired (see Chapters 17 and 20). This can be accomplished via an arthroscopic or mini-open approach, depending upon the surgeon's preference and level of experience. If care was taken to make longitudinal incisions in the rotator cuff, a complete repair can usually be accomplished with side-to-side sutures alone. If the removal of a calcium deposit requires extensive debridement at the insertion sit of the cuff tendon, suture anchors or bone tunnels should be used to allow for a direct repair to bone.

POSTOPERATIVE MANAGEMENT

Postoperative management begins with pendulum and early range-of-motion exercises as tolerated. If the integrity of the rotator cuff has been maintained, the patient is allowed to begin active range of motion immediately. A rotator cuff strengthening program is begun 6 weeks after surgery and progressed as tolerated. If a rotator cuff repair was performed in addition to the debridement, the patient is restricted to passive range of motion of the shoulder for 6 weeks. Active range-of-motion and strengthening protocols are then added to the therapy regimen. Most patients are able to resume full, unrestricted activities by 8 to 12 weeks following surgery if a debridement alone was performed. When there was a concomitant rotator cuff repair, full recovery may take 6 months to a year.

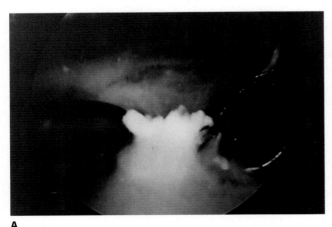

A

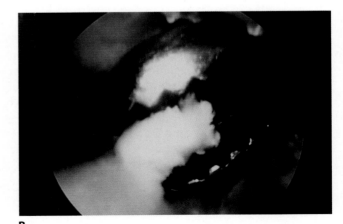

B

FIGURE 21.5. Arthroscopic photographs of the subacromial space viewed from a posterior portal. If the calcium deposit is large enough to require a formal excision, the rotator cuff can be incised along the line of its fibers directly over the deposit. (A) Use of a curette mobilizes the deposit by separating it from the supraspinatus tendon. (B) Removing the deposit from the subacromial space with a simple arthroscopic grabber.

RESULTS/OUTCOME SUMMARY

In 1991 Snyder and Eppley described satisfactory results in 13 of 13 patients with calcific tendonitis treated arthroscopically.[2] These authors raise the issue of whether acromioplasty is necessary and conclude that it should be performed when radiographic evidence of impingement is present. In 1992 Ark et al. demonstrated the efficacy of arthroscopic treatment of calcific tendonitis in 23 patients. These authors reported good or satisfactory results in 20 of the patients.[3] In 1993 the French Society of Arthroscopy published a multicenter review of 112 patients treated with either an isolated arthroscopic excision of the calcium deposit or excision accompanied by arthroscopic acromioplasty.[4] There were no statistical differences between the two groups, with overall 61% excellent, 24% very good, 7% good, and 5% fair results. The most important predictor of a successful outcome was complete excision of the calcium deposits. In 1998 Jerosch et al. evaluated 48 patients who underwent arthroscopic excision of calcific deposits.[5] Postoperative constant scores were significantly improved in this group of patients. No benefit from arthroscopic acromioplasty was noted. These authors also noted the importance of removing the entire deposit. To assist in this process Rupp et al. described a technique of preoperative ultrasonographic mapping of calcium deposits to facilitate localization during arthroscopic surgery.[6] In an appropriately equipped facility, this technique can be of significant assistance. These studies demonstrate the efficacy of the arthroscopic approach in treatment of the traditional open approach, without the attendent of the morbidity. As such, the success of arthroscopic excision of calcium deposits is highly dependent on the surgeon's ability to visualize the subacromial space, address the necessary pathology, and perform any indicated repairs.

New advances in arthroscopic surgery, accompanied by widespread familiarity with basic shoulder arthroscopy, have made arthroscopic debridement the primary surgical option in the treatment of calcific tendonitis. The success of this procedure is based on adequate visualization, a complete excision of the calcific deposit and, when necessary, successful restoration of the integrity of the rotator cuff.

COMPLICATIONS

Intraoperative complications are uncommon and usually are associated with the technical aspects of the surgery. The majority of the procedure is performed in the subacromial space, and the major neu-

rovascular structures of the shoulder are anatomically remote. Failure of the procedure usually arises from incomplete excision of the deposit. This can result in a continuation of preoperative symptomatology. Failure to recognize whether classical impingement is a component of the patient's symptoms can lead to an inadequate decompression and residual pain. An overaggressive debridement of the deposit can lead to significant injury to the rotator cuff. Structural defects need to be repaired at the time of surgery, and a weakened rotator cuff should be protected during healing.

References

1. Uthoff H, Loehr J. Calcifying tendinitis. In: Rockwood C, Matsen F, eds. *The Shoulder.* Vol 2. Philadelphia: WB Saunders; 1997;989–1008.
2. Eppley RA, Synder SJ, Brewster S. Arthroscopic removal of subacromial calcification. Presented at the Annual meeting of the Arthroscopy Association of North America, San Diego, California, April 1991.
3. Ark JW, Flock TJ, Flatlow EL, Bigliani LU. Arthroscopic treatment of calcific tendinitis of the shoulder. *Athroscopy.* 1992;8:183–188.
4. Mole D, Kemppf JF, Gleyze P, et al. Resultats du traitement arthroscopique des tendinopathies non-rompues de la coiffe des rotateurs. 2. Calcifications de la coiffe. *Rev Chir Orthop Reparative Appat Mot* 1993;79:532–541.
5. Jerosch J, Strauss JM, Schmiel S. Arthroscopic treatment of calcific tendonitis of the shoulder. *J Shoulder Elbow Surg* 1998;7(1):30–37.
6. Rupp E, Seil R, Kohn D. Preoperative ultrasonographic mapping of calcium deposits facilitates localization during arthroscopic surgery for calcifying tendinitis of the rotator cuff. Athroscopy. 1998;14:540–542.

Recommended Reading

Henningan S, Romeo A. Calcifying tendonitis. In: Iannotti J, Williams Jr G, eds. *Disorders of the Shoulder.* Philadelphia: Lippincott; 1999;129–157.
Loew M, Sabo D, Wehrle M, Mau H. Relationship between calcifying tendonitis and subacromial impingement: a prospective radiography and magnetic resonance imaging study. *J Shoulder Elbow Surg* 1996;5(4):314–319.
Pfister J, Gerber H. Chronic calcifying tendonitis of the shoulder—therapy by percutaneous needle aspiration and lavage: a prospective open study of 62 shoulders. *Clin Rheumatol* 1997;16(3):269–274.
Postel J, Goutallier D, Lambotte J, Duparc F. Treatment of chronic calcifying or postcalcifying shoulder tendonitis by acromioplasty without excision of the calcification. In: Gazielly D, Gleyze P, Thomas T, eds. *The Cuff.* Paris: Elsevier; 1997;159–163.

Resch H, Povacz P, Seykora P. Excision of calcium deposit and acromioplasty. In: Gazielly D, Gleyze P, Thomas T, eds. *The Cuff*. Paris: Elsevier; 1997;169–171.

Rompe JD, Zoellner J, Nafe B. Shock wave therapy versus conventional surgery in the treatment of calcifying tendonitis of the shoulder. *Clin Orthop* 2001;(387):72–82.

Vebostad A. Calcific tendonitis in the shoulder region. A review of 43 operated shoulders. *Acta Orthop Scand* 1997;46:205–210.

Wang CJ, Ko JY, Chen HS. Treatment of calcifying tendonitis of the shoulder with shock wave therapy. *Clin Orthop* 2001;(387):83–89.

Acromioclavicular Joint

22

Arthroscopic Distal Clavicle Resection: The "Indirect" Subacromial Approach

Robert Sellards, Augustus D. Mazzacca, and Anthony A. Romeo

The acromioclavicular (AC) joint, a common source of discomfort in the shoulder, can be affected by a variety of disorders including osteoarthritis, posttraumatic arthritis, and distal clavicle osteolysis. Conservative management of these conditions with activity modification and medication are often successful in relieving the pain. When nonoperative management fails, the orthopedic surgeon must consider distal clavicle resection.

Treatment of this condition with distal clavicle resection was reported separately in 1941 by Mumford[1] and Gurd.[2] Mumford, who excised the distal clavicle in patients with persistent subluxation and degenerative changes, emphasized the need for coracoclavicular ligament reconstruction when the distal clavicle is noted to be unstable. Open excision of the distal clavicle was the procedure of choice until the late 1980s and early 1990s. It was during this period that arthroscopic technology improved to the point of allowing the distal clavicle to be removed without a formal, open incision. Potential disadvantages of open distal clavicle resection include joint instability and muscle weakness.[3] The open approach violates the deltotrapezial fascia and can weaken the surgically treated extremity.[4]

The several advantages of arthroscopic resection of the distal clavicle include (1) avoiding detachment of the deltoid and trapezius muscles, (2) allowing a shorter postoperative recovery time and more rapid return to premorbid activities, and (3) protecting many of the supporting AC joint ligaments and decreasing the chance of distal clavicle instability. Arthroscopic AC joint resection does however require a technically skilled surgeon who is adept at shoulder arthroscopy.

This chapter illustrates the steps necessary to resect the AC joint arthroscopically through the indirect subacromial approach. This approach permits the arthroscopist to address not only the AC joint, but also other concomitant subacromial procedures such as decompression or rotator cuff repair.

INDICATIONS/CONTRAINDICATIONS

A number of conditions can affect the AC joint, leading to persistent pain. Distal clavicle excision is indicated when symptoms are attributable to the joint and conservative treatment is unsuccessful.

Distal Clavicle Osteolysis

Distal clavicle osteolysis is postulated to result from repetitive overloading of the joint and its articular cartilage. This can cause in the AC joint an inflammatory, localized condition that is aggravated with activity and is typically seen in weight-lifting athletes. The end result of this series of events is resorption of the distal clavicle.

Traumatic

Injuries to the AC joint are common. In 1942 Thorndike and Quigley showed that 9% of shoulder girdle injuries involved injuries to the AC joint.[5] The spectrum of trauma ranges from AC joint sprains, which may be treated conservatively, to fracture/dislocations that require immediate surgical management. Pain following traumatic injury is more common than that associated with primary osteoarthritis.

Distal clavicle resection is undertaken as a salvage procedure for persistent pain following acromioclavicular dislocation, or as treatment of degenerative or osteolytic acromioclavicular joint arthrosis. Outcome reports indicate a high rate of success, although poorer results have been found in patients with fractures or instability.

Osteoarthritis

Primary osteoarthritis (OA) is another common cause of pain in the AC joint. This disorder is more common than OA of the glenohumeral joint.[4] The onset is gradual. Radiographic changes often occur before clinical symptoms. Radiographic findings include narrowing of the AC joint, the formation of superior and inferior osteophytes of the distal clavicle, sclerosis, and cyst formation. The differential diagnosis includes rotator cuff tears, impingement syndrome, biceps tendonitis, and glenohumeral arthritis.

Despite the prevalence of OA radiographically, symptoms associated with the disorder are uncommon.[4–8] In one study of elderly patients, radiographs demonstrated evidence of degenerative arthritis in 54 to 57% of the AC joints.[6] DePalma found degenerative changes in the majority of AC joint specimens obtained from 151 patients.[7] Treatment must be based on the clinical findings rather than the results of radiographic evaluation alone.

Rheumatoid Arthritis and Other Disorders

Other potential causes of AC joint pain include rheumatoid arthritis, crystal-induced arthritis (gout and pseudogout), septic arthritis, and hyperparathyroidism. Ganglia and cysts of the AC joint, which can be symptomatic, are often associated with massive rotator cuff tears. Musculoskeletal tumors must also be included in the differential diagnosis of AC joint pain. Patients presenting with pain in the joint at night or at rest must be carefully evaluated. Examples of neoplastic lesions include Ewing's sarcoma in the child and multiple myeloma in the adult.[8]

Contraindications

In cases of preexisting distal clavicle instability, resection of the AC joint may lead to persistent symptoms postoperatively.[9,10] Patients with a history of trauma to the AC joint must be carefully evaluated to avoid this potential complication. A second contraindication is a set of symptoms for which the AC joint is not clearly responsible. Selected preoperative injections are important to determine the contribution of the AC joint to the patient's symptoms. If the joint is not a clear source of pain, AC resection should not be undertaken.

PREOPERATIVE PLANNING

In addition to the history and physical examination, the surgeon must obtain appropriate radiographic data to substantiate the diagnosis and rule out other sources of pathology.

Presentation

Individuals with AC joint pathology complain of pain at the superior or anterior aspect of the shoulder. Symptoms can be associated with certain activities of daily living, such as reaching across the body toward the opposite axilla, hooking a brassiere, or reaching to get a wallet out of the back pocket. A history of athletic participation, such as weight lifting, golfing, swimming, or overhead throwing, may exacerbate the symptoms.

Physical Examination

Visual inspection may reveal AC joint prominence. Palpation, tenderness, and/or painful crepitation may be elicited with manipulation. Pain referred to the AC joint is often produced with the cross-body adduction maneuver (Figure 22.1).

Radiographs

Routine radiographs include the scapular anteroposterior (AP), outlet, and axillary views. The scapular AP view assesses AC joint narrowing as well as superior and inferior osteophytic changes. The outlet view il-

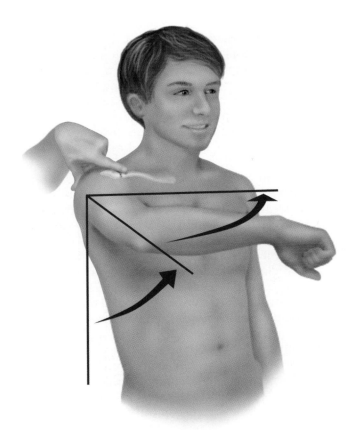

FIGURE 22.1. Cross-arm adduction test: pain to palpation of the AC joint with cross-arm adduction.

lustrates inferior clavicular osteophytes and subacromial changes, such as a prominent anterior acromial spur. The axillary view can reveal anterior/posterior displacement of the clavicle and joint space narrowing. It is also helpful in assessing the amount of clavicle resected after surgery.

Especially useful in the identification of AC joint pathology is the Zanca view, which allows imaging of the AC joint with less soft tissue or bony overlay from the scapular spine. It is obtained by tilting the x-ray tube 10 to 15° cephalad and decreasing the routine kilovoltage used for a standard glenohumeral exposure by half.[11]

When one is evaluating the radiographs, joint space narrowing is probably the least important finding because it is commonly seen with aging. Osteophyte formation, subchondral cysts, and sclerosis are more diagnostic of arthritis. In distal clavicle osteolysis, radiographs reveal osteoporosis, loss of subchondral bone detail, and cystic changes in the distal part of the clavicle.[12] There may also be a tapering of the distal clavicle with a resultant widening of the joint space.

Bone Scan

When radiographic changes are not evident on plane films, bone scan can demonstrate pathology such as idiopathic osteolysis and other inflammatory arthritides.[12]

Magnetic Resonance Imaging

In the presence of a normal physical examination, positive MRI findings are not diagnostic of AC joint pathology. In a 25-month period, one facility documented a 12.5% incidence of abnormally increased T2 signal in the distal clavicle.[13] The authors demonstrated that this is not an uncommon finding on MRI and in most cases it is of no clinical importance. However, if radiographs demonstrate no abnormalities and pain persists, T2-weighted images may aid in the diagnosis of early distal clavicle osteolysis.

SURGICAL TECHNIQUE

Positioning/Setup

The patient may be placed under general anesthesia for the operative procedure. This can be performed with endotracheal intubation or a laryngeal maintained airway (LMA), depending on the preference of the anesthesiologist. Endotracheal intubation is preferred because the airway is more easily maintained during the procedure when the head is covered under the operative drapes. When more than one procedure is to be performed, such as a rotator cuff repair, an interscalene block may be used in combination with the general anesthesia to lessen the postoperative pain.

The patient is placed in the beach chair or lateral position based on surgeon preference. For beach chair positioning, the patient is pulled to the side of the bed with the ipsilateral buttock partially hanging over the edge of the bed. This will keep the patient lateral on the bed for access to the posterior aspect of the shoulder. Using the bed controls, the patient is positioned first into "reflex," which flexes the waist. The legs are then dropped to a 30° angle with the horizontal, and the back of the bed is elevated to bring the torso upright. A lateral post can be placed beneath the axilla to prevent the patient from sliding over the edge of the bed. The neck is positioned in neutral, and the head is secured by tape to the bed. The contralateral arm is positioned across the patient's lap. All pressure points are padded. The arm is then prepped and draped in the usual sterile fashion.

For the lateral position, the patient must be placed on a beanbag. With assistance, the patient is positioned laterally and the bag is exhausted with suction to make the beanbag rigid. A roll is placed in the patient's axilla, and the lower extremities are padded to prevent undue pressure. Sufficient support is placed under the patient's head to maintain the neck in a neutral position.

Instrumentation

1. *Pump* The surgeon must monitor the pressure to avoid soft tissue extravasation. Epinephrine may be added to the inflow bags to help with hemostasis and improved visualization. Each 3 L bag should have one ampule of 1:1000 concentration epinephrine added.
2. *Shaver* A 4.5 or 5.5 mm shaver for debridement of the soft tissue.
3. *Burr* A 5.5 mm round or oval burr for bone excision.
4. *Electrocautery* Unipolar or bipolar devices can be used for soft tissue excision and hemostasis.
5. *Arthroscope* A 30° lens for visualization.
6. *Outflow cannula* A 4 mm cannula.

Surgical Technique

All pertinent anatomy is drawn out on the patient's skin with a marker, including the acromion, the clavicle, the AC joint, and the coracoid process. The portal locations are also drawn on the shoulder, including a posterior, a lateral, and an anterior portal (Figure 22.2). All portals are injected with 0.5% marcaine with epinephrine. This helps to prevent excessive bleeding

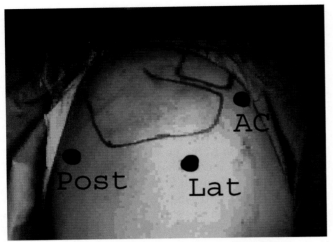

FIGURE 22.2. Scope portals: posterior, lateral, and anterior AC joint portals.

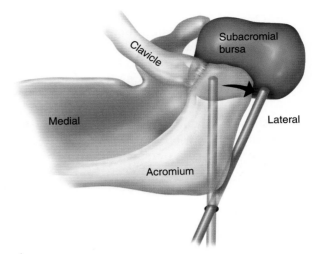

FIGURE 22.3. To enter the subacromial bursa, an anterior structure, a medially directed trocar is passed laterally.

at the portal sites. If medically permissible, the systolic blood pressure must be maintained at around 100 mmHg to minimize bleeding.

A posterior portal is established in the "soft spot," approximately 3 cm inferior and 1 cm medial to the posterolateral corner of the acromion. Another method used to find this portal is shifting the humeral head anterior to posterior, to palpate the location of the glenohumeral joint. Correct identification of this "soft spot" guards against placing the arthroscope in the joint in a position that is either too medial or too lateral.

The skin is incised longitudinally, and the arthroscope is inserted into the glenohumeral joint with a blunt trocar. A diagnostic arthroscopy is performed, and an anterior portal in the rotator interval. The skin incision for this portal is created in line with the AC joint, which permits direct access to this joint.

When the glenohumeral portion of the case is complete, the arthroscope is introduced into the subacromial space (Figure 22.3). The acromion can be palpated with the tip of the blunt trocar to double-check the location of the arthroscope sheath. The coracoacromial (CA) ligament can also be palpated with the tip of the blunt trocar. The tip of the trocar is placed beneath the CA ligament and out through the anterior incision. A 4 mm cannula is placed over the tip of the trocar and introduced into the subacromial space. The goal of this maneuver is to provide a "room with a view." The tips of both cannulas should converge within the subacromial bursa. The bursa lies in the anterolateral aspect of the subacromial space. Location of the arthroscope is initially confirmed without inflow, preventing fluid extravasation and disruption

of the tissue planes. When the camera is seen to be within the bursa, flow is initiated.

The lateral portal is placed approximately two fingerbreadths below the lateral edge of the acromion at the point where an imaginary line bisecting the center of the clavicle intersects. This portal can be used for bursectomy, rotator cuff repair, subacromial decompression, and distal clavicle resection. A spinal needle is inserted into the subacromial space to verify the correct location of the portal (Figure 22.4). Once the correct position has been identified, the skin is incised horizontally along the lines of Langer.

With the scope posterior, a shaver through the lateral portal is used to perform a bursectomy. If necessary, the anterior edge of the acromion can be cleared of soft tissue and a subacromial decompression can be performed. Using electrocautery, the anterior edge of the acromion and the acromioclavicular joint are de-

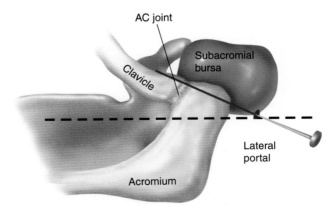

FIGURE 22.4. Lateral portal placement in line with the posterior AC joint approximately 2 cm laterally.

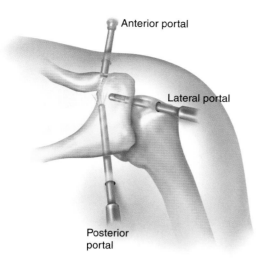

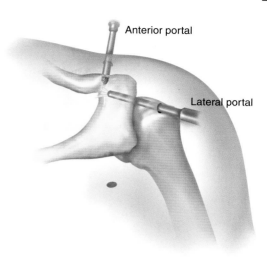

FIGURE 22.5. The arthroscope in the posterior portal with the shaver in the lateral portal cleaning up any debris under the AC joint. An electrocautery ablation device could be used in this instance because there is quite a bit of vascularity in this region.

FIGURE 22.7. The arthroscope is kept in the lateral portal and the burr is placed in the anterior portal; no outflow is placed in the posterior portal.

brided of soft tissue to clarify the anatomy (Figure 22.5). The arthroscope is then removed from the posterior portal and placed into the lateral portal. From this position, the end of the clavicle can be seen "head-on" when manual pressure is applied to the superior end of the distal clavicle (Figure 22.6). Remaining soft tissue is debrided with a shaver or electrocautery inserted through the anterior portal. The bursal tissue

is more vascular in the medial aspect of the subacromial space, necessitating vigilant hemostasis.

Bony resection of the distal clavicle is started with the 5.5 mm burr through the anterior portal, while the arthroscope remains in the lateral portal (Figure 22.7). Ideally, the burr should be parallel to the AC joint. Removal of the inferior AC joint capsular ligaments facilitates resection of the distal clavicle (Figure 22.8).

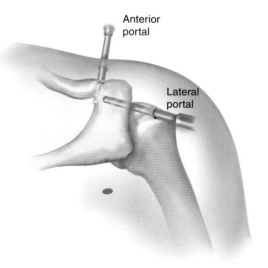

FIGURE 22.6. The arthroscope has been moved to the lateral position, with the shaver/burr positioned anteriorly. With downward pressure, the distal clavicle is delivered into the operative field for resection under direct vision.

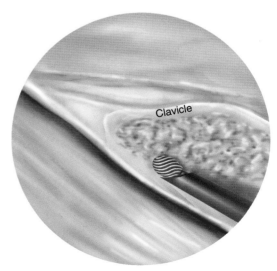

FIGURE 22.8. Arthroscopic view of the burr coming in from the anterior portal, looking from the lateral portal.

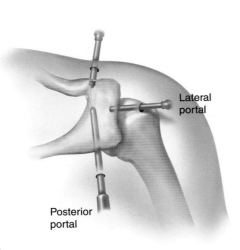

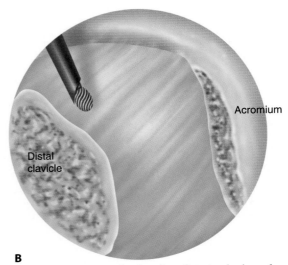

FIGURE 22.9. (A) Arthroscope placed in the posterior portal with the burr placed in the anterior portal and outflow in the lateral portal. (B) Arthroscopic view with the arthroscope in the posterior portal, outflow in the lateral portal, and the burr in the anterior portal.

If resection has not been performed, inferior acromial osteophytes must be removed to promote visualization. The inferior third of the clavicle is removed.

A this point, the arthroscope may be repositioned in the posterior portal. With the camera looking up, the burr is focused on the lateral edge of the clavicle and the resection is completed (Figure 22.9). Work should progress in an anterior-to-posterior, inferior-to-superior direction. The goal is to excise the bone completely while leaving a periosteal tube behind. Errors made during the resection include leaving bone either superiorly or posteriorly. The superior capsule of the AC joint must be protected to prevent destabilization of the joint.

Using the 5.5 mm tip of the burr as a guide allows the accurate removal of 1.0 cm of distal clavicle, which can then be checked arthroscopically. The arthroscope should also be placed in the anterior portal to verify that the distal clavicle has been completely excised (Figure 22.10). The space is thoroughly irrigated of osseous debris, and the portals are injected with Marcaine and closed with suture.

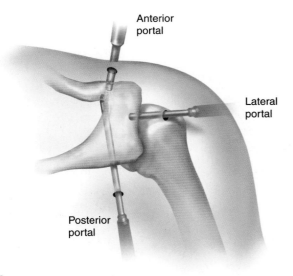

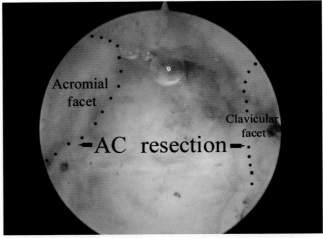

FIGURE 22.10. (A) The arthroscope placed in the anterior portal with the burr placed for final check of the resection in the posterior portal and outflow in the lateral. (B) Photoarthroscopic view of final resection with scope anteriorly.

POSTOPERATIVE MANAGEMENT

After the procedure, the patient's arm is placed in a sling for comfort. From the first postoperative day until the sutures are removed, around postoperative day 7 to 10, the patient should perform pendulum exercises and elbow/wrist range-of-motion exercises five times a day. From weeks 1 to 4, the following protocol is used. Range of motion is advanced from passive to active assisted, and then to active as tolerated. Cross-body adduction is avoided until 8 weeks following resection. Range-of-motion goals during this period are 140° of forward flexion and 40° of external rotation at the side. Abduction and rotation is not done until 4 to 8 weeks after surgery. The sling is discontinued at 1 to 2 weeks after surgery and used only when the patient is sleeping, if needed. Heat is used before physical therapy and ice is used after therapy.

For weeks 4 to 8, active range of motion is increased in all directions, with passive stretching at end ranges to maintain shoulder flexibility. The goals are changed to 160° of forward flexion and 60° of external rotation at the side. Light isometric exercises are instituted with the arm at the side for the rotator cuff and the deltoid. The patient is later advanced to Therabands as tolerated.

For weeks 8 to 12, the strengthening is advanced from Therabands to weights, 10 reps per set for the rotator cuff, deltoid, and scapular stabilizers. These exercises should be limited to three times a week to avoid rotator cuff tendinitis. Range of motion is increased to full with passive stretching at the end ranges. Eccentrically resisted motions, plyometrics, and closed-chain exercises are also advanced as tolerated.

RESULTS/OUTCOME SUMMARY

Outcomes of arthroscopic distal clavicle resection using the indirect subacromial approach compare favorably with those for open procedures. The studies illustrating this vary slightly with regard to study design, number of patients, diagnosis, procedures performed, duration of follow-up, methods of evaluation, and amount of distal clavicle removed.

Snyder et al. treated fifty patients for AC joint pain with arthroscopic distal clavicle resection (DCR).[14] Preoperatively, all patients had pain on palpation and 80% had a positive cross-body adduction test. There were no intraoperative complications, and an average of 14.5 mm of distal clavicle was resected. At 2 years of follow-up, there were 94% good-to-excellent results

according to the UCLA shoulder score and the subjective patient satisfaction questionnaire. There were calcifications at the site of resection in 16% of patients at follow-up. The authors concluded that this procedure had low associated morbidity and high patient satisfaction.

Kay et al. reported 10 successful results in patients treated with arthroscopic DCR.[15] They concluded that in experienced hands, arthroscopic distal clavicle excision is an excellent substitute for the "open" procedure. Gartsman reported the results of 20 patients treated with arthroscopic DCR at 2 years of follow-up.[16] There were only 3 unsuccessful results, and all were treated with open resection. Auge and Fisher reported their results of arthroscopic distal clavicle resection in 10 weight lifters with osteolysis.[17] At an average of 18.7 months of follow-up, all patients were found to have returned to their sport in an average of 3.2 days. The patients were asymptomatic and had increased their activity postoperatively over preoperative levels. The authors felt that this procedure permitted weight lifters to return quickly to their sport as well as improving their cosmesis in comparison to open surgery.

The indirect subacromial approach for distal clavicle excision has also been successful when combined with arthroscopic subacromial decompression (SAD). Martin et al. performed a retrospective analysis of combined arthroscopic SAD and DCR in 32 shoulders.[18] At an average follow-up of 4 years and 10 months, 26 patients had no pain and 6 had some pain with activity. All patients were satisfied with their result, and isokinetic strength testing of both upper extremities failed to demonstrate any weakness of the involved shoulder. The authors concluded that these results were excellent and compared favorably with those from an open approach.

Levine et al. performed a retrospective review of combined arthroscopic SAD and DCR procedures.[19] At an average of 32.5 months of follow-up, the 24 patients in their study had 17 excellent results, there were 4 good results and 3 failures. The authors, who had removed an average of 5.4 mm of distal clavicle, concluded that as long as the bone end was smooth, even, and completely excised, the amount of bone removed did not affect the outcome.

A retrospective study was performed comparing the results of patients who had a SAD performed with or without violation of the AC joint.[20] There were no postoperative sequelae associated with the AC joint in patients who had no violation of the AC joint or in those who had a formal distal clavicle excision. However, 39% of patients with intraoperative violation of the AC joint (without distal clavicle excision) had postoperative pain attributed to the AC joint at an average of 8.4 months after surgery. The authors recommended an all-or-none approach regarding treatment of the AC joint.

COMPLICATIONS

Diagnostic error can lead to persistent pain after the procedure. AC joint pain can present like impingement syndrome, a rotator cuff tear, a SLAP (superior labrum, anterior and posterior) lesion, and biceps tendonitis. It may also present alone or in combination with these other diagnoses. A careful history, physical examination, and radiographic evaluation can minimize this avoidable complication. A review of 20 arthroscopies done after a distal clavicle resection (Mumford) revealed 15 SLAP lesions that were missed during the index procedure.[21] These patients were young, with an average age of 37 years, and 14 of the 15 patients had had a specific traumatic event leading to the pain. The authors felt that SLAP lesions should be considered in the differential diagnosis of AC arthrosis in young patients with a traumatic history, and a diagnostic glenohumeral arthroscopy was recommended in this population.

Inadequate distal clavicle resection is one of the most common technical causes of persistent pain after surgery. Failure to remove the posterior aspect of the distal clavicle can lead to posterior abutment against the acromion.[22] Arthroscopic procedures have a greater chance of inadequate bone resection in comparison to the open counterpart, particularly with retained posterior cortical ridges or uneven resection.[23,24]

Instability of the AC joint after distal clavicle resection may also lead to persistent symptoms postoperatively. A retrospective review attempted to compare clavicle motion in the anterior–posterior plane with patient outcomes after DCR.[10] The average motion after resection was 8.7 mm (anterior to posterior) in the operative shoulders and 3.2 mm in the unoperated shoulder. Amount of translation and the visual analog score did not correlate with the amount of bone resected. There was a correlation between the amount of translation and the postoperative visual pain score. The authors concluded that poor outcomes can be associated with excessive anteroposterior clavicle motion after resection.

Flatow et al. reported the results of 41 patients treated with distal clavicle excision via the superior, or direct approach.[9] At an average follow-up of 31 months, there were 18 excellent, 16 good, and 7 poor results. The poor results were associated with shoulders with previous grade II AC joint separations or AC

hypermobility. Total amount of bone did not correlate with success as long as the bone cut was even. The authors recommended that this procedure not be performed in patients with subtle AC instability, given the high failure rate in these individuals (42%).

Another potential complication following DCR is heterotopoic ossification (HO). Although a recognized sequela of AC joint trauma, HO is rarely symptomatic in affected individuals. One study characterized the patients at risk for this complication.[25] A review of patients treated with SAD or DCR by open or closed means revealed an incidence of 3.2% in 40 patients. An association was noted in patients with chronic pulmonary disease ($p < 0.05$). There was no predilection for either open or closed procedures. Postoperative radiographs taken within 8 weeks of the procedure revealed no bone fragments, leading the authors to conclude that the bone formation occurred de novo. They recommended that patients at risk for HO formation (those with hypertrophic pulmonary osteoarthropathy or active spondylitic arthropathy) be treated with prophylaxis to prevent this complication.

References

1. Mumford EB. Acromioclavicular dislocation—a new treatment. *J Bone Joiint Surg* 1941;23:799–802.
2. Gurd FB. The treatment of complete dislocation of the outer end of the clavicle. *Ann Surg* 1941;113:1094–1098.
3. Corso SJ, Furie E. Arthroscopy of the acromioclavicular joint. *Orthop Clin North Am* 1995;26:661–670.
4. Henry MH, Liu SH, Loffredo AJ. Arthroscopic management of the acromioclavicular joint disorder. A review. *Clin Orthop* 1995;316:276–283.
5. Thorndike A, Quigley TB. Injuries to the acromioclavicular joint: a plea for conservative treatment. *Am J Surg* 1942;55:251–261.
6. Horvath F, Kery L. Degenerative deformations of the acromioclavicular joint in the elderly. *Arch Gerontol Geriatr* 1984;3:259–265.
7. DePalma AF. The role of the disks of the sternoclavicular and the acromioclavicular joints. *Clin Orthop* 1959;13:222–233.
8. Shaffer BS. Painful conditions of the acromioclavicular joint. *J Am Acad Orthop Surg* 1999;6:176–188.
9. Flatow EL, Duralde XA, Nicholson GP, Pollock RG, Bigliani LU. Arthroscopoic resection of the distal clavicle with a superior approach. *J Shoulder Elbow Surg* 1995;4:41–50.
10. Blazar PE, Iannotti JP, Williams GR. Anteroposterior instability of the distal clavicle after distal clavicle resection. *Clin Orthop* 1998;348:114–120.
11. Zanca P. Shoulder pain: involvement of the acromioclavicular joint. Analysis of 1,000 cases. *AJR Am J Roentgenol* 1971;112:493–506.
12. Cahill BR. Osteolysis of the distal part of the clavicle in male athletes. *J Bone Joint Surg Am* 1982:64:1053–1058.

13. Fiorella D, Helms CA, Speer KP. Increased T2 signal intensity in the distal clavicle: incidence and clinical implications. *Skeletal Radiol* 2000;29:697–702.

14. Snyder SJ, Banas MP, Karzel RP. The arthroscopic Mumford procedure: an analysis of results. *Arthroscopy* 1995;11:157–164.

15. Kay SP, Ellman H, Harris E. Arthroscopic distal clavicle excision. Technique and early results. *Clin Orthop* 1994;301:181–184.

16. Gartsman GM. Arthroscopic resection of the acromioclavicular joint. *Am J Sports Med* 1993;21:71–77.

17. Auge WK II, Fischer RA. Arthroscopic distal clavicle resection for isolated atraumatic osteolysis in weight lifters. *Am J Sports Med* 1998;26:189–192.

18. Martin SD, Baumgarten TE, Andrews RJ. Arthroscopic resection of the distal aspect of the clavicle with concomitant subacromial decompression. *J Bone Joint Surg Am* 2001;83:328–335.

19. Levine WN, Barron OA, Yamaguchi K, Pollock RG, Flatow EL, Bigliani LU. Arthroscopic distal clavicle resection from a bursal approach. *Arthroscopy* 1998;14:52–56.

20. Fischer BW, Gross RM, McCarthy JA, Arroyo JS. Incidence of acromioclavicular joint complications after arthroscopic subacromial decompression. *Arthroscopy* 1999;15:241–248.

21. Berg EE, Ciullo JV. The SLAP lesion: a cause of failure after distal clavicle resection. *Arthroscopy* 1997;13:85–89.

22. Neer CS II: *Shoulder Reconstruction.* Philadelphia: WB Saunders; 1990;433–436.

23. Tolin BS, Snyder SJ. Our technique for the arthroscopic Mumford procedure. *Orthop Clin North Am* 1993;24:143–151.

24. Jerosch J, Steinbeck J, Schroder M, Castro WHM. Arthroscopic resection of the acromioclavicular joint (ARAC). *Knee Surg Sports Traumatol Arthrosc* 1993;1:209–215.

25. Berg EE, Ciullo JV. Heterotopic ossification after acromioplasty and distal clavicle resection. *J Shoulder Elbow Surg* 1995;4:188–193.

Recommended Reading

Bell RH. Arthroscopic distal clavicle resection. *Instr Course Lect* 1998;47:35–41.

Bergfeld JA, Andrish JT, Clancy WG: Evaluation of the acromioclavicular joint following first and second degree sprains. *Am J Sports Med* 1978;6:153–159.

Bigliani LU, Nicholson GP, Flatow EL. Arthroscopic resection of the distal clavicle. *Orthop Clin North Am* 1993;24:133–141.

Branch TP, Burdette HL, Shahriari AS, Carter FM 2nd, Hutton WC. The role of the acromioclavicular ligaments and the effect of distal clavicle resection. *Am J Sports Med* 1996;24:293–297.

Buford D Jr, Mologne T, McGrath S, Heinen G, Snyder S. Midterm results of arthroscopic co-planing of the acromioclavicular joint. *J Shoulder Elbow Surg* 2000;9:498–501.

Cook FF, Tibone JE. The Mumford procedure in athletes: an objective analysis of function. *Am J Sports Med* 1988;16:97–100.

Cox JS. The fate of the acromioclavicular joint in athletic injuries. *Am J Sports Med* 1981;9:50–53.

Eskola A, Santavirta S, Viljakka HT, Wirta J, Partio TE, Hoikka V. The results of operative resection of the lateral end of the clavicle. *J Bone Joint Surg Am* 1997;79:633–634.

Fukuda K, Craig EV, An KN, et al. Biomechanical study of the ligamentous system of the acromioclavicular joint. *J Bone Joint Surg Am* 1986;68:434–440.

Gartsman GM, Combs AH, Davis PF, Tullos HS. Arthroscopic acromioclavicular joint resection. An anatomical study. *Am J Sports Med* 1991;19:2–5.

Klimkiewicz JJ, Williams GR, Sher JS, Karduna A, Des Jardins J, Iannotti JP. The acromioclavicular capsule as a restraint to posterior translation of the clavicle: a biomechanical analysis. *J Shoulder Elbow Surg* 1999;8:119–124.

Lee KW, Debski RE, Chen CH, Woo SL, Fu FH. Functional evaluation of the ligaments at the acromioclavicular joint during anteroposterior and superoinferior translation. *Am J Sports Med* 1997;25:858–862.

Matthews LS, Parks BG, Pavlovich LJ Jr, Giudice MA. Arthroscopic versus open distal clavicle resection: a biomechanical analysis on a cadaveric model. *Arthroscopy* 1999;15:237–240.

Novak PJ, Bach BR Jr, Romeo AA, Hager CA: Surgical resection of the distal clavicle. *J Shoulder Elbow Surg* 1995;4:35–40.

O'Brien SJ, Pagnani MJ, Fealy S, McGlynn SR, Wilson JB. The active compression test: a new and effective test for diagnosing labral tears and acromioclavicular joint abnormality. *Am J Sports Med* 1998;26:610–613.

Petersson CJ. Resection of the lateral end of the clavicle. A 3- to 30-year follow-up. *Acta Orthop Scand* 1983;54:904–907.

Zawadsky M, Marra G, Wiater JM, Levine WN, Pollock RG, Flatow EL, Bigliani LU. Osteolysis of the distal clavicle: long-term results of arthroscopic resection. *Arthroscopy* 2000;16:600–605.

23

Acromioclavicular Resection: Direct "Superior" Approach

Suzanne L. Miller, Ken Shubin Stein, and Evan L. Flatow

Acromioclavicular (AC) joint pain is a common shoulder problem that can often be effectively treated by resecting the distal end of the clavicle.[1-3] Because AC joint pathology often occurs in association with other shoulder disorders, resection not uncommonly accompanies other procedures.[1,4] In cases of isolated AC joint pathology unresponsive to nonoperative treatment, open or arthroscopic techniques are both effective operative strategies. Quantitative comparisons have demonstrated that an adequate amount of bone resection can be achieved by either arthroscopic or open means.[5,6] The direct "superior" and indirect "bursal" approaches are the two main options for arthroscopic AC joint resection.

First described by Johnson,[7] the direct, or superior approach, involves direct resection of the joint through arthroscopic portals on the superior aspect of the joint, targeting the pathology directly. With appropriate patient selection, there are several advantages of this technique over the indirect approach. The variable angle of inclination of the AC joint in the coronal plane[8] can cause the clavicle to override the acromion, inhibiting adequate resection through a bursal approach unless an acromioplasty is performed first—which is unnecessary with isolated AC joint pathology. The superior approach is ideal for acromioclavicular joints that are inclined medially and are therefore difficult to reach from the bursal side. Patients with isolated AC joint pathology such as osteoarthritis or osteolysis of the distal clavicle are well suited because this approach limits collateral injury to surrounding structures, preserving AC joint capsule integrity, and avoiding subacromial space and bursa violation. In addition, the superior approach affords precise visualization, which allows uniform resection of bone and preserves the acromioclavicular ligamentous complex.

In comparison to open approaches, both outpatient arthroscopic techniques permit a relatively quick rehabilitation protocol, with return to full activity 3 to 4 months earlier than those patients undergoing an open procedure.[6] Finally, arthroscopic techniques certainly minimize the risk of deltoid compromise and weakness[6,9] in comparison to open approaches.

INDICATIONS/CONTRAINDICATIONS

Patient selection is critical for the successful application of this technique. Osteolysis of the distal clavicle and osteoarthritis of the AC joint, either primary or secondary, are the main indications for the direct superior approach. This approach is contraindicated in patients whose AC joint pathology is not isolated, such as those with concomitant bursal or rotator cuff pathology, patients in whom the joint space is too narrow to permit introduction of even the small (2.7 mm diameter) arthroscope, and those with acromioclavicular instability, which can be seen after grade II AC joint separations.

PREOPERATIVE PLANNING

Physical Exam

Acromioclavicular joint tenderness and swelling are the most sensitive clinical indicators of AC joint pathology. Physical exam findings include pain with forced horizontal adduction of the arm across the body and internal rotation of the shoulder (Figure 23.1). Although these are sensitive tests for acromioclavicular pathology, they are not necessarily specific, inasmuch as other shoulder disorders (posterior capsular stiffness, early frozen shoulder, impingement, etc.) may also cause pain with these maneuvers. Look for these tests to reproduce pain specifically in the vicinity of the AC joint as a more reliable indicator of AC joint pathology. In addition, O'Brien's test for superior labral pathology can cause pain in the AC joint area.

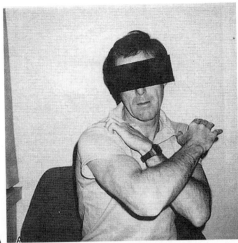 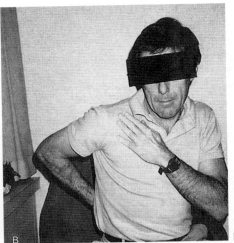

FIGURE 23.1. (A) Horizontal adduction of the arm across the body drives the scapula toward the sternum and compresses the acromioclavicular joint. (B) Internal rotation of the shoulder twists and compresses the acromioclavicular joint, producing pain in patients with osteolysis of the distal clavicle.

Diagnostic Tests

There are many diagnostic tests that assist the surgeon in making the diagnosis of AC joint pathology. Injecting the AC joint with lidocaine is an easy and quick method of diagnosing AC joint problems, as well as indicating the potential efficacy of future joint resection. In addition to a local joint injection, many imaging studies are useful. A radiographic shoulder series including an anteroposterior (AP) view in the scapular plane in both internal and external rotation, an outlet view, and an axillary view, can demonstrate AC joint pathology as well as assisting in diagnosing any additional pathology. An AP radiograph with a 10 to 15° cephalic tilt with reduced voltage can reveal subtle changes in the distal clavicle, as well as the true inclination of the AC joint. Additionally, magnetic resonance imaging (MRI) can be done to evaluate cuff pathology, encroaching osteophytes on the bursa or cuff, and acromioclavicular synovitis. However, MRI tends to show significant changes in a high percentage of patients and is probably not a very reliable test. Used in combination with a careful physical exam, these diagnostic tests allow for the accurate diagnosis of AC joint pathology.

SURGICAL TECHNIQUE

Positioning

The patient is positioned in a modified beach chair position with the arm draped free. We prefer interscalene regional anesthesia, but general anesthesia can be used.

Instrumentation

Instruments used for this procedure include a 2.7 mm arthroscope, a 2.0 mm synovial resector, a 2 or 3.5 mm burr, and an 8 mm rasp.

Surgical Technique

To start, the bony anatomical landmarks of the distal clavicle and acromion are outlined. To assist with localization, two or three 22-gauge spinal needles are placed anterosuperiorly, anteroposteriorly, and in the center of the joint (Figure 23.2A). The joint is then insufflated and the portals are injected with 1% lidocaine with epinephrine, to obtain capsular hemostasis and to minimize skin bleeding. Next, anterosuperior and posterosuperior portals are made in line with the AC joint, 0.75 cm anterior and posterior to the joint, respectively (Figure 23.2B). A no. 11 blade scalpel is used to incise the skin and the capsule of the acromioclavicular joint both anteriorly and posteriorly. Normal saline with epinephrine (1:300,000) is used for irrigation during the procedure. If the AC joint is narrow, a 2.7 mm arthroscope is placed in the posterior portal and a small shaver is placed in the anterior portal, and resection of the meniscal remnant and joint debris is initiated under direct visualization. Next a small burr is used to begin the bony resection.

Following the initial resection, a 4 mm arthroscope is inserted into the posterior portal, providing a panoramic view and high inflow. Electrocautery is used to subperiosteally "shell out" the distal clavicle while preserving the acromioclavicular ligaments superiorly and inferiorly. The resection of the distal clavicle can be completed by using a large burr (Figure

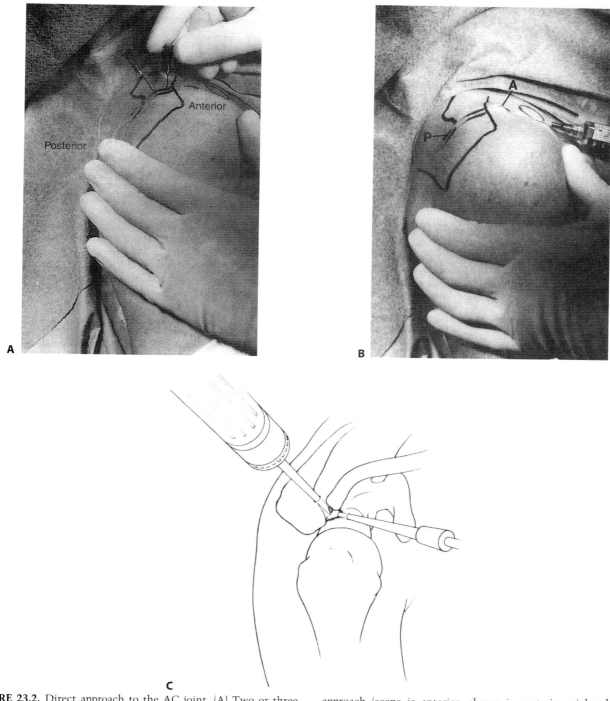

FIGURE 23.2. Direct approach to the AC joint. (A) Two or three 22-gauge needles are used to precisely locate the AC joint, determining the superior–inferior obliquity and anteroposterior inclination. (B) The portal sites are made in the line with the joint and are injected with 1% lidocaine with epinephrine to diminish bleeding. (A, anterior; B, posterior.) (C) Schematic superior view of the direct approach (scope is anterior, shaver is posterior; right shoulder). (Reprinted with permission from Flatow EL, Cordasco FA, Bigliani LU. Arthroscopic resection of the clavicle from a superior approach: a critical, quantitative, radiographic assessment of bone removal. *Arthroscopy* 1992;8:55–64.)

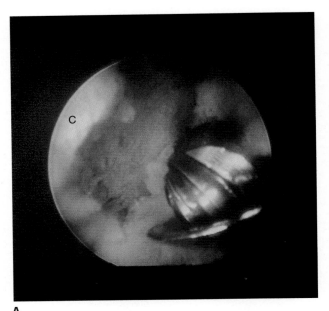

A

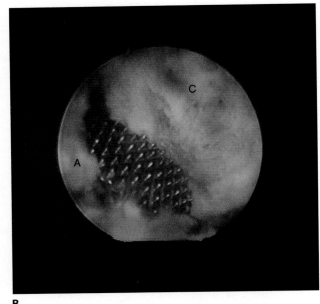

B

FIGURE 23.3. (A) While viewing from the posterior portal, a burr from the anterosuperior portal is used to resect and sculpt the outer end of the clavicle under direct visualization. (B) While viewing from the anterosuperior portal, the surgeon uses a rasp from the posterior superior portal (right shoulder) to perform the final con-touring and to assess the space between the clavicle and the acromion (A, acromium; C, clavicle). (Reprinted with permission from Flatow EL, Cordasco FA, Bigliani LU. Arthroscopic resection of the clavicle from a superior approach: a critical, quantitative, radiographic assessment of bone removal. *Arthroscopy* 1992;8:55–64.)

23.3A). Next the burr and arthroscope are exchanged to facilitate uniform resection of bone. Special attention should be paid to the most anterior portion of the clavicle, taking care not to leave retained ridges or edges that could abut the acromion, causing recurrence of pain. Final beveling of the clavicle can be accomplished with an arthroscopic rasp (Figure 23.3B). When the bony part of the operation is complete, the joint is carefully examined, and any remaining debris or soft tissue is removed. The joint is then insufflated with a long-acting local anesthetic, and the arthroscopic portals are closed with absorbable subcuticular sutures.

Pearls

In standard open distal clavicle resections, 1.0 to 2.5 cm of bone is removed to prevent the clavicle from abutting against the acromion, especially with overhead motion. Arthroscopic resection offers the advantages of preserving the AC ligaments and capsule, thus providing greater stability, and requiring only 5 to 6 mm of bone resection to prevent impingement.[10,11] Biomechanical studies comparing axial compression of the acromioclavicular joint after open and arthroscopic acromioclavicular resection confirm intraoperative observations that the joint is main-tained after resection of 5 to 6 mm of bone, provided the ligaments are intact.[12,13]

Retained cortical ridges can cause recurrent symptoms and therefore should be carefully removed (Figure 23.4A). Ridges are most often left at the joint margins where the capsule inserts, especially posterior

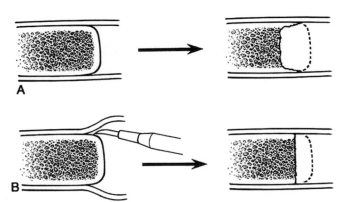

A

B

FIGURE 23.4. (A) Uneven resection of the distal clavicle may leave bone peripherally, which can lead to continued pain. (B) The problem can be avoided by using electrocautery to first shell out the distal clavicle from the intact AC joint capsule, thus allowing even resection of bone. (Reprinted with permission from Flatow EL. Arthroscopic resection of the distal clavicle from a superior approach. In: Torg JS, Shepard RJ, eds. *Current Therapy in Sports Medicine.* 3rd ed. St. Louis, MO: CV Mosby; 1995; 189.)

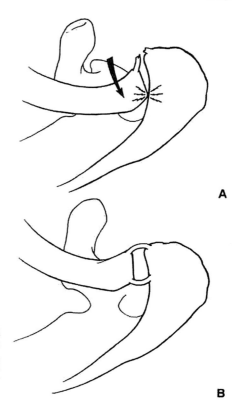

FIGURE 23.5. (A) Incompetence of the acromioclavicular joint ligamentous complex can lead to excessive posterior translation of the distal clavicle stump and painful abutment against the acromion. (B) Preservation of the soft tissue complex avoids potential abutment. (Reprinted from Flatow EL. The biomechanics of the acromioclavicular, sternoclavicular, and scapulothoracic joints. In: Heckman, ed. *Instructional Course Lectures.* American Academy of Orthopaedic Surgeons, 1993;42:237–245.)

superior. These must be removed by "shelling out" (subperiosteally exposing) the distal clavicle with electrocautery, then resecting the bone with the burr (Figure 23.4B). To avoid destabilizing the distal clavicle, care should be taken to preserve the capsuloligmen- tous envelope (Figure 23.5). Although intraoperative x-rays may be useful during one's learning curve, we do not routinely find these aids necessary, although we do obtain postoperative films to ensure the adequacy of our resection (Figure 23.6).

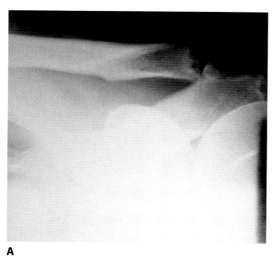
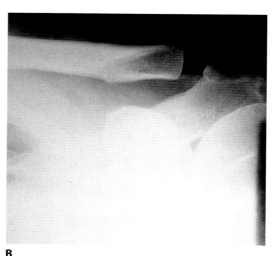

A **B**

FIGURE 23.6. (A) Preoperative radiograph showing a degenerative acromioclavicular joint. (B) Postoperative radiograph showing even re- section of the distal clavicle.

POSTOPERATIVE MANAGEMENT

Postoperatively, the patient wears a sling for comfort for 1 to 2 days. Passive and assistive motion is started immediately, progressing to active motion as soon as comfort allows (usually postoperative day 3 to 5). Early emphasis is placed on regaining full range of motion and strength, with early return to preoperative levels of activity.

RESULTS/OUTCOME

Arthroscopic distal clavicle resection, from either a bursal, indirect approach or a superior, direct approach, yields predictable results in the majority of patients. Flatow et al.[14] have reported 93% excellent or good results at 31 months after distal clavicle resection through a superior approach in patients with osteolysis of the distal clavicle or acromioclavicular arthritis. These patients had resolution of pain and return to full activity without restriction. Patients with previous instability from a grade II acromioclavicular separation had only only 58% successful results, and the authors recommend formal ligament stabilization (in addition to distal clavicle resection) in this group of patients.

COMPLICATIONS

Few complications are associated with this technique. When poor outcomes do occur, they are due to retained cortical ridges caused by uneven resection, or to treatment of patients with unstable clavicles, such as patients with a previous grade II AC joint separation.

References

1. Mumford EB. Acromioclavicular dislocation: a new operative treatment. *J Bone Joint Surg* 1941;23:799–801.
2. Neer CS. *Shoulder Reconstruction*. Philadelphia: WB Saunders; 1990;433–436.
3. Petersson J. Resection of the lateral end of the clavicle. *Acta Orthop Scand* 1983;54:904–907.
4. Ellman H. Arthroscopic subacromial decompression: analysis of one to three year results. *Arthroscopy* 1987; 3:173–181.
5. Gartsman GM, Combs AH, Davis PF, et al. Arthroscopic acromioclavicular joint resection: an anatomical study. *Am J Sports Med* 1991;19:2–5.
6. Flatow EL, Cordasco FA, Bigliani LU. Arthroscopic resection of the outer end of the clavicle from a superior approach: a critical, quantitative, radiographic assessment of bone removal. *Arthroscopy* 1992;8(1):55–64.
7. Johnson LL. *Diagnostic and Surgical Arthroscopy*. St. Louis: CV Mosby; 1981.
8. Urist M. Complete dislocation of the acromioclavicular joint: the nature of the lesion and effective methods of treatment with an analysis of 41 cases. *J Bone Joint Surg* 1946;28:13.
9. Cook FF, Tibone JE. The Mumford procedure in athletes: an objective analysis of function. *Am J Sports Med* 1988;16:97–100.
10. Flatow EL, Bigliani LU. Arthroscopic acromioclavicular joint debridement and distal clavicle resection. *Oper Tech Orthop* 1991;1:240–247.
11. Bigliani LU, Nicholson GP, Flatow EL. Arthroscopic resection of the distal clavicle. *Orthop Clin N Am* 1993;24(1):133–141.
12. Matthews LS, Parks BG, Pavlovich LJ et al. Arthroscopic versus open distal clavicle resection: a biomechanical analysis on a cadaveric model. *Arthroscopy* 1999;5(3): 237–240.
13. Branch TP, Burdette HL, Shahriari AS, Carter FM II, et al. The role of the acromioclavicular ligaments and the effect of distal clavicle resection. *Am J Sports Med* 1996;24:293–297.
14. Flatow EL, Duralde XA, Nicholson GP, et al. Arthroscopic resection of the distal clavicle with a superior approach. *J Shoulder Elbow Surg* 1995;4:41–50.

Recommended Reading

Branch TP, Burdette HL, Shahriari AS, Carter FM II, et al. The role of the acromioclavicular ligaments and the effect of distal clavicle resection. *Am J Sports Med* 1996;24: 293–297.

Cook FF, Tibone JE. The Mumford procedure in athletes: an objective analysis of function. *Am J Sports Med* 1988;16: 97–100.

Flatow EL, Cordasco FA, Bigliani LU. Arthroscopic resection of the outer end of the clavicle from a superior approach: a critical, quantitative, radiographic assessment of bone removal. *Arthroscopy* 1992;8(1):55–64.

Post M, Flatow EL, Bigliani LU, Pollock RG. *The Shoulder: Operative Technique*. Baltimore: Williams & Wilkins, 1998:239–241.

Rehabilitation

24

Rehabilitation Following Operative Shoulder Arthroscopy

W. Ben Kibler

Advances in understanding the principles and appropriate implementation of arthroscopy for the shoulder have resulted in greater success in defining and restoring the anatomical lesions associated with shoulder dysfunction. Similarly, advances in understanding and implementation of rehabilitation principles for the shoulder have resulted in greater success in restoring the physiological and biomechanical alterations associated with shoulder dysfunction.

Arthroscopy, by providing (often less traumatic) restoration of anatomy, has allowed earlier implementation of functional rehabilitation protocols. This can lead to the creation of "accelerated" rehabilitation programs that can restore more complete function in shorter time frames.

This chapter discusses the role of the operative arthroscopist in shoulder rehabilitation, presents the basic science in physiology and biomechanics that provides the basis for shoulder rehabilitation, and offers guidelines and clinical practices that implement the accelerated protocols.

THE OPERATIVE ARTHROSCOPIST'S ROLE IN REHABILITATION

The operative arthroscopist plays several roles in shoulder rehabilitation. The first is to establish the complete and accurate diagnosis of the anatomical, biomechanical, and physiological alterations that may be present in shoulder injury and dysfunction. Preoperatively, this requires knowledge of the functional anatomy of the shoulder, and how to clinically examine the shoulder. It also requires some knowledge of how the shoulder functions in relation to the other segments of the kinetic chain. Intraoperatively, the surgeon needs both the skills to identify the intra- and extra-articular pathology and the techniques to assure adequate repair or reconstruction to optimize the anatomy. The surgeon also needs to be able to determine

the inherent stability and safe limits of motion for the repair. The ability to optimize the anatomical restoration does not guarantee functional restoration, but it does create the foundation by which rehabilitation can restore function.

The second role is to determine the timing of entry into and exit from the rehabilitation program. In many cases, entry into rehabilitation should be started before surgery. This will allow correction of flexibility and strength deficits in distant parts of the kinetic chain as well as an early start on restoring strength and flexibility in the shoulder area. This is similar to the protocol for preop preparation in injuries to the anterior cruciate ligament (ACL).

Postoperative entry into rehabilitation may be quite early, while the shoulder is still protected. Kinetic chain rehabilitation of the legs, trunk, and scapula may be started early, and closed-chain range of motion may be started in safe ranges determined at the time of surgery.

Exit from rehabilitation should be based not only on healing of the anatomical lesion, but on normalization of physiology and biomechanics to allow functional return to the demands of the sport or activity. This requires reassessment as rehabilitation proceeds, and evaluation of key functional components such as range of motion, balanced strength, and intact kinetic chain.

The third role is to guide the "pace" of the rehabilitation protocol. In the early stages, this will be determined by the anatomical diagnosis and integrity of the anatomic repair. In later stages, it will be determined by the progressive acquisition of components of normal kinetic chain function, normal flexibility, normal strength, and sport- or activity-specific functions. This requires periodic reassessment of the patient and frequent precise communication with the therapist. Rehabilitation should be viewed as a "flow" of exercises that will vary according to stages of healing and reestablishment of key points of muscle and joint function. This flow is indicated in the rehabili-

TABLE 24.1. Rehabilitation Flow Sheet: Weeks and Stages Estimated.

	Weeks at stages									
	Acute			Recovery				Functional		
Guideline	1	2	3	4	5	6	7	8	9	10
1. Diagnosis	X	X								
2. Proximal segment control										
Step up/step down	X	X	X							
Lunges	X	X	X				X	X		
Squats	X	X	X	X			X	X		
Hip extension/trunk rotation	X	X	X	X	X	X	X	X		
3. Scapular rehabilitation										
Pectoral minor/up trap stretch	(X)	(X)	X	X						
Posterior joint mobilization	(X)	(X)	X	X	X					
Hip/trunk extension: scapular retraction:		X	X	X	X	X				
Diagonal rotation: scapular retraction		X	X	X	X	X	X	X		
Pinches	X	X								
Scapular clock	(X)	(X)	X	X	X					
Low row	(X)	(X)	X							
Shoulder dumps			X	X	X	X	X	X		
Punches				X	X	X	X	X	X	
Table push-up		X	X	X						
Normal push-up plus					X	X	X	X		
4. Glenohumeral rehabilitation										
Weight shifts		(X)	(X)	X						
Scapular clock	(X)	(X)	X	X	X					
Wall washes				(X)	X	X	X			
Rotation diagonal					X	X	X	X	X	
Isolated rotator cuff						X	X			
5. Plyometrics										
Lower extremity				X	X	X	X	X	X	
Medicine ball						X	X	X	X	X
Rotation diagonals						X	X	X	X	X
Dumbbell rotations						X	X	X	X	X

a(X) designates activity that may be performed if indicated by tissue healing.

tation flow sheet (Table 24.1). In most cases, it is not appropriate to abdicate the responsibility or involvement in rehabilitation by marking "evaluate and treat." Even though the operative arthroscopist does not actually provide the details of the exercises, the surgeon must be an integral part of the team that provides the rehabilitation protocol.

BASIC SCIENCE

Rehabilitation is sometimes difficult in the shoulder, whose complex function involves not only local anatomical and biomechanical integrity, but also biomechanical and physiological contributions from distant body segments. The distant segment contribu-

tions are key components of the sequential activation of body segments that is necessary to accomplish any athletic activity. The activation sequence is termed a kinetic chain. The kinetic chain harmonizes the interdependent segments to produce a desired result at the distal segment. The shoulder does not function in isolation, but functions as a link in kinetic chain activity that optimizes shoulder function. Alterations in any of the other links of the kinetic chain can affect the shoulder, and alterations in the shoulder can affect the other links in the kinetic chain. The existence of this interaction has two implications for shoulder rehabilitation. First, the evaluation and identification process preceding shoulder treatment and rehabilitation should include more than just local shoulder structures. The evaluation process should result in a complete and accurate diagnosis of all the altered structures throughout the kinetic chain. Second, optimum restoration of shoulder function requires activation of all the kinetic chain segments to reestablish the interactions that existed before injury.

The biomechanical model for striking and throwing sports is an open-ended kinetic chain of segments that work in a proximal-to-distal sequence.[1-3] The goal of the kinetic chain activation sequence is to impart maximum velocity or force through the distal segment (the hand) to the ball, racquet, or other implement. The ultimate velocity of the distal segment is highly dependent on the velocity of the proximal segments. The proximal segments accelerate the entire chain and sequentially transfer force and energy to the next distal segment.[1,2,4-6] Because of their large relative mass, the proximal segments are responsible for the majority of the force and kinetic energy that is generated in the kinetic chain.[3] As a result, lower extremity force production is more highly correlated with ball velocity than is upper extremity force production.[7]

The physiological model for throwing and striking sports is a motor program.[8] Motor programs activate muscles in coordinated sequences to create joint movements that simplify and perform movement tasks. These programs are of two types.[9] Length-dependent patterns operate locally at one joint, are responsible for resisting joint perturbations, and result in cocontraction force couple activation. An example would be deltoid–supraspinatus activation to control the humeral head in the glenoid socket. Force-dependent patterns harmonize motions of several joints, create coordinated joint motions, and use agonist–antagonist force couple activation to generate force. An example would be latissimus dorsi–lower trapezius activation to simultaneously retract/stabilize the scapula and internally rotate the arm. In combination, these result in motor programs for voluntary upper extremity movements that are task oriented and include lower extremity and trunk muscle activation prior to and during arm motion.[10] In addition to generating and transferring force to the distal segments, these programs create a stable proximal base for voluntary arm movements, so that the rapid arm movements will not disturb body equilibrium during throwing or striking.[10,11]

The motor programs rely upon specific sensory and proprioceptive feedback for integration and activation.[9,12] Rehabilitation protocols must be position specific, motion specific, and function specific, and they must include gravity resistance and joint integration to stimulate the proprioceptive feedback that will cue the appropriate functional patterns.[13,14]

GUIDELINE 1: COMPLETE AND ACCURATE DIAGNOSES

The actual shoulder injury is the primary factor that determines treatment and rehabilitation. This may involve tendon injury or tear, instability, and/or joint internal derangement, whose overt clinical symptoms can be evaluated by standard diagnostic methods. However, both nonovert local alterations and distant alterations are frequently associated with shoulder clinical symptoms and dysfunction. The most common local alterations are decreased shoulder internal rotation,[15,16] which creates altered glenohumeral translations,[16,17] altered strength,[16,18] and alterations in scapular motion and position (scapular dyskinesis)[16,19-24] which disrupt the normal smooth coupling of scapulohumeral motions in voluntary activation,[25] and are present in a majority of patients with shoulder impingement.[20,26] Distant alterations include lumbar muscle inflexibility and muscle weakness,[27] and hip and knee inflexibility.[16]

Because these alterations are common findings in shoulder injury, ranging from 34% (hip tightness)[16] to nearly 100% (glenohumeral internal rotation deficit and scapular dyskinesis),[15,16,20,21] they need to be assessed through a screening process in the clinical evaluation. This requires a "victims and culprits" approach.[28] The site of symptoms is the "victim," but the "culprits" may include alterations at other sites.

Practice

The clinical evaluation should include some screening tests for hip/trunk posture and functional strength. Our screening exam includes standing posture evaluation of legs, lumbar, thoracic, and cervical spine, bilateral hip range-of-motion assessment, trunk flexibility assessment, and a one-leg stability series (Figure 24.1), which assesses control of the trunk over the leg. Any abnormalities can be evaluated in more detail.

Scapular evaluation can be accomplished from behind the patient.[19] It should assess resting position and note any asymmetries in definition of the bony landmarks. The most common differences are prominence of the inferior medial border, which is associated with anterior rotatory tilting of the coracoid and acromion, prominence of the entire medial border, which simulates classical scapular winging, or superior translation of the entire scapula, which results in prominence of the superior medial border. Dynamic motion screening involves evaluation of the same asymmetries of scapular control with arm abduction and forward flexion, in both ascent and descent. Mus-

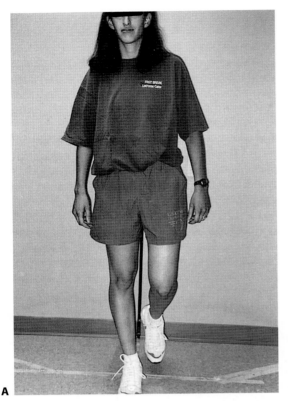

A

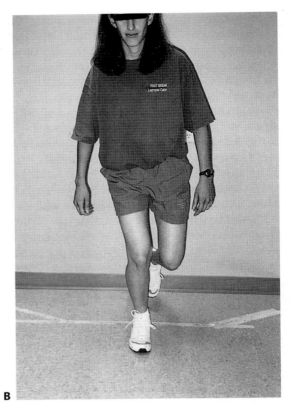

B

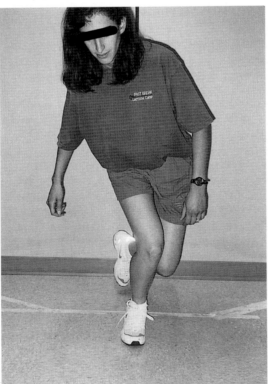

C

FIGURE 24.1. One-leg stability series: (A) one-leg stance, (B) one-leg squat, and (C) "corkscrew" with hip varus and rotation due to loss of hip control.

cular strength screening is accomplished through wall push-ups and the lateral scapular slide test.[19]

Shoulder joint evaluation should include the standard battery of tests for instability, rotator cuff injury, and joint internal derangement. The acromioclavicular (AC) joint should be evaluated for arthrosis or instability. Glenohumeral internal/external rotation, which is the biomechanically important component of shoulder rotation, should be screened by bilaterally assessing humeral rotation on the stabilized scapula. Internal rotation assessment by the "thumb on the spine" method has 7 degrees of freedom inherent in the test and has no correlation with goniometrically measured glenohumeral rotation.[29]

GUIDELINE 2: PROXIMAL SEGMENT CONTROL

If the proximal segments of the kinetic chain—the legs, pelvis, and spine—are altered in posture, flexibility, or strength, they should be corrected in the early stages of rehabilitation. Early in rehabilitation, the inhibited scapular muscles or the injured or inhibited shoulder muscles require a large degree of facilitation of their activation, so the role of proximal segment control and activation is increased. These exercises may be started in the early stage of rehabilitation, even in the preoperative stage, since they do not rely on shoulder motion or loading. They may even be done with the arm in a sling.

All exercises are started with the feet on the ground and involve hip extension and control. The patterns of activation are both ipsilateral and contralateral. Diagonal motions involving trunk rotation around a stable leg simulate the normal patterns of throwing. As the shoulder heals and is ready for motion and loading in the intermediate or recovery stage of rehabilitation, the patterns can include arm motion as the final part of the exercise.

Practice

Specific exercises include step up/step down with trunk extension, front and side lunges, one-leg and two-leg squats, and hip flexions and extensions with trunk rotations (Figure 24.2). These may be done on a stable surface and may progress to unstable surfaces for added difficulty and proprioceptive input.

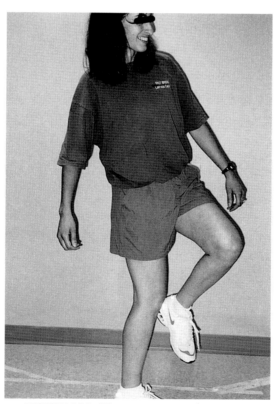

FIGURE 24.2. Hip extension: trunk rotation.

GUIDELINE 3: SCAPULAR REHABILITATION

Optimal scapular muscle activation allows proper scapular motion and position while maintaining the glenohumeral instant center of rotation throughout arm motion.[19,30,31] Scapular muscle activation proceeds and facilitates rotator cuff activation in the throwing or striking sequence,[32] so this should be instituted before emphasis on rotator cuff activation.

Loss of scapular control, or "scapular dyskinesis," noted early and very frequently associated with shoulder injury,[19,20–22,26] is caused by inhibition of coupled muscle activation needed to elevate, depress, retract, and protract the scapula and for subsequent substitute patterns of muscle activation.[19,32,33] The lower trapezius and serratus anterior appear to be most affected by inhibition, and the upper trapezius most commonly becomes overactivated. This creates the most common manifestation of scapular dyskinesis, lack of effective retraction with a tendency to protraction. Owing to its anatomical position on an ellipsoid thorax, the protracted scapula also tends to tilt anteriorly, with acromial depression, glenoid antetilting, and resultant external and internal impingement,[16,21,26] and increases the strain on the anterior-inferior glenohumeral ligament.[34]

Practice

Hip and trunk extension patterns are used to initiate and facilitate scapular control. Scapular control exercises can be started in the preoperative or early healing stages of rehabilitation because they do not require shoulder or arm movement. Early-stage exercises to regain scapular retraction control include ipsilateral and contralateral hip/trunk extension with scapular retraction, diagonal hip/trunk rotation with scapular retraction (Figure 24.3), and isometric scapular pinches. These can all be done even with the arm in a sling.

When arm motion is safe, or in nonoperative or preoperative situations, an extremely effective exercise for initiation of scapular retraction and depression is a "low row" (Figure 24.4), which includes trunk extension, scapular retraction, and shoulder extension

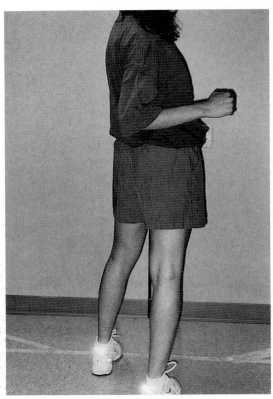

FIGURE 24.3. Hip/trunk rotation: scapular retraction.

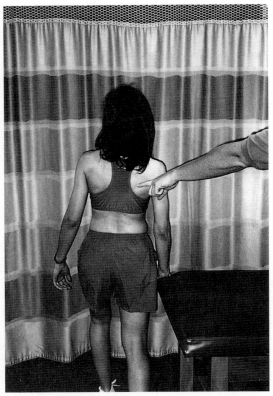

FIGURE 24.4. "Low row"–hip/trunk extension: shoulder extension. The muscle contraction should be felt at the inferior medial scapular tip.

with the arm at the side. These may be started in isometric fashion, and progressed to isotonic, concentric, and eccentric work with rubber tubing.

Scapular exercises that may be done when the shoulder is mobile include scapular clock (Figure 24.5), these elevation/depression and retraction/protraction exercises are performed with the hand on a wall or a movable object. Other advanced scapular exercises include shoulder "dumps," a trunk rotation/scapula retraction/shoulder extension exercise, and punches with dumbbells or tubing, which load the

serratus anterior and posterior shoulder musculature. Push-ups with a plus, or full protraction, is also an advanced scapular exercise. They may be done originally on a table, and then advanced to normal style.[35]

These exercises require muscular flexibility and joint mobility. The upper trapezius and pectoralis minor are common sites of myofascial tightness, and shoulder internal rotation is frequently decreased.[15,16] Manual stretching, massage techniques, and joint mobilizations must be used to normalize these alterations.

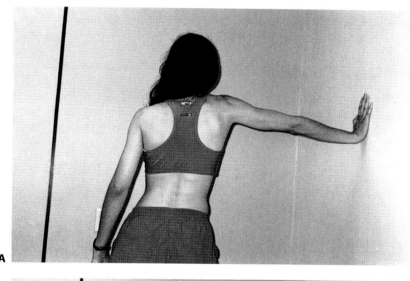

A

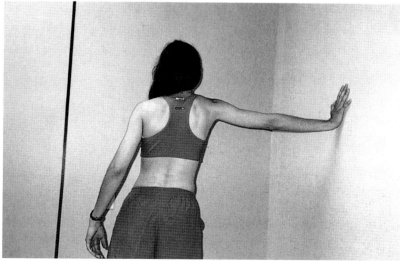

B

FIGURE 24.5. Scapular "clock": (A) elevation/depression, 12 o'clock/6 o'clock, and (B) retraction/protraction, 3 o'clock/9 o'clock.

GUIDELINE 4: GLENOHUMERAL REHABILITATION

The two major glenohumeral rehabilitation problems are dynamic joint stability and rotator cuff deficiencies; often those are interdependent. Dynamic glenohumeral stability can be improved by eliminating joint mobility deficits, thereby decreasing abnormal joint translations in the midrange of shoulder motion, by positioning and moving the glenoid socket in a "ball on a seal's nose" relation to the moving humerus so that concavity/compression of the joint is maintained,[19] and by active rotator cuff contraction.

In this stability role, as well as its role in humeral head depression, the rotator cuff is essentially operating as a "compressor cuff." Rotator cuff activation is coupled with and follows scapular muscle activation[25,32] so that the rotator cuff muscles work from a stabilized and optimally positioned base, are physiologically activated, and are mechanically placed in an optimal length–tension arrangement to create appropriate joint stiffness.[30,34]

Since functional rotator cuff activation is integrated within its component parts and with the kinetic chain[25,32] and results in the rotator cuff functioning as a compressor cuff, "closed-chain" protocols involving axial loading from distal to proximal are the most physiological way to simulate normal rotator cuff function.[13,14,22,36,37] Isolated rotator cuff exercises do not integrate muscle activation, potentially create shear across the joint, and are usually performed in nonphysiological positions.

Practice

Closed-chain exercise practices may be started in early rehabilitation stages with the hand in a relatively fixed position, below shoulder level on a table. Weight shifts on a table or balance board are safe in this position. When the arm may be raised toward shoulder height, the patient may begin axial loading rotator cuff exercises, which place the hand on unstable surfaces and apply an axial load through the moving hand. A good axial load exercise is the "wall wash" (Figure 24.6). This may be done initially with the arm close to the body, progressing with arm extension as strength improves. An advanced axial loading exercise that shades into open chain activity is the internal/external rotation diagonal (Figure 24.7), with the shoulder moving through 90° of abduction and using rubber tubing resistance. This may also start with the arm close to the body, with the hand being moved farther away for more strength. Isolated rotator cuff exercises may be used if any local deficit is still present. Internal and external rotation strengthening should be done at the functional position of 90° abduction.

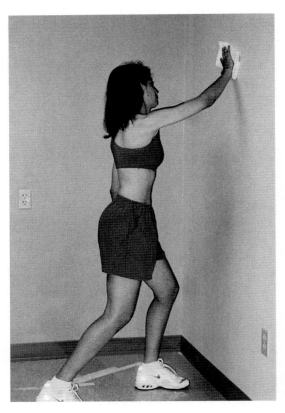

FIGURE 24.6. "Wall washes": axial loading with resistance to moving arm.

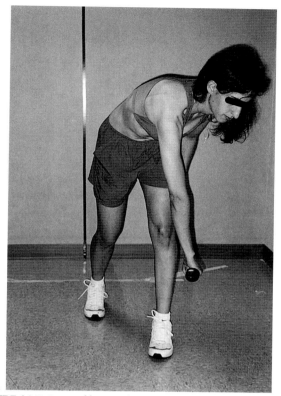
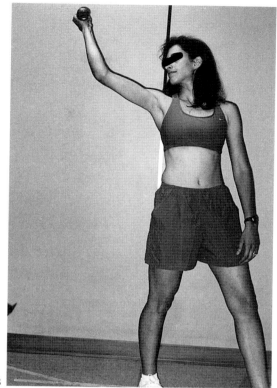

FIGURE 24.7. Internal/external rotation diagonal. This exercise connects all of the kinetic chain segments in functional arcs. (A) Internal rotation. (B) External rotation.

GUIDELINE 5: PLYOMETRIC EXERCISES

Power is required for shoulder function in throwing or striking. Plyometric training, through activation or stretch/shortening responses in muscles, is the most effective method of power development.[38] Since power is generated in the entire kinetic chain, plyometric training should be done in every segment. Plyometrics can be instituted in noninjured areas early in rehabilitation but must be deferred to later stages in injured areas, owing to the large range of required motions and the large forces developed.

Practice

Lunges, vertical jumps, depth jumps, slides, and fitter exercises are some methods of lower extremity plyometrics.[39] Trunk and upper extremity plyometrics include rotation diagonals, medicine ball rotations and pushes, and dumbbell rotations.

GUIDELINES FOR PROGRESSION

Since this type of rehabilitation program focuses on functional return of kinetic chain patterns, there is less emphasis on specific stages or pathways or specific isolated exercises and more emphasis on flow and overlap between the acquisition of function of the various segments. This requires periodic close reassessment for progressions. The program must be flexible enough to be applied over a wide range of the individual aptitudes. New exercises are instituted when the segment function is appropriate. This is illustrated by the flow sheet diagram of Table 24.1, which represents estimated times and sequences for the exercises.

Several key points should be checked as markers for safe progression (Table 24.2). These may be

TABLE 24.2. Key Points for Progression in Rehabilitation and Return to Play.

Pelvis control over the planted leg (negative Trendelenburg sign)

Effective hip and trunk extension

Scapular control, especially of retraction

Normal glenohumeral rotation

No substitutions for these functions

"Readiness to play"

Functional progressions of throwing or striking

"Return to play"

checked by the operative arthroscopist at the re-assessment exam. Normal pelvis control over the planted leg (negative Trendelenburg sign) is a prerequisite for proximal segment control. Effective hip and trunk extension is required for proximal segment facilitation of scapula and arm activation. Scapula control, especially of retraction, allows coupled shoulder motion and coupled rotator cuff muscle activation. Normal glenohumeral rotation, especially in internal rotation, is required to decrease joint translation. If the patient exhibits substitute activities for those normal functions, or cannot progress because of alterations in these functions, more detailed investigations should be done before rehabilitation is resumed.

GUIDELINES FOR RETURN TO PLAY

Return to play requires not only anatomical healing of the injured part, but also, restoration of the physiological patterns and biomechanical motions in the appropriate kinetic chain of function. "Readiness to play" is indicated by clinical evidence of anatomic healing and completion of the "key points" listed in Table 24.2. The patient may exit from rehabilitation at this point. Functional progressions of throwing or striking may be started from the readiness-to-play functional base. Return to play is dependent upon completion of the functional progressions.[13,36,39]

SUMMARY

The operative arthroscopic surgeon has a unique opportunity to participate in accelerated rehabilitation protocols that show promise in early return of shoulder function. This is the result of the ability to preoperatively and intraoperatively establish the complete and accurate anatomical, physiological, and biomechanical diagnosis to repair or reconstruct the anatomic lesion with less tissue damage, stiffness, and pain, and to evaluate the integrity of the repair. These advantages allow early entry into functional rehabilitation protocols, establishment of a safe "pace" of progression through the protocols, and sequential progression through the flow of rehabilitation exercises.

This framework for rehabilitation is consistent with the proximal-to-distal kinetic chain biomechanical model and applies current concepts of motor control and closed-chain exercises. This framework approaches the final goal—glenohumeral motion and function—through facilitation by scapular control, and scapular control through facilitation by hip and trunk activation.

This chapter supplies both guidelines for rehabilitation and practices to implement the guidelines that have proven effective in our hands. Other protocols may be effective, as long as they adhere to several basic concepts of kinetic chain based shoulder rehabilitation:

1. Functional shoulder rehabilitation requires that the muscle activations and joint motions follow a proximal-to-distal pathway along the appropriate kinetic chain.
2. Muscles around the shoulder function in an integrated fashion and should be rehabilitated in integrated patterns. Specific muscles may need isolated activation, but this activation should be facilitated by placing the proximal segments in a facilitating function.
3. Scapular control and coupled rotator cuff activation are vital to normal shoulder function.
4. Closed-chain axial loading exercises are the primary means of early shoulder rehabilitation and are the mainstays of functional rehabilitation protocols.

References

1. Putnam CA. Sequential motions of body segments in striking and throwing skills: descriptions and explanations. *J Biomech* 1993;25:125–135.
2. Feltner ME, Dapena J. Three-dimensional interactions in a two-segment kinetic chain. Part I: General model. *Int J Sport Biomech* 1989;5:403–419.
3. Kibler WB. Biomechanical analysis of the shoulder during tennis activities. *Clin Sports Med* 1995;14:79–86.
4. Elliott BC, Marshall R, Noffal G. Contributions of upper limb segment rotations during the power serve in tennis. *J Appl Biomech* 1995;11:443–442.
5. Toyoshima S, Hoshikawa T, Miyashita M. Contribution of body parts to throwing performance. *Biomechanics IV*. Baltimore: University Park Press; 1974:169–174.
6. Fleisig GS, Barrentine SW, Escamilla F. Biomechanics of overhand throwing with implications for injuries. *Sports Med* 1996;21:421–437.
7. Kraemer WJ, Triplett NT, Fry AC. An in-depth sports medicine profile of women college tennis players. *J Sports Rehabil* 1995;4:79–88.
8. Shumway-Cook A, Woollacott MH. Theories of motor control. In: *Motor Control Theory and Practical Applications*. Baltimore, Williams & Wilkins, 1995:3–18.
9. Nichols TR. A biomechanical perspective on spine mechanics of coordinated muscular action. *Acta Anat* 1994;15:1–13.
10. Zattara M, Bouisset S. Posturo-kinetic organization during the early phase of voluntary upper limb movement. *J Neurol Neurosurg Psychiatry* 1988;51:956–965.

11. Cordo PJ, Nashner, LM. Properties of postural adjustments associated with rapid arm movements. *J Neurophysiol* 1982;47:287–308.

12. Lephart SM, Pinciuero DM, Giraldo JL. The role of proprioception in the management and rehabilitation of athletic injuries. *Am J Sports Med* 1997;25:130–137.

13. Lephart, SM, Henry TJ. The physiological basis for open and closed kinetic chain rehabilitation for the upper extremity. *J Sport Rehabil* 1996;5:71–87.

14. Wilk KE, Harrelson GL, Arrigo C. Shoulder rehabilitation. In: Andrews JR, Harrelson GL, Wilk KE, eds. *Physical Rehabilitation of the Injured Athlete*. Philadelphia: WB Saunders; 1998:478–553.

15. Silliman FJ, Hawkins RJ. Current concepts and recent advances in the athlete's shoulder. *Clin Sports Med* 1991;10:693–705.

16. Burkhart S, Morgan CD, Kibler W,. The dead arm revisited. *Clin Sports Med* 2000;19:125–158.

17. Harryman ET, Sidles JA, Clark JM. Translation of the humeral head on the glenoid with passive glenohumeral motions. *J Bone Joint Surg* 1990;72:1334–1343.

18. Kibler WB, McQueen C, Uhl TL. Fitness evaluations and fitness findings in competitive junior tennis players. *Clin Sports Med* 1988;7:403–416.

19. Kibler WB. The role of the scapula in athletic shoulder function. *Am J Sport Med* 1998;26:325–337.

20. Warner JJP, Micheli LJ, Arslanian LE. Scapulothoracic motion in normal shoulders and shoulders with glenohumeral instability and impingement syndrome. *Clin Orthop* 1992;285:199–215.

21. Paletta GA, Warner JJP, Warren RF. Shoulder kinetic with two-plane x-ray evaluation in patients with anterior instability or rotator cuff tears. *J Shoulder Elbow Surg* 1997;6:516–527.

22. Paine RM, Voight, M. The role of the scapula. *J Orthop Sports Phys Ther* 1993;18:386–391.

23. Bagg SD, Forrest WJ. Electromyographic study of the scapular rotators during arm abduction in the scapular plane. *Am J Phys Med* 1986;65:111–124.

24. Bagg SD, Forrest WJ. A biomechanical analysis of scapular rotation during arm abduction in the scapular plane. *Am J Phys Med* 1988;67:238–245.

25. Happee R, Van der Helm FC. Control of shoulder muscles during goal directed movements, an inverse dynamic analysis. *J Biomech* 1995;28:1179–1191.

26. Lukasiewici AC, McClure P, Michener L. Comparison of three-dimensional scapular position and orientation between subjects with and without shoulder impingement. *J Orthop Sports Phys Ther* 1999;29:574–586.

27. Young JL, Herring SA, Press JM. The influence of the spine on the shoulder in the throwing athlete. *J Back Musculoskeletal Rehabil* 1996;7:5–17.

28. MacIntyre JG, Lloyd-Smith DR. Overuse running injuries. In: Renstrom P, ed. *Sports Injuries, Principles of Prevention and Care*. London: Blackwell; 1993:139–160.

29. Delcomyn SMB, Ha MH, Fletcher JP. The relationship between posterior reach and its component movements at the shoulder joint during active range of motion. Poster presented at: American Physical Therapy Association Annual Meeting; March 2000; New Orleans.

30. Perry J. Anatomy and biomechanics of the shoulder in throwing, swimming, gymnastics, and tennis. *Clin Sports Med* 1983;2:247–270.

31. Inman T, Saunders M, Abbott LC. Observations on the function of the shoulder joint. *J Bone Joint Surg* 1944;20:1–31.

32. Speer KP, Garrett WE. Muscular control of motion and stability about the pectoral girdle. In: Matsen FA, Fu FH, Hawkins RJ, eds. *The Shoulder: A Balance of Mobility and Stability*. American Academy of Orthopedic Surgeons; Rosemont, IL: 1994:159–173.

33. McQuade KJ, Dawson J, Smidt GL. Scapulothoracic muscle fatigue associated with alterations in scapulohumeral rhythm kinematics during maximum resistive shoulder elevation. *J Orthop Sports Phys Ther* 1998;5:71–87.

34. Weiser WM, Lee TQ, McMaster WC. Effects of simulated scapular protraction on anterior glenohumeral stability. *Am J Sports Med* 1999;27:801–805.

35. Moseley JB, Jobe FW, Pink MM, et al. EMG analysis of the scapular muscles during a shoulder rehabilitation program. *Am J Sports Med* 1992;20:128–134.

36. Wilk KE. Closed and open kinetic chain exercise for the upper extremity. *J Sport Rehabil* 1996; 5:88–102.

37. Dillman CJ, Murray TA, Hintermeister RA. Biomechanical differences of open and closed chain exercises with respect to the shoulder. *J Sports Rehabil* 1994;3:228–238.

38. Wilk KE, Voight ML, Keirns MA. Stretch–shortening exercises for the upper extremity: theory and clinical application. *J Orthop Sports Phys Ther* 1993;17:225–239.

39. Kibler WB, Livingston B, Bruce R. Current concepts of shoulder rehabilitation. *Adv Oper Orthop* 1995;3:249–299.

Complications

25

Complications in Shoulder Arthroscopy

Benjamin S. Shaffer and James E. Tibone

Complications following shoulder arthroscopy are relatively uncommon. In 1986 Small first reported 40 complications in a review of over 14,000 procedures, for an overall complication rate of 0.28%.[1] In 1988 he noted a slightly higher rate among experienced arthroscopists, 0.78% of 1184 cases reviewed.[2] Most complications were due to staple use, reflex sympathetic dystrophy, and hemarthrosis. Subsequent studies have suggested the complication rate is probably higher. Berjano et al. in 1998 reporting an incidence of 10.6% in their 179 cases.[3] Complications can be generally divided into those that occur during any shoulder arthroscopy and those that are are procedure specific. This chapter reviews complications of shoulder arthroscopy, with emphasis on how to avoid them.

GENERAL COMPLICATIONS

General complications include swelling and fluid extravasation, bleeding and problems with visualization, infection, iatrogenic damage/instrument breakage, nerve injury, and anesthetic or medical-related complications.

SWELLING

Swelling of the soft tissues can be alarming. This is particularly true in today's environment in which the arthroscopic pump is so frequently used. Multiple punctures of the glenohumeral joint capsule predisposes to soft tissue extravasation. The subacromial arch is not a truly confined space, and readily permits extravasation as well. Although compartment syndrome has never been reported to occur in the shoulder, accumulation of fluid can certainly jeopardize one's ability to complete the procedure arthroscopi-

cally, or makes conversion to an open procedure more difficult. Studies have shown that pressure elevations in the deltoid are transient, and usually return to baseline within minutes of the procedures' completion. Swelling/fluid extravasation can be minimized by 1) avoiding unnecessary glenohumeral capsule punctures, 2) attention to maintaining intra-articular portal position, 3) attention to pump flow, pressure, and outflow, and 4) expeditious completion of the procedure.

BLEEDING/VASCULAR INJURY

Vascular problems are rare, and most commonly occur during subacromial decompressions, in which bleeding compromises visualization. Inadvertent injury to the acromial branch of the thoracoacomial artery can create a challenge for even an experienced arthroscopist. Clear visualization during arthroscopic subacromial decompression is enhanced by 1) maintaining a relatively low systolic blood pressure, preferably less than 100mmHg (if not medically contraindicated), 2) proper flow mechanics with sufficient pressure and inflow, 3) use of Epinephrine (1:100,000 per 3 L bag of normal saline), 4) availability of cautery device as necessary, 5) pre-injection of subacromial bursa with Marcaine with epinephrine, and 6) avoidance of vascular tissue beneath the AC joint.

Arterial injury is rare but has been reported. A more common risk is to the cephalic vein, particularly if using an inferior "5 o'clock" portal during anterior shoulder stabilization. Pearsall et al. cautioned against use of a "5 o'clock" portal because of risk to the nearby cephalic vein, which in their cadaveric study averaged only 2mm from the portal.[4] Davidson and Tibone have also observed the proximity of the cephalic vein and anterior humeral circumflex artery to their "5 o'clock" portal, but have encountered no complications in clinical use.[5]

INFECTION

Superficial and deep infections are uncommon. D'Angelo and Ogilvie-Harris reported on nine cases of septic arthritis (of 4,000 cases of shoulder and knee arthroscopies), for an overall deep infection rate of 0.23%.[6] All resolved with arthroscopic irrigation, debridement, and intravenous antibiotics. Small also noted this complication, but it occurred in only two of over fourteen thousand procedures.[1] Infection risk can be minimized through appropriate pre-operative antibiotic administration and gentle soft tissue handling.

IATROGENIC INJURY/INSTRUMENT AND IMPLANT BREAKAGE/ TISSUE REACTION

Iatrogenic injury can occur with any technique or device. Such damage probably most commonly occurs to the articular cartilage, where scuffing due to inadvertent trauma from the scope or instrumentation occurs. Failure to establish portals that permit accurate targeting leads to unnecessary cannula manipulation and to stress on drill sleeves and drills, insertion devices, and implants; there are also risks of instrumentation failure and damage to the articular cartilage. Injury can also be caused by overly aggressive debridement of cuff or labral tissue, unnecessary "repair" of normal variants, or violation of normal joints [e.g., coplaning of the acromioclavicular (AC) joint during subacromial decompression].

With the advent of bioabsorbable implants, occasional adverse tissue reactions are seen, initially described with the Suretac device (Figure 25.1). Any of these biological devices, however, can elicit an intensive synovial reaction or an exuberant foreign body reaction. Unfortunately, preoperative identification of the patient at risk is currently impossible.

Intraoperative equipment breakage or failure is relatively rare, estimated by Small at 0.1%. The risks depend on the procedure performed and are greatest for stabilization/repair procedures in which multiple devices and implants are used. Iatrogenic trauma can best be avoided by familiarity with normal anatomy and appropriate, careful surgical technique. Minimize stress on equipment such as drill sleeves and insertion devices, and avoid inappropriate placement of implants. Instruments should be inspected preferably before removal, and always afterward, to ensure that nothing has been left behind. Anchors can be proud or become loose, so one must ensure proper seating and tensioning at the time of insertion. Special instruments, including arthroscopic graspers and a "golden retriever" device for removal of metallic frag-

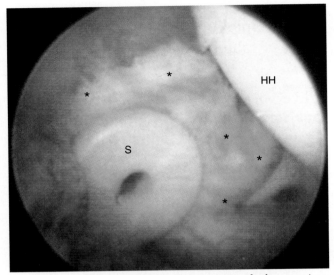

FIGURE 25.1. Arthroscopic view demonstrating the hyperemic response elicited in a patient at approximately one month following implantation of a Suretac device for labral fixation. Following implant removal and joint irrigation, the intense synovitic response abated and symptoms resolved. The labrum was sufficiently healed to require no further surgical intervention: HH, humeral head; S, Suretac device; *, synovitis.

ments should be available. Disposable cannulas can leave debris and must be handled with care. Finally, remember to consider backup instrumentation to avoid having to abort or compromise the procedure.

NERVE INJURY

Nerve injury, the most common complication associated with shoulder arthroscopy, varies in incidence from 0 to 30%. The vast majority of these injuries are neuropraxias, and most resolve. The most common injuries are to the cutaneous nerves during portal placements, occurring as a mild (but permanent) sensory deficit in 3.3% of patients undergoing shoulder arthroscopy.[7] These can be avoided by incising only the skin and then bluntly spreading the underlying soft tissue.

Portals must be established in described "safe zones" that permit glenohumeral and subacromial access and instrumentation without risk of injury. There are vulnerable nerves in the vicinity of each portal. The traditional posterior scope portal, located approximately 1 to 3 cm inferior and 1 cm medial to the posterolateral acromion edge, is approximately 2 to 4 cm superior to the axillary nerve and approximately 1.5 cm lateral to the suprascapular nerve. Care must be taken to ensure appropriate orientation to avoid these structures (Figure 25.2). The anterior portal is relatively safe unless one strays too far medially (Figure 25.3). This can occur when one is using an "inside-

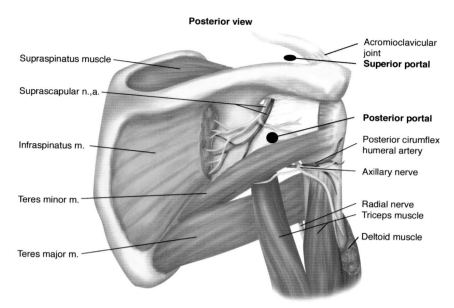

FIGURE 25.2. The posterior scope portal is approximately 2 to 4 cm superior to the axillary nerve and approximately 1.5 cm lateral to the suprascapular nerve. Attention to anatomy will preclude inadvertent injury to these important structures.

out" approach to establish the anterior portal and inadvertently allows the Wissinger rod to exit medial to the coracoid process. Marking out the location of the coracoid in advance can prevent this errant move.

Other less common causes of injury include excessive traction to the arm (and thus the brachial plexus), inappropriate positioning (reported in both beach chair and lateral decubitus position), and injuries due to specific procedures. The role of traction in brachial plexus strains has been emphasized by several authors, who have documented measurable neurological changes with shoulder traction. This emphasis probably accounts for the rarity of traction injuries, which usually occur as a consequence of excessive weight. In fact, "traction" during the lateral decubitus position might more appropriately be considered to be "suspension" because there should be merely sufficient weight to "suspend" the arm in the

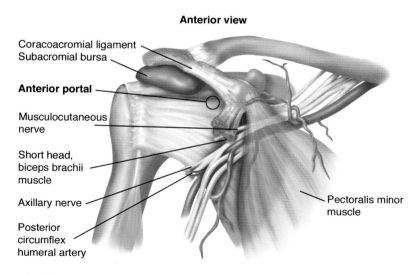

FIGURE 25.3. Relationship between the anterior portal and the brachial plexus, which lies medial to the coracoid process. Staying lateral to the coracoid will prevent any untoward plexus injuries.

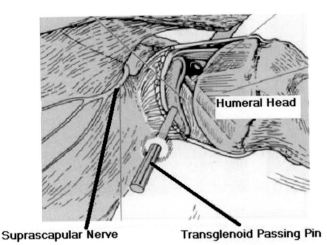

FIGURE 25.4. The passing pin used during a transglenoid Bankart repair must be angled laterally enough to avoid injury to the suprascapular nerve, which travels a mere 1.5 cm medial to the glenoid rim.

appropriate position of approximately 30 to 50° of abduction and 20° of forward elevation. Rarely is more than 10 lb necessary. Limiting the duration of traction will also decrease risk of undue strain to the brachial plexus. In the lateral decubitus position, one must also remember to use an axillary roll and to pad the downside extremity. A proposed advantage of the "beach chair" position is the lack of brachial plexus strain, since no traction is used. However, care must also be taken to ensure protection against cervical or brachial plexus due to positioning. One transient hy-

poglossal nerve injury after a combined arthroscopic/open reconstruction in the beach chair position has been reported.[8] The authors speculated that an intraoperative table position change led to nerve injury. Permanent quadriparesis has also been reported.[9]

Nerve injuries can also be procedure related, specific to the particular procedure being performed. The suprascapular nerve is at risk with the transglenoid approach to Bankart repair (Figure 25.4) and may also be compromised during biceps tenodesis if the passing pin technique is used. Guidelines have been developed emphasizing care and accuracy in Beath pin passage during this technique to avoid nerve injury. The pin must be aimed lateral to avoid the nerve. During arthroscopic cuff repair, care must be taken in cuff mobilization between the superior glenoid and the supraspinatus, since the suprascapular nerve is vulnerable a mere 1.5 cm medial to the glenoid rim.

Another portal that puts the axillary and musculocutaneous nerve potentially at risk is the "5 o'clock portal" for access to the anterior-inferior glenoid during anterior stabilization procedures. Recent examination of the anterior-inferior portal has shown it to be safe when accessing is performed correctly. However, the relationship of this portal to the musculocutaneous (average distance 22.9 mm) and axillary (average distance 24.4 mm) nerves mandates attention to detail during the establishment of this portal.[5] To avoid nerve injury, care must be taken to ensure that the portal is lateral to the conjoint tendon (Figure 25.5).

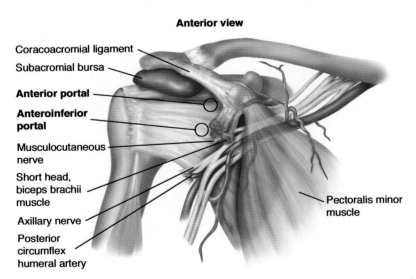

FIGURE 25.5. The "five o'clock" portal, useful in establishing a more inferior portal during arthroscopic Bankart repair, is safe as long as it is established lateral to the conjoint tendon.

STIFFNESS/RESTRICTED MOTION/ADHESIVE CAPSULITIS

Stiffness is an uncommon complication following arthroscopic shoulder surgery, but it has been reported, particularly following stabilizations. Some patients have experienced considerable and prolonged disability as a consequence. Adhesive capsulitis has also been described and probably occurs more often than has been reported, especially when unrecognized as the true cause of presumed "subacromial impingement."

ANESTHETIC COMPLICATIONS

Complications due to anesthesia are relatively uncommon, occurring in only 0.2% of all arthroscopic procedures according to Small's survey of nearly 400,000 cases in 1986.[1] Of these 63 complications, 18 were due to cardiac arrhythmias, 10 due to pnemonia, 4 due to aspiration pnemonia, and 31 to other "minor" untoward events. Most anesthetic complications are recognized and treated successfully.

Interscalene block anesthesia has proven a safe and effective alternative and/or adjunct in providing satisfactory anesthesia and postoperative pain relief. The risks with this procedure are not insignificant, however, and include hematoma, phrenic nerve blockade, vasovagal event, pneumothorax, total spinal anesthesia (with respiratory distress), hoarseness, Horner's syndrome, and cardiac arrest. Fortunately, such complications are uncommon and rarely permanent, and with a dedicated anesthesia effort, decrease with experience and technical mastery. Nevertheless, permanent nerve injury to the brachial plexus has been reported, with a permanent neurological injury rate estimated at 3.6%.[10] Understandably this has somewhat dampened enthusiasm for this type of anesthesia, at least in some centers.

MEDICAL COMPLICATIONS

Reported medical complications include spontaneous pneumothorax, reflex sympathetic dystrophy (RSD), deep venous thrombosis (DVT) of the upper extremity, coma, blindness, and reversible renal failure. Such complications are best avoided by careful preoperative screening for "at risk" patients and avoiding excess local anesthetic.

PROCEDURE-SPECIFIC COMPLICATIONS

Perhaps the most common complications of all are procedure specific. Complications in this context include not only adverse events (nerve injury, poor visualization, iatrogenic trauma), but the much more common complication of procedure failure. Because complications inherent with each procedure have been discussed in the relevant chapters, here we briefly address the most common problems associated with each procedure.

Synovectomy/Debridement for Osteoarthritis/Inflammatory Arthritis

Failure to relieve symptoms is the most common problem associated with debridement for glenohumeral arthritis. When debridement is carefully performed, most patients have some pain relief, but improvement in pain and function can be expected in this difficult-to-manage population only with careful patient selection.

SLAP Repair

The most common complication of SLAP repair is inappropriate labeling of a normal "central detachment"-type superior labral variant as a pathological finding (Figure 25.6). This reflects both the unnecessary

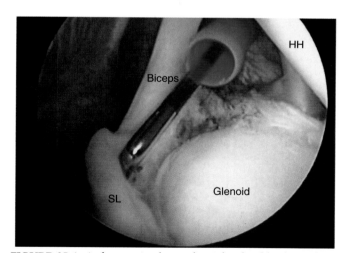

FIGURE 25.6. Arthroscopic photo of a right shoulder (view from posterior portal, lateral decubitus position) demonstrating a normal "central detachment" type of superior labral variant: the probe is placed from the anterior portal (disposable blue cannula) and is elevating the superior labrum from the glenoid. Notice the normal transition of tissue from the superior glenoid articular margin to the smooth undersurface of the labrum. Although the superior labrum may appear to be "loose," it is in fact attached peripherally quite soundly and did not account for this patient's symptoms: HH, humeral head; SL, superior labrum.

overtreatment of many superior labral variations and failure to recognize the true cause of a patient's symptoms. Familiarity with normal and variational anatomy will preclude this unnecessary exercise.

Biceps Tenodesis

Failure to recognize significant pathology can lead to the unfortunate complication of postarthroscopy long head rupture. Ruptures following debridement, use of thermal devices, or performance of other arthroscopic shoulder procedures also reportedly have led to this complication. The most significant risks to recently developed arthroscopic approaches to tenodesing the long head include failure to secure adequate fixation, failure to restore appropriate tension, and risks to the axillary and suprascapular nerve if a passing pin technique is used. Attention to detail and evolution away from the pin will decrease and possibly eliminate this risk.

Subacromial Decompression

Perhaps the most common indication for shoulder arthroscopy today, decompression remains a technically challenging procedure that requires expertise and experience. Preoperative films will permit surgical planning with respect to acromial morphology and thick-

ness, and will also allow recognition of os acromiale when it occurs (Figure 25.7). Attention to proper fluid control, availability of a cautery device to ensure a clear field, and appropriate surgical technique with respect to acromial resection will minimize complications (Figure 25.8).

AC Joint Resection

Complications during AC joint surgery can occur with failure to adequately resect sufficient distal clavicle, or as a result of overgenerous resection. Whether by a direct or indirect approach, AC joint decompression should ensure a smooth and adequate resection, avoiding the most common problem of residual posterior distal clavicle abutment. Naturally, the preoperative exam, with selective anesthetic injections as necessary, remains the best opportunity to identify and address AC pathology. Failure to recognize concomitant AC joint symptoms remains one of the more common reasons for persistent pain following subacromial surgery.

Cuff Repair

Arthroscopic repair of the rotator cuff has evolved from the treatment of partial tears to small and medium tears to repairs, now, of the subscapularis and

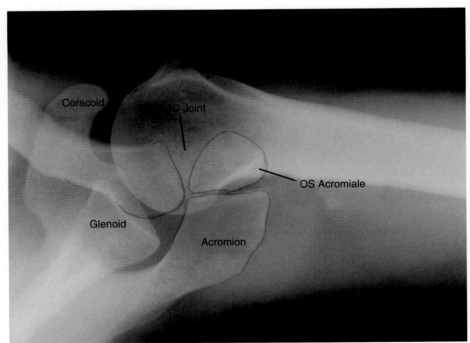

FIGURE 25.7. Axillary view of os acromiale in which the anterior acromion has failed to attain complete fusion. It is important to obtain such films preoperatively, to avoid both intraoperative surprise and inappropriate acromial resection.

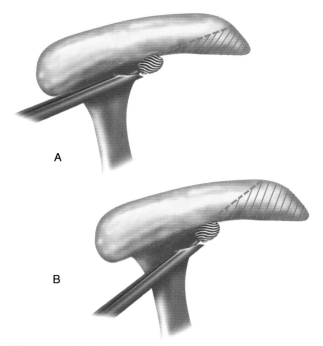

FIGURE 25.8. Outlet views. (A) A satisfactory approach to subacromial decompression, resecting the anterior inferior acromial spur. (B) Demonstration that the "cutting block" technique is not necessarily foolproof and, if oriented too vertically, can lead to an inappropriate resection of the anterior acromion.

massive tears. These latter entities require substantial arthroscopic shoulder expertise and pose considerable risk for the uninitiated surgeon (and patient). Although experienced surgeons believe that arthroscopic evaluation permits a better appreciation of the tear pattern and mobilization opportunities than conventional open strategies, the casual arthroscopist or his or her patients may not benefit. Opportunities for complications abound with this procedure, including those associated with subacromial decompressions, failure to adequately repair the cuff, and problems associated with new and untested implants. Recent evidence suggests that clinical outcomes following arthroscopic cuff repair compare favorably to its open counterpart, but may have no higher rate of "success" when evaluated by postoperative imaging studies.

Capsular Release for the Stiff/Frozen Shoulder

Failure to adequately restore normal motion is the most common complication of arthroscopic release. Chondral injury in tight and restricted spaces is a common problem. Attention to detail will decrease the risk of injury to the axillary nerve, which is proximate to instrumentation during inferior capsular release.

Arthroscopic Stabilization

Arthroscopic stabilization has the highest reported complication rate of any arthroscopic shoulder procedure. This is true even among experienced arthroscopists (where the overall rate of complication is 3.3% according to a review by Neal Small in 1988.)[2] The most common complication is that of recurrent instability, which varies according to technique and technician. Despite the potential advantages of cosmesis, preservation of motion, and improved function, outcomes following arthroscopic stabilization have lagged expectations, with recurrence rates consistently higher than the 2 to 5% failure rate following open repairs. Other complications, including nerve injury, articular damage, stiffness, loose and migrating hardware, and foreign body reactions are much less frequent and rarely result in permanent disability. Complications are frequently technique specific and can be prevented by familiarity with the common pitfalls inherent in each particular arthroscopic repair procedure. Complications can be further minimized through familiarity with normal, variational, and pathological shoulder anatomy. Because the preceding chapters have discussed the specific complications inherent in their respective techniques (fixation tack vs suture anchor vs thermal vs knotless anchor device), we present stabilization pitfalls that are common to all repair techniques. Factors that contribute to recurrent instability following arthroscopic repair can be classified according to *when*, relative to the procedure, the error occurs. These factors can occur during the preoperative, intraoperative, or postoperative period.

PREOPERATIVE FACTORS

Preoperative factors include errors in diagnosis, patient selection, and surgical preparation. Diagnostic inaccuracy is a common pitfall in the treatment of shoulder instability. This preventable error can be minimized through careful clinical evaluation, including a thorough history and physical and radiographic examination to identify the underlying instability direction (anterior, posterior, inferior, bidirectional, or multidirectional) and cause (posttraumatic dislocation with Bankart lesion vs atraumatic subluxation with generalized ligamentous laxity). Although simplistic classification schemes are available, many shoulder instability patterns may elude easy categorization, reflecting the continuum of overlapping glenohumeral patholaxity seen in the spectrum of instability.

Poor patient selection has been implicated in the relatively higher rates of failure following arthroscopic (versus open) stabilization. The optimal patient seems to be one with recurrent posttraumatic unidirectional instability, a discrete Bankart lesion, good-quality tissue, negligible Hill–Sachs lesion, and no bony Bankart. Relative contraindications include the absence of a Bankart lesion, an engaging large Hill–Sachs lesion, significant capsular laxity, evidence of multidirectional instability, poor-quality glenohumeral ligament tissue, poor voluntary component, and noncompliance.

Because arthroscopic shoulder stabilization is technically demanding and technologically intensive, it requires appropriate support personnel and satisfactory equipment. This procedure is not for the casual arthroscopist, and the surgeon must be thoroughly familiar with shoulder arthroscopy, normal portal anatomy, and conversant with the specific instrumentation and technical steps necessary in this surgical exercise.

INTRAOPERATIVE FACTORS

Failure to Accurately Assess Instability

Failure to accurately identify the true cause of instability is a common and often preventable cause of failure following arthroscopic stabilization. Diagnostic accuracy depends upon familiarity with normal and variational shoulder anatomy. Understanding the anatomy and orientation of the anterior inferior glenohumeral ligament complex (AIGHLC) is mandatory. The most common arthroscopic finding in posttraumatic anterior instability is a Bankart lesion, in which the AIGHL, either with or without the labrum, is detached from the anterior inferior glenoid rim (3 to 6 o'clock in a right shoulder). In contrast, patients with multidirectional instability usually have no true Bankart lesion, with findings limited to a capacious and redundant axillary pouch. A "drive-through" sign, in which the arthroscope can be easily negotiated from the superior aspect of the joint inferiorly into the axillary pouch, sweeping under the humeral head, is also usually present.

Recent evidence suggests that even patients with Bankart lesions often have some component of capsular injury *in addition to the labral detachment*. Failure to recognize and address this capsular component has been implicated as the most common cause of failure following arthroscopic shoulder stabilization. Recognizing capsular laxity, however, is sometimes difficult. Even experienced arthroscopists may have difficulty discerning the degree to which capsular laxity is "pathological." Wolf has pointed out that recognizing this particular component is the "single most difficult aspect to arthroscopic shoulder stabilization".[11] Recent experimental evidence by Dettling et

al. has suggested that the amount of irrecoverable deformation within the anterior band of the inferior glenohumeral ligament following failure at the glenoid margin is approximately 0.8 mm.[12] This small amount of deformation calls into question both the importance of associated laxity and the need for capsular reduction procedures, but the authors acknowledge the possibility that recurrent instability may contribute to further laxity.

The surgeon must also be familiar with variations in glenohumeral pathology, including lesions other than the "Bankart" glenoid labral detachment. These include the "ALPSA" lesion coined by Neviaser, referring to an anterior labroligamentous periosteal sleeve avulsion.[13] This variant, in which the entire labrum and AIGHL–labrum complex slips medially and inferiorly along the glenoid neck, may be less dramatic in its appearance because there is no visible "detachment" from the rim per se. Another variant is midsubstance AIGHL rupture or detachment from its humeral insertion. Known as "HAGL" (**h**umeral **a**vulsion of the **g**lenohumeral **l**igament) lesions, humeral side detachments of the AIGHL complex have been recognized since first described by Nicola in 1942[14] and later observed arthroscopically by Bach,[15] Wolf,[16] and others.[17] Savoie writes that since becoming aware of this lesion, he has "noted lateral capsular injuries to be relatively common in patients in whom the transglenoid technique failed."[18] Field and coauthors have reported on five cases in which the anterior inferior glenohumeral ligament failed on both the glenoid and the humeral side.[19] Oberlander has recently added "BHAGL" lesion to the repertoire of observed pathology, coining the term to reflect a **b**ony **h**umeral **a**vulsion of the **g**lenohumeral **l**igament.[20]

A final cognitive limitation in arthroscopic stabilization involves the "deficient" rotator interval, between the supraspinatus and subscapularis. "Insufficiency" of this region has been touted as contributing to inferior, posterior, and multidirectional instability.[21–23] Definitive treatment of interval lesions has been recommended during open[24,25] and arthroscopic repair.[26] However, despite its probable importance, there are no guidelines by which to judge interval deficiency. Further complicating assessment is the routine establishment of arthroscopic stabilization portals up to 8 mm in diameter within the interval itself. Techniques for accurate arthroscopic assessment and indications for closure of the rotator interval remain elusive.

Poor Tissue Quality

Excellent visualization and technical skills will not overcome the disadvantages associated with poor-quality tissue. Variability of the quality and the type of injury to the anterior inferior glenohumeral ligament has been recognized by a number of authors,[27–29] some of whom have developed classification schemes intended to identify lesions that are amenable to arthroscopic repair.[27,28,30–32] Several studies have demonstrated a clear relationship between tissue quality and clinical outcome. Anterior inferior glenohumeral ligaments that are not discrete and robust, or are degenerative, are probably inappropriate targets for arthroscopic stabilization and are better treated by open means.

Inadequate Ligamentous/Labral Mobilization

Most authors recommend mobilization of the AIGHL–labrum complex inferiorly to the 6 o'clock position to eliminate inferior capsular laxity. Such mobilization requires considerable effort. In one cadaveric study, adequate mobilization of the AIGHL–labrum complex to close the Bankart lesion required stripping from the glenoid neck medially by 2 cm.[33] Bony Bankart lesions may be difficult to mobilize.

Inadequate Glenoid Preparation

Because tissue healing relies on biological fixation, preparation to expose bleeding bone along the rim and neck of the glenoid is crucial. Failure to do so risks effective healing.

Inadequate Bankart Reattachment

No amount of glenoid preparation or tissue mobilization will compensate for inadequate fixation. Factors that are thought to influence fixation security include failure to reapproximate tissue to the anatomic glenoid margin, failure to repair the tissue inferiorly along the less accessible 5 to 6 o'clock position, inadequate implant fixation strength, and poor surgical technique.

Failure to Reapproximate Tissue Anatomically to the Glenoid Margin

Several arthroscopic surgeons emphasize the importance of anatomically restoring the AIGHL–labrum complex to its normal site of attachment along the glenoid's articular margin. Harryman has shown the importance of restoring this labral "buttress" in controlling translation.[34] The degree to which failure to reapproximate the AIGHL–labrum directly to the rim, however, is unknown. Embryonic studies have demonstrated that AIGH ligament insertion medial to the rim may be normal in up to a third of shoulders.[35] Further complicating the issue is the technical difficulty inherent in targeting the glenoid rim to permit some precise implant purchase. The Suretac device,

for example, usually requires placement along the medial neck rather than on the rim itself.

Failure to Repair Inferiorly

The importance of repairing the *entire* Bankart lesion *down to the inferior 6 o'clock position* is a recognized and important step in the open repair literature. Yet surprisingly, little importance has been conferred on the same principle during arthroscopic repair. Though virtually every arthroscopic technique emphasizes complete tissue mobilization and glenoid preparation down to the 6 o'clock position, few stress the importance of *fixation* at this site. This is probably a consequence of difficulty of routinely targeting this somewhat inaccessible region by means of traditional anterior arthroscopic portals. Many arthroscopic surgeons have emphasized placing the inferior of the anterior portals as low as possible for inferior glenoid targeting purposes.[36–38] Located immediately above the subscapularis tendon, this low anterior portal still does not permit implant placement below 5 o'clock unless placed directly within the anterior inferior glenoid articular cartilage (which is a strategy recommended by some shoulder arthroscopists). Difficulties in inferior glenoid targeting have led several developers to develop alternative anterior portals to achieve better access inferiorly. Davidson and Tibone, in a cadaveric and clinical study, described the safe zones for placement of an inside-out "5 o'clock" portal, through which the anterior inferior glenoid could be easily and safely targeted.[5] Resch et al. described their lab and clinical experience using an "anterior inferior portal" through which the anterior inferior glenoid could be targeted for placement of an extra-articular staple.[39] Recent support for the importance of achieving fixation at the 6 o'clock position was provided by Black et al., who demonstrated significant decrease in anterior and inferior glenohumeral translation following labral detachment and repair with an inferior (6 o'clock) point of fixation in a cadaver model.[40]

Harryman described anterior inferior targeting through a technique in which a drill guide was used to place sutures from a posterior-superior portal.[34] This novel concept permitted accurate targeting and fixation along the entire site of detachment. However, clinical outcome data on the success of this interesting and safe technique have yet to be published.

Inadequate Initial Security of Fixation

Security of initial fixation depends on the implant design, surgical repair technique, and bone quality. Variability in implant design has received the greatest attention. Implant strength has been predominantly evaluated by load-to-failure testing, which depends not only on the anchor or implant but on the methodology by which it is tested. Barber et al., have shown that any construct whose pullout strength exceeds 30 lb (133.4 N) is probably sufficient to sustain the physiological stresses on the repair during the postoperative period.[41–43] Nearly all implants are thought to provide sufficient strength at the time of insertion to ensure adequate fixation. Once this threshold has been reached, other factors influence fixation security, including the strength of the anchoring system to the soft tissue (through which failure usually occurs), the tensile strength of the soft tissue itself, and the strength of the construct *over time*.

Inadequacy of Technique

The implant's inherent strength is of little relevance if implantation has been improper. The implant must be secured such that it captures and approximates the tissue in the manner in which it was designed. Failure to do so will build "slack" into the construct. Examples of this pitfall have been described with virtually every arthroscopic technique. Warner showed that failure to coaptate the capsule between two Suretac devices predisposed to a weak construct.[33] Transglenoid technique fixation over a soft tissue bridge distended with extravasated fluid has been implicated by many authors, some of whom have modified the technique to improve fixation security. Incomplete seating of an anchor can make for direct predisposition to recurrent instability.

Procedures that rely on arthroscopic knot tying for fixation are at risk of insecurity because of known technical difficulties with this technique. Most attention in the literature has been placed on the importance of "knot security," avoiding unraveling or slippage of the initially thrown knot, and using knots of sufficient strength. However, Burkhart has recently pointed out that of even greater potential significance is "loop security."[44] Failure to establish a secure initial "loop" of suture, in which the soft tissues are snugly approximated against the glenoid, compromises repair security regardless of how effectively the subsequent knots are thrown.

Inadequate Bone Quality

Because most patients undergoing arthroscopic shoulder reconstruction are young, implant failure due to poor bone quality is unlikely. However, a study published in 1998 demonstrates measurable bone density differences in the glenoid, with a significant decrease in cortical thickness from superior to inferior glenoid locations.[45] This difference directly influenced failure properties of the implants. Anchor placement at the inferior 5:30 position (right clock face) was found to

have lower ultimate pullout strength than placement in the 2:00 o'clock position. The authors speculated that the lower strength of fixation along the inferior glenoid might have clinical significance both in the presence of relative weakness at the time of implantation and under conditions of cyclic loading.

Inadequate Maintenance of Fixation

Regardless of implant strength at the time of initial fixation, failure to *maintain* strength or tissue apposition in the postoperative period may jeopardize even the best-repaired labrum. Implant fatigue properties under conditions of cyclic loading, more closely approximating the clinical situation, have received recent attention. Roth et al. found that cycling at submaximal loads resulted in implant cutout through the cancellous bone of the glenoid.[45] Calculations of ultimate fatigue life revealed a dramatic decrease in fixation strength, with a maximum load of less than 50% of the ultimate pullout load-to-failure strength. Cyclic loading shifted the mode of failure from suture/soft tissue failure to implant migration/pullout. The implication is that any construct subjected to cycling jeopardizes normal tissue coaptation, regardless of initial strength or security. On this basis, Roth et al. recommend intraoperative cycling of the implant before suture tying. In their experience, most anchors settled almost completely if the surgeon "repeatedly (up to 10 times) pulled on the suture with the same force that was initially used to ensure placement and/or engagement of the device."

Monofilament sutures, such as Prolene and polydioxanone sulfate (PDS), commonly used during shoulder stabilization procedures, are at risk of stretching out, with a reported 30% stretch when subjected to cyclic loading, and greater cyclic displacements than braided suture.[46] Gerber et al. demonstrated development of 5 to 10 mm "gaps" at the repair site even under low-level cyclic loading, due to elasticity of the material.[47] On this basis, some authors have recommended use of braided suture rather than monofilament in arthroscopic repairs.

This issue of maintenance of strength over time is particularly relevant when one is using implants whose material properties change with degradation. This is true for suture (PDS) as well as implants, whose characteristics are largely determined by their chemical composition. Bioabsorbable implants, unlike metal anchors and braided sutures, undergo degradation with loss of strength over time.[48,49] For example, the Suretac device (Smith and Nephew Dyonics, Andover, MA), molded from a synthetic copolymer identical to that used in Maxon sutures (Davis and Geck, Danbury CT), has a rapid rate of degradation, with loss of 50% of its strength by 2 weeks, and 95% of its strength by 3 weeks.[50,51] Most implants are made of polyglutamic acid, polylactic acid, or combinations thereof, with specific degradation rates that in large part depend on their composition.

Poor Surgical Technique

Surgical technique has been shown to have a great impact on outcome of arthroscopic repairs. Some authors, in reviewing their failures, have observed poor technique as the principal reason for failed repairs. The literature clearly reflects a higher failure rate in the early part of the "learning curve" than in later efforts. Complications have been reported even among experienced and trained arthroscopists.[2]

Postoperative Factors

Noncompliance with immobilization, inappropriate rehabilitation, or return to activity premature constitute fairly common and preventable cause of recurrent instability following arthroscopic stabilization. Several authors have found higher failure rates in patients inadequately immobilized postoperatively, and on this basis they justify current protocols recommending 3 to 6 weeks of immobilization. Very few protocols permit early postoperative recovery without enforced sling use. Conversely, some surgeons feel that arthroscopic repairs should be managed similarly to open repairs, allowing early-protected motion. Rarely are patients permitted to return to sport before 3 months, with contact or collision athletes usually restricted for 4 to 6 months.

SUMMARY

Complications associated with arthroscopic shoulder surgery are relatively common. Excluding recurrent instability, however, complications are infrequent and rarely disabling. Current statistics undoubtedly underestimate the true incidence. Many complications, including neurovascular injuries and articular damage, are preventable and can be minimized through familiarity with anatomy, proper surgical technique and instrumentation, and clinical experience. Nevertheless, despite these efforts, a small percentage of complications persists. With careful clinical indications, improved surgical techniques and increased experience, the surgical risks associated with arthroscopic shoulder surgery will remain low.

References

1. Small NC. Complications in arthroscopy: the knee and other joints. *Arthroscopy* 1986;2:253–258.
2. Small NC. Complications in arthroscopic surgery performed by experienced arthroscopists. *Arthroscopy* 1988;4:215–221.
3. Berjano P, Gonzalez BG, Olmedo JF, Perez-Espana LA, Munilla MG. Complications in arthroscopic shoulder surgery. *Arthroscopy* 1998;14(8):785–788.
4. Pearsall AW, Holovacs TF, Speer KP. The efficacy and safety of a low anterior portal established with an "outside-in" technique for arthroscopic shoulder surgery. Paper presented at: 17th Annual Meeting of the Arthroscopy Association of North America; May 1998; Orlando, FL.
5. Davidson PA, Tibone JE. Anterior inferior (5 o'clock) portal for shoulder arthroscopy. *Arthroscopy* 1995;5:519–525.
6. D'Angelo GL, Ogilvie-Harris DJ. Septic arthritis following arthroscopy, with cost/benefit analysis of antibiotic prophylaxis. *Arthroscopy* 1988;4(1):10–14.
7. Segmuller HE, Alfred S, Zilio G, et al. Cutaneous nerve lesions of the shoulder and arm after arthroscopic shoulder surgery. *J Shoulder Elbow Surg* 1995;4:254–258.
8. Mullins RC, Drez D, Cooper J. Hypoglossal nerve palsy after arthroscopy of the shoulder and open operation with the patient in the beach-chair position. *J Bone Joint Surg Am* 1992;74:137–140.
9. Stanish WD, Peterson DC. Shoulder arthroscopy and nerve injury: pitfalls and prevention. *Arthroscopy* 1995;11(4):458–466.
10. Arciero, RA, Taylor DC, Harrison SA, et al. Interscalene anesthesia for shoulder arthroscopy in a community-sized military hospital. *Arthroscopy* 1996;12(6):715–719.
11. Wolf EM. Arthroscopic shoulder stabilization using suture anchors: technique and results. Instructional Course 201. Presented at: 15th Annual Meeting of the Arthroscopy Association of North America; April 1996; Washington DC.
12. Dettling JR, Sandusky MD, McMahon PJ, et al. Shoulder instability: strain characteristics of the anterior band of the inferior glenohumeral ligament. *Orthop Trans* 1997;21(1):289–290.
13. Neviaser TJ. The anterior labroligamentous periosteal sleeve avulsion lesion: a cause of anterior instability of the shoulder. *Arthroscopy* 1993;9:17–21.
14. Nicola T. Anterior dislocation of the shoulder. The role of the articular capsule. *J Bone Joint Surg* 1942;24:614–616.
15. Bach B, Warren RF, Fronek J. Disruption of the lateral capsule of the shoulder. A cause of recurrent dislocation. *J Bone Joint Surg Br* 1988;70:274–276.
16. Wolf EM, Cheng JC, Dickson K. Humeral avulsion of glenohumeral ligaments as a cause of anterior shoulder instability. *Arthroscopy* 1995;11:600–607.
17. Taylor DC, Arciero RA. Pathologic changes associated with shoulder dislocations: arthroscopic and physical examination findings in first-time, traumatic anterior dislocations. *Am J Sports Med* 1997;25(3):306–311.
18. Savoie FH, Miller CD, Field LD. Arthroscopic reconstruction of traumatic anterior instability of the shoulder: the caspari technique. *Arthroscopy* 1997;13(2):201–209.

19. Field LD, Bokor DJ, Savoie FH III. Humeral and glenoid detachment of the anterior inferior glenohumeral ligament: a cause of anterior shoulder instability. *J Shoulder Elbow Surg* 1997;6(1):6–10.

20. Oberlander MA, Morgan BE, Vistosky JL. Case report: the BHAGL lesion: a new variant of anterior shoulder instability. *Arthroscopy* 1996;12(5):627–633.

21. Nobuhara K, Ikeda H. Rotator interval lesion. *Clin Orthop* 1987;223:44–50.

22. Harryman DT, Sidles JA, Harris LS, et al. The role of the rotator interval capsule in passive motion and stability of the shoulder. *J Bone Joint Surg Am* 1992;74:54–66.

23. Schwartz E, Warren RR, O'Brein SJ. Posterior shoulder instability. *Orthop Clin North Am* 19897;18:409–419.

24. Behr C, O'Brien SJ, Field L, et al. Anterior shoulder stabilization using a rotator interval approach. Paper presented at: Meeting of American Orthopaedic Society for Sports Medicine; June 1997; Sun Valley, ID.

25. Field LD, Warren RF, O'Brien SJ, et al. Isolated closure of rotator interval defects for shoulder instability. *Am J Sports Med* 1995;23:556–563.

26. Treacy SH, Field LD, Savoie FH. Rotator interval capsule closure: an arthroscopic technique. *Arthroscopy* 1997;13(1):103–106.

27. Green MR, Christensen KP. Arthroscopic Bankart procedure: two- to five-year follow-up with clinical correlation to severity of glenoid labral lesions. *Am J Sports Med* 1995;23(3):276–281.

28. Hayashida Kengi, Yoneda Minoru, Nakagawa S, et al. Arthroscopic Bankart suture repair for traumatic anterior shoulder instability: analysis of the causes of a recurrence. *Arthroscopy* 1998;14(3):295–301.

29. Pagnani MJ, Anderson AF, Warren RF, et al. Patient selection for arthroscopic shoulder stabilization. *Arthroscopy* 1996;12(3):373–374.

30. Arciero RA, Wheeler JH, Ryan JB, et al. Arthroscopic Bankart repair versus nonoperative treatment for acute initial anterior shoulder dislocations. *Am J Sports Med* 1994;22(5):589–594.

31. Kirkley A, Griffin S, Richards C, et al. Prospective randomized clinical trial comparing the effectiveness of immediate arthroscopic stabilization versus immobilization and rehabilitation in first-time traumatic anterior dislocations of the shoulder. Presented at: Arthroscopy Association of North America Specialty Day Meeting; March 1998; New Orleans.

32. Wolf EM. Arthroscopic capsulolabral reconstruction using suture anchors. Presented at: Arthroscopy Association of North America Specialty Day Meeting; February 1994; New Orleans.

33. Warner JJP, Miller MD, Marks P. Arthroscopic Bankart repair with the Suretac device. Part II: Experimental observations. *Arthroscopy* 1995;11(1):14–20.

34. Harryman DT II, Ballmer FT, Harris SL, et al. Arthroscopic labral repair to the glenoid rim. *Arthroscopy* 1994;10:20–30.

35. Uhthoff HK, Piscopo M. Anterior capsular redundancy of the shoulder: congenital or traumatic. *J Bone Joint Surg Br* 1985;67:363.

36. Wolf EM. Arthroscopic anterior shoulder capsulorrhaphy. *Tech Orthop* 1998;3:67–73.

37. Warner JJP, Warren RF. Arthroscopic Bankart repair using a cannulated absorbable fixation device. *Oper Tech Orthop* 1991;1:192–198.

38. Pagnani MJ, Warren RF. Arthroscopic shoulder stabilization. *Oper Tech Sports Med* 1993;1:276–284.

39. Resch H, Povacz P, Wambacher M, et al. Arthroscopic extra-articular Bankart repair for the treatment of recurrent anterior shoulder dislocations. *Arthroscopy* 1997;13(2):188–200.

40. Black KP, Schneider DJ, Yu JR, et al. A biomechanical evaluation of the relationship between labral fixation site and shoulder translation during a bankart reconstruction. Paper presented at: Annual Meeting of American Orthopaedic Society for Sports Medicine; March 1998; New Orleans.

41. Barber FA, Cawley P, Prudich JF. Suture anchor failure strength—an in-vivo study. *Arthroscopy* 1993;9:647–652.

42. Barber FA, Herbert MA, Click JN. The ultimate strength of suture anchors. *Arthroscopy* 1995;11:21–28.

43. Barber FA, Herbet MA, Click JN. Suture anchor strength revisited. *Arthroscopy* 1996;12:32–38.

44. Burkhart SS, Wirth MA, Simonick M, et al. Technical note: loop security as a determinant of tissue fixation security. *Arthroscopy* 1998;14(7):773–776.

45. Roth CA, Bartolozzi AR, Ciccotti MG, et al. Failure properties of suture anchors in the glenoid and the effects of cortical thickness. *Arthroscopy* 1998;14(2):186–191.

46. Loutzenheiser TD, Harryman DT II, Ziegler DW, et al. Optimizing arthroscopic knots using braided or monofilament suture. *Arthroscopy* 1998;14(1):57–65.

47. Gerber C, Schneberger AG, Beck M, et al. Mechanical strength of repairs of the rotator cuff. *J Bone Joint Surg Br* 1994;76:371–380.

48. Blasier RD, Bucholz R, Cole W, Johnson LL, Makela E. Antero bioresorbable implants: applications in orthopaedic surgery. *Instr Course Lect* 1997;46:531–546.

49. Athanasiou KA, Agrawal CM, Barber FA, et al. Current concepts: orthopaedic applications for PLA-PGA biodegradable polymers. *Arthroscopy* 1998;14(7):726–737.

50. Warner JJP, Miller MD, Marks P, et al. Arthroscopic Bankart repair with the Suretac device. Part I: Clinical observations. *Arthroscopy* 1995;11(1):2–13.

51. Speer KP, Warren RF. Arthroscopic shoulder stabilization. A role for biodegradable material. *Clin Orthop* 1993;291:67–74.

Recommended Reading

Brown R, Weiss R, Greenberg CP, et al. Interscalene block for shoulder arthroscopy: comparison with general anesthesia. 1993;9(3):295–300.

McGinty JB. Complications of arthroscopy and arthroscopic surgery. In: McGinty JB, Caspari RB, Jackson RW, Poehling, eds. *Operative Arthroscopy.* New York: Lippincott-Raven; 1996; Chap. 7.

Nottage WM. Arthroscopic portals: anatomy at risk. *Orthop Clin North Am* 1993;24(1):19–26.

Rodeo S, Forster RA, Weiland AJ. Current concepts review: neurological complications due to arthroscopy. *J Bone Joint Surg Am* 1993;75(6):917–926.

Stanish WD, Peterson DC. Shoulder arthroscopy and nerve injury: pitfalls and prevention. *Arthroscopy* 1995;11(4):458–466.

Index

ISBN 0-387-95363-9